PROGNOSTICS

PROGNOSTICS

A science in the making surveys and creates the future

BY FRED. L. POLAK

ELSEVIER PUBLISHING COMPANY Amsterdam/London/New York, 1971

THIS MONOGRAPH IS A TRANSLATION OF THE ABRIDGED EDITION OF PROGNOSTICA, PUBLISHED BY Æ. E. KLUWER, DEVENTER, 1969.

ELSEVIER PUBLISHING COMPANY
335 JAN VAN GALENSTRAAT
P.O. BOX 211, AMSTERDAM, THE NETHERLANDS

ELSEVIER PUBLISHING CO. LTD.
BARKING, ESSEX, ENGLAND

AMERICAN ELSEVIER PUBLISHING COMPANY, INC.
52 VANDERBILT AVENUE
NEW YORK, NEW YORK 10017

LIBRARY OF CONGRESS CARD NUMBER: 71-135482

ISBN 0-444-40879-7

PRINTED IN THE NETHERLANDS

TO THE DOVES AND THE SEEKERS AFTER CLARITY
TO THE HAWKS AND THE HEAVEN-STORMERS

Contents

X

Foreword

Fred Polak is well enough known; he needs no foreword from another. But since he has asked me to introduce this book, I shall try to formulate my opinion of his work. The significance of this work has been disputed. It has been said that it is not a science. And it does in fact display characteristics that can be criticized along those lines; Dijksterhuis has pointed this out as well. But science cannot flourish without the explorers, the pioneers, to indicate new fields for future attention. Moreover, in many cases the most important advances in our knowledge and capabilities have been made because the terra incognita between the provisionally demarcated areas already known to us was trodden by people of wider vision. And vision is characteristic of Polak. He is now extending one major line that he has drawn before. In his "The Image of the Future" he pointed not only to the causal links between past and future but also to the importance of a vision of the future to culture. At the same time he felt himself obliged to state that the absence of such a vision in the social and cultural sphere is spreading ever wider. I interpreted this chiefly as an analysis. Polak has now turned to policy. In terms of today his new work is a presentation of scientific policy, and of more; it is also a preamble to a political policy.

Two properties of his mind are very much in the forefront of his work. He has an encyclopedic knowledge of the most varied developments in thought and a capacity for association that is of very great importance in the reconnoitring and formulating of new fields of thought. In addition he has a rare gift for delineation and a mastery in word play. This he has in common with Bolland. Although this has the drawback mentioned by Dijksterhuis that concepts tend to become blurred, it also has the advantage of mental gymnastics and of a dramatic elucidation of the situation; a situation that is always hazy at first from afar.

In keeping with the growing tendency of specialists in many fields to ask themselves what their field will look like in the future, and what must be tackled first, Polak advocates above all a similar attitude among the social sciences too, because when all is said and done it is there that the contributions of the specialized fields must be blended into a harmonious whole directed towards the future well-being of mankind. Accordingly he suggests programs of research and training, and also programs of information. One of his questions is "Why shouldn't there be as many professors teaching about the future as there are professors of history?" Many of his questions and suggestions are extremely fascinating and challenging. They deserve a wide audience.

J. TINBERGEN

Prognostics: what, why, which way, whither?

It is always a most precarious business to evaluate contemporary events rightly. As history shows all too clearly, the man on the spot is always exposed to a treacherous one-sidedness, which may yield the dual danger of ultimate error in one direction or the other. Either he is typically inclined to underestimate or even neglect irregular phenomena, occurring at a given moment and regarded as innocuous, which might on occasion be the heralds of a lasting renovation with considerable repercussions in due course. Or conversely he is tempted to overrate their symptomatic importance, which might prove after the event to have been of a transitory nature and to have caused no more than a quickly dying ripple in the infinite sea of the time continuum.

In such cases, therefore, one cannot say that forewarned is forarmed. The contemporary spectator should be very well aware of these two antipodes of optical illusion and of the danger of misrepresentation that is always lying in wait to mislead him and those around him. Nevertheless, I believe that I may — indeed must — say that the signs of the time, as omens, truly point in the direction of a spectacular acceleration as the prelude to a complete swing. The difficulties that I have mentioned are accordingly further intensified. It is not only contemporary events that we are evaluating here; the future is already being discounted in the process. I am convinced that later historians, i.e. operating at a greater distance, will mark this sharp and significant dividing-line, which is still practically masked today for most observers, although it is nevertheless already running right through our own time here and there. Perhaps they will speak of a revolution or a transformation, in the same way as we today, with the last doubts having finally evaporated, recognize as large-scale renovations in world history the French Revolution or the first industrial revolution, both transplanted to America with their essential traits after the rebellious Declaration of Independence cleared the way, and re-exported with renewed vigor to Europe.

Now, although doubtless there is a close connection, I do not mean here so much that we have now entered into the age of a *second* industrial revolution thanks to a considerably further-reaching scientific and technological development going ahead with still stronger drive. In my opinion that is quite definitely the case in itself, especially as the result of the process of automation spreading with such great rapidity. Automation is making a most important and on some points even decisive contribution towards the breakthrough to a new era. True, as such and including its ramifications, it is also reaching to the deeper intellectual roots of the present processes of revolution, partly on account of a permanent interaction. Taken in a narrower sense, however, it does not fully explain the origin and existence of the specific dividing-line referred to above, which forms an unmistakable demarcation between our present day and a differing future.

The dividing-line which I believe I can perceive does not, after all, lie just in the technical or material plane, but equally intersects and churns up the *mental* plane. For in my opinion our generation is gradually distinguishing and separating itself from preceding generations, though this is not an entirely conscious, let alone a fully planned process. The change to which I refer is being both revealed and performed thanks to a new mode of thought and attitude of mind that is slowly but surely crystallizing. This new mental approach relates — not exclusively but largely so — to a changed and still drastically changing attitude towards the *future*. Conversely the future, which is itself subject to such pronounced change, is also influencing our attitude in that connection. To an increasing extent, both quantitatively and qualitatively, the future seems to be forming an essential element in our present-day thinking, and specifically the future with a continuously extended time dimension, but equally the future with renewed and at the same time more clearly defined objectives. The purposive projection of the future on an increasingly long term, with related ideal targets to be achieved in due course, is arousing an increasingly intensive interest, which is being converted into an enhanced and effectively directed energy. More and more the need for a usefulness of long-term forecasts and also long-term tasks aiming at social reform are beginning to penetrate from the top of society to subordinate groups and strata of the population. The awareness is dawning that a well-considered, activated choice between possible alternative futures will have to be made in good time.

As we shall see, this kind of prospectivistic, long-term attitude of mind with relation to the future-dimension to be breached was first advocated with vigor in France during the 1950's. At first it related to a new philosophical trend of thought. Perhaps reinforced by a preceding successful renewal of economic thought, and certainly also to a not inconsiderable extent with a rationale rehabilitating the future, this new approach took a practically opposite stand to the existentialism of the style of Sartre, which was flourishing greatly at that time in that very country. For the latter deliberately featured the present day or the present time always with us by definition as an eternally unchangeable and therefore fundamentally and permanently hopeless category. Crossing the ocean to America was only a step for a future-orientation systematically differing from this somber view and offering meaningful renovation.

In America this long-term future-thinking, consciously applied and very concretely adjusted to reality there, like the application of the renewed economic theory, almost automatically acquired a reinforced pragmatic strain matching the American national character. It proved indispensable (e.g. for the brain trusts in the military sector), particularly useful (e.g. in certain parts of the civilian government sector) and — last but not least, I shall be returning to this — it offered an advantage of which grateful use was made: it evidently paid for itself twice over (especially in large industrial concerns).

Moreover, both inside and outside America insight developed into by origin purely idealistic objectives or world policy which gradually likewise won ground partly in a pragmatic direction. According to this new, matured view such objectives as those of the preservation of world peace and of appropriate development aid will no longer be soluble in the future, or at least not adequately so, without purposive, systematic, long-range thought procedures.

Such purposive future-thinking began to expand in particular in the course of the present decade and to converge into an international phenomenon also characterizing other fields of progressive human endeavor. The Soviet Union soon followed America in this direction, from both the political-doctrinaire and academic-scientific points of view. In a number of countries behind the Iron Curtain greatly increased interest has developed in recent years in particular in concentrated future-thinking, whether or not connected with the central economic planning in those countries. In Poland, Hungary and Czechoslovakia, for example, the authorities are now on the point of setting up future-research institutes specifically equipped for that purpose.

In Japan, which characterizes itself as the most inquisitive nation in the world, vigorous attempts to catch up in this same field cannot be noted, after observation of and the collection of information on this current trend. It is not impossible that, as has already happened there before in considerable areas of technology, this country will do everything to overtake its predecessors in this prognostic field too, throwing in the necessary generous financing and manpower.

Europe viewed as a whole has without any doubt not been able to keep up with this accelerated process of development at present. There are, however, a few promising outposts to be seen, for example in Britain, Germany and Austria, and also in Italy. Despite its praiseworthy pioneering spirit, France has no longer been able to keep up with the new, greater pace in all respects. The Benelux countries, Scandinavia and Switzerland have, with the exception of the odd forerunner in a more pointed or pronounced direction, remained practically neutral and non-committal; they are virgin territory with regard to exploring and tackling the future. These arrears, which are growing with relative rapidity, are beginning to assume alarming forms.

The more so because elsewhere two major developments have set in which have detached themselves from the initially purely philosophical reflection as the royal mother of scientific knowledge and ability. On the one hand there is the beginning of a development towards a separate, scientifically founded knowledge of the future, often still designated in that early stage as "futurology". On the other hand, in part detached from this, the development of an operational future-technique or future-methodology. The future-research performed along these lines serves above all for approaching and also controlling, or at least adjusting, expected future processes of development.

So far there is no such thing as a true and independent *future-science*. That should be explicitly stated here and now. At present understandable doubt still exists as to whether and in what way such a science could exist. Can any science really logically have as its subject something that does not yet exist: the future? Or does it instead relate to reflection on, reconnaissance and approach of the future? The present work concerns itself in detail with this problem. Subject to certain conditions and provisos it arrives at a result which is affirmative in principle. A great deal of attention will also have to be devoted to the question of the extent to which the future-thinking now feeling its way forward and the corresponding new attitudes towards the future will, with an almost Einsteinian mental leap forward, take off in principle from what was formerly long regarded as customary. In that case, what was proclaimed by way of self-evident tradition or axiom in a preponderantly dogmatic sphere as exclusively valid and valuable everywhere, and therefore usually adhered to uncritically, would be shaken to its foundations and acceptably reformed.

In addition, as already stated, a specific future-technique — not or only very partly based on a theoretical basis or one recognized as scientific, and already anticipating the latter — has now developed, especially in America. A still constant elaboration and refinement, continued with tremendous push, is now going on there. A surprising number of different long-term prognostic techniques are concerned. If a separate future-science could in fact form, or even in certain circumstances be obliged to develop, the fanning spectrum of such modern (not only economic and technological, but also socio-dynamic and cultural) prognostic methods would certainly form the heart of it. If only for that reason — others will be discussed later — there is much to be said for giving the whole of these new scientific approaches to the future the joint title of *prognostics*. In the broad sense prognostics covers *all* the variants and methods of scientific future-thinking, i.e. also the many older ones.

XVI

It is to be expected that this developing prognostics will tend to extend its ambitions over a gradually wider plane. Whilst initially, as outlined above, it started as a new philosophical view of the future, its sphere of interest has widened to cover every field — perhaps tangentially — of social science, of socio-practical application and of social policy. In the American team-work, set up for long-term research into the future, the practitioners of *all* social sciences are generally called upon to assist as much as possible. In addition to economics, which had already been earning its spurs in this field for decades, one finds sociology, psychology, politicology, the science of history, didactics, etc. Even theology, which formerly had increasingly reflected existentialism, right down to its pessimistic traits, is now also coming into contact with this more optimistically oriented prospectivism — I should perhaps say, having regard to its originally eschatological, though for a long time mainly transcendental vision of the future, coming into contact again. This time directly interested in and oriented towards human society on earth.

It also proves that modern psychiatry, not in the last place on account of the needs of the younger generation, but equally on account of the gener ally increasing neurotic uncertainty about what the future will bring, is adopting this new reasoning and the prospects that it is opening. A further clear trend is that this new orientation is appealing, and will presumably appeal still more, to many branches of university education. This leads to contact with the revolutionary development which in fact is now breaking through on every plane of education, whether of young people or of adults. For there too a striking shift has been started (it was, incidentally, urgently required), turning away from the ossified past-present line and moving towards the fluid "shape of things to come". At the same time this shift is reflected in the plans being formulated everywhere by the progressive student movement for the foundation of a "critical university" and for a say on their part in the subject-matter taught, which in their opinion should be renewed or widened, and also a say in the appointment of teachers, in part to teach the new material.

At present there are interesting indications in a variety of fields of such a switch in the mental plane consciously re-oriented towards the future. Opinions may differ about their respective importance. In America, still the Mecca of entrepreneurical private production (though somewhat watered down to less pure mixed forms) increasing attention is consequently being paid to an equally revolutionary process, especially in business. This process of development, which originated in strategic military planning, has been borrowed by the industrial and commercial giants at the top of the economic pyramid, and is now beginning to filter through to the medium-sized firms and even to the relatively smaller ones. A steadily swelling flood of literature is accompanying and reinforcing this expansion.

Characteristic of the mental advance towards and opening of a quite different span of time is the change of front in America (which, as has been stated, is taking place in a pre-eminently pragmatic fashion) as it can be notably derived from the new typical definition of the properties required for an optimum policy by industrial top management. For in what Americans mean in practice by this new philosophy we again find the same shift forward in time, i.e. towards a conscious future-orientation. A top industrial manager now devotes a preponderant part of his time and that of his staff, specially selected on a qualitative basis for that purpose, to deep consideration of the long-term problems of the future which have penetrated to the heart of business policy and of decision-making.

In Europe and in much of European business there is still far too little awareness of the true nature of the much-discussed technological gap in respect of America. In its deepest essence — as I hope to show — this is largely caused by a "forecasting gap". With the aid of purposive long-range future-research and national, purposive modes of thought tying in with this, American big business is capable of achieving a considerable lead and of steadily increasing it. There is an ever-deeper rooted realization in America — and it is repeatedly proved to be correct — that turnover and profits can be multiplied thanks to new products and diversification in new lines selected as priorities for investment by executive management on the strength of systematic future-research. In economic theory the conviction has long prevailed that the implicit future-expectations of businessmen determine their investment policy. But now these future-expectations are being institutionalized and organically integrated by the businessmen themselves and consequently are explicitly becoming future-determinants to a considerably enhanced degree. Not only for industrial investment, but moreover for the whole of economic growth and an entirely new type of economic development of and for the developed countries. Industrial future-policy determines the trend and the character of the "wave of the future". A modern top manager of this new successful type is at the top above all as a future-manager. In this way a revolution of industrial policy is beginning to be delineated and to continue in accelerated fashion. The result is a break-through of a mentality which is entirely different from the prevailing old one (still extant in Europe). A mentality which is positive, indeed little short of aggressive, in its approach to the future, and which therefore "makes" this future itself. Partly as a result of this, large industrial concerns are gaining in intensified expansionistic drive; through this mental restructuring they are again acquiring monopolistic traits. And in addition new industrial forces, using this future-stategy, are rising to the top. They are spreading all over the world, and also penetrating Europe from the outside.

If we finally manage to break through this intellectual defense and mental repression — which are sometimes still very powerful — in Europe, and of course elsewhere too, this could be of particular importance, indeed of great and fruitful influence on progress inside and equally outside Europe.

I therefore do not simply mean — although its necessity and importance can hardly be denied — that for instance Europe could make up industrial arrears and could again bring up to par a gradually weakening competitive position, where necessary with the use of the same weapons.

This work will in addition spotlight three other aspects which I regard as being of world-embracing importance. All three relate to the cardinal question of how we are to arrive at a different and better society in the future. It is the same fundamental question that is contained in the subtitle of this work, where, however, it has already been answered in a positive sense: *a science in the making surveys and creates the future.* Needless to say — to obviate any misunderstanding forthwith — we are in no sense concerned here with a scientific monopoly, nor even less with a dictate, but with a creative contribution, which on the other hand must do all within its power to help to fulfil an essential mission to mankind. The mission of continuing to pose and approach forward-looking future-ideals. Of creating the future and our future destiny in our own image. The medium is the image!

As regards the *first* main point, the social sciences (except in recent decades economics in particular, of which more later) have with a few shades of difference and relatively solitary exceptions incurred a tremendous and still growing lag practically everywhere, above all if they are compared with the development of science and technology. This lag has led to the occurrence of a steadily growing gulf. Sir C. P. Snow has given this antithesis the new current name of "the two cultures". This phenomenon may be regarded from different points of view, with varying degrees of disquiet. One thing that is certain is that the social sciences have not followed the tremendously accelerated growth rate and phenomenal expansion of the natural sciences. It is precisely these sciences, taken in the broadest sense, that have completely changed the face of the world and will continue to change it in an unrestrained, increasingly stepped-up tempo into what may well be complete metamorphoses. However, the social sciences have not only lagged behind the tremendous proportions assumed by their "natural" sister sciences, which would on the whole simply be of comparative scientific importance. They have also been equally overtaken — and this is of almost inestimable social importance — by the rate, impact and range of these kaleidoscopic shifting images of social configurations and patterns.

The social sciences and their practitioners are in essence powerless, mainly passive and, to tell the truth, practically apathetic in their attitude towards this radical intervention in social events with, it may be expected, fundamental structural changes constantly urged ever further onward. They have lost their grip on this social dynamics, stirred up more and more vigorously by uncontrolled forces, in their turn urged on chiefly by series after series of scientific and technological applications and inventions put into practice. As a result a serious and possibly in the long fatal disturbance of equilibrium has come into being between these motorial forces and, in comparison with this tremendous drive, counterforces deployed inadequately if at all or a potential for conducting it into the right channels which is not effective in this respect. The social sciences have stated, in dignified fashion, with a rationalization after the event, that their negativism or asceticism in respect of this lost handhold is completely in accordance with their intentions and should therefore be regarded as a good thing for their theoretical work. After all, they want to restrict themselves to actually observable reality and not allow themselves to be tempted into all kinds of subjective and unverifiable speculations about what might possibly happen or not happen as a result of incalculable impulses and inventions. The possible social effect or the anticipating appraisal of the latter does not, they say, concern them for the time being, and from the scientific point of view is not relevant to a well-founded interpretation. However, it remains an equally indisputable "fact" that the *future* social reality is now being determined essentially and one-sidedly in the force field of applied natural science and technical development, without those sciences which have selected this same social reality (once it has become the compressed present day) as their field of study having the slightest say in things or even displaying real interest. This does indeed point to a pretty dreadful breakdown in communication, which may perhaps have catastrophic consequences for that future development of society which for the time being is being abandoned or made light of. It need therefore occasion no surprise, although this is a paradoxical situation, that precisely in the circle of natural scientists the dissatisfaction at and the veiled or open criticism of this aloofness are steadily growing. Especially when the ball — quite wrongly on the whole — is returned to their court, with the urgent request to natural scientists to refrain henceforth from further new inventions or applications that might perhaps be even more harmful to society. The "question of guilt" comes into play here, but unfortunately not a rational, effective and cooperative solution for a crisis which is gradually becoming more dangerous.

In the *second* place, in close collaboration with and elaboration of the preceding point, this bridging of positions which have grown further away from each other, almost on a basis of enmity, and now are antithetically fixed on both sides, is no longer still possible without more ado on the outside or the surface. We shall now have to dig deeper to expose the innermost core and the intrinsically active divisive force of the dilemma, clearly noted above the surface. There is no escaping the fact that the essentials of a sound scientific procedure in general and of its search for truth in particular with regard to the social dynamics will again have to be submitted to a fundamental examination. A renaissance of the social sciences and of their thought springing up again constructively and purposively, which would then, as in the natural sciences, be oriented consciously and positively towards the future, can no longer be achieved by a simple change of course. This revival requires, after a painstaking, thorough weighing-up, nothing less than a drastic, if necessary total revision of a number of scientific values anchored in the prevailing social methodology and as a rule still undisputed. The already mentioned, long-awaited "Einsteinian mental leap forward" — even though we lack a magic formula comparable to $E = mc^2$. Only such a fundamental renewal with a parallel emancipation can liberate the social sciences from the confining, isolated position into which they have gradually manoeuvred themselves and can enable them to reassume their vacated place on the globus scientiarum with honor. In that case — and here the second phase of research develops — paralysing antithesis may be converted into fertile synthesis. Hence too — apart from other equally important motives towards the same end to be explained later — the coordinative, pre-eminently *interdisciplinary* nature of this work.

For the sake of good order I may already point out here en passant — subject to a later detailed elaboration — that it is not for the first time in the history of the social sciences that an attempt has been made to develop them pari passu and to raise them to the level of the natural sciences. On the contrary, as we shall see, this has often been pursued too greatly, too servilely and, partly as a result, often in the wrong way. Nor have the social sciences in the past lacked certain high-flown, indeed sometimes rather distorted visions of the future. However, these forms and intellectual trends of a still primitive future-thought had to be successively abandoned again, with a deep frustration leading to bitterness or aversion, and swallowed whole. Not infrequently the baby was thrown out with the bath-water. If we are to succeed this time it is necessary first to attempt an analysis of the causes of the many former failures. One of these socio-scientific future-endeavors, contained in the key concept: to know = to predict has, as we shall see, still tried to maintain itself here and there down to our time. Unfortunately without this having resulted so far in the systematic development of an operationally usable prognostics. However, the renewed shot at a modern prognostics may possible form a welcome and, in the opinion of the present author, also tenable reason, this time of an extremely urgent and therefore more coercive character, for achieving that aim.

Here, as a doubt which will be further discussed, a kind of chicken or the egg problem will be passed over. For it is the question whether purposive restructuring and modernization of the social sciences do in fact form a sine qua non for this development of prognostics, or whether it could and should if necessary develop independently in its own way. In any case this cuts both ways. The active endeavor to develop a prognostics can certainly form a not inconsiderable stimulus towards revision of stereotyped socio-scientific norms and procedures. Conversely, a too long continued ossification and haughty aloofness of the social sciences can equally foster the autonomous secession and build-up of prognostics. The system of challenge and response can operate here in two directions, without it being possible for the time being to predict with a well-founded prognosis the resultant of this interplay of forces.

However, one thing we can say for certain is that "the hour of truth" is definitely at hand now and "a parting of minds" could ultimately prove inescapable. The barricade of the present-day order erected on the mental plane forms only an illusory protection, gives a false sense of security, against coming revolutions. There is no other way open to us than to leap over the threshold of contemporary events deliberately and without too much delay, so as to meet unafraid and fruitfully the new eon breaking ground with irresistible force.

In the *third* place — and this again cannot be detached from the two preceding points — conscious future-thinking as such and in its many variants has long formed part of the most valuable European intellectual heritage. It is true that through various historical causes merging together, which will be further analysed, opposition to it has gradually grown. However strongly this may now have hardened and lodged, the course of development of Western thought (incidentally fructified by older Oriental influences) continues to stand at the cradle of all centuries-long inspiring positive images of the future. Christian eschatology, Greek philosophy, the humanistic Renaissance, idealistic and enlightened philosophy, utopianism, early socialism and orthodox Marxism, the optimism of progress, etc., form not only illustrative types of future-thinking but at the same time milestones of the "European Spirit". The refounding of future-thinking to be elevated to a science will therefore definitely not be unbecoming to Europe.

Three remarks will be made to conclude this introductory survey. None of these remarks is original, but they are all three taken from future-thinkers, who have likewise rather apologetically sought some cover beforehand, or have applied a further qualifying restriction of their range or aims. Without attempting to elevate myself to their level, I may take warning from their words.

J. M. Keynes began the Foreword to his collected "Essays in Persuasion" as follows: "Here are collected the croakings ... of a Cassandra who could never influence the course of events in time. The volume might have been entitled "Essays in Prophecy and Persuasion", for the *Prophecy*, unfortunately, has been more successful than the *Persuasion*. But it was in a spirit of persuasion that most of these essays were written, in an attempt to influence opinion. They were regarded at the time, many of them, as extreme and reckless utterances". Keynes adds: "... this was because they often ran directly counter to the overwhelming weight of contemporary sentiment and opinion ..." Fortunately, we now realize all too well that Keynes achieved more not only in his prophecy but later in his persuasion too than he himself could ever have dreamed. An therefore, despite his prophetic genius, Keynes gave an incorrect prognosis of his own powers of persuasion. I must submit the destiny of prognostics to the decisive opinion of the future; in *that* respect I shall refrain from any kind of prognosis.

Sir George Thomson, who was awarded the Nobel Prize for physics, writes the following in a short Foreword to his "The Foreseeable Future": "In some of what follows I have gone outside the studies of which I can claim any professional knowledge. For this rash act I ask forgiveness of those into whose coverts I have trespassed. If some of the game I have reported exists only in my imagination, at least this kind of poaching does no harm to the rightful owners, while the onlooker may occasionally see something that is both unexpected and real." I should like to associate myself with these sentiments, with the proviso that I must ask myself whether I myself may claim any specific professional knowledge. That is why, too, I must apologize in advance with all the greater emphasis for my systematic yet unavoidable transgression of all specialized fields foreign to me, and I shall accept all resultant deserved rebukes.

In the third place I should like to borrow a figure of speech from my friend Kenneth Boulding, who in the Foreword to his well-known economic textbook warns his readers that he is not going to pour them full, creamy milk but intends principally to give them a teething ring to chew on. In the absence of the usual textbooks the present work could without pretension serve as a specimen textbook or systematic manual for beginners. However, it is only a first acquaintanceship with and groping exploration of something which does not yet exist in all its completeness. An exploration of the budding scientific exploration of the future, and also of the many obstacles encountered en route. Dogmatic criticism — one of these obstacles — will confirm my arguments, undogmatic criticism will elucidate my views. Both are therefore equally welcome.

Boekelo, March 1967.   F. L. P.

By way of justification

La dernière chose qu'on trouve en faisant
un ouvrage est de savoir celle qu'il faut
mettre la première

PASCAL, PENSEES

This work consists of two main parts, presented under the titles of Dogmatics and Prognostics. I naturally have given some thought to whether it might not be preferable to publish these two parts as completely separate works.

An argument in favor of this would be the fact that — quite apart from a doubling of the contents caused by placing them in one work and thus a reduced clarity of the whole — there are numerous differences and also dissimilarities or even contrasts between these two parts.

However, there is also considerable similarity, precisely on one point of particular importance here. First let me explain why the latter argument finally decided me to combine the two parts.

The first part is devoted exclusively to a discussion of *that dogmatic* attitude of mind and thought which at all times has always existed or been adopted in one special respect — the same is true of our present day — towards the *future* in particular. That part therefore does not aim at a comprehensive treatment of dogmatics or the dogmatic attitude of mind as such, however interesting such an attempt would be. It deals exclusively — something which to the best of my knowledge has *never* happened before in this way — with what could be further defined as future-dogmatics. The term future-dogmatics should thus for the time being be taken to mean the forcing of all thought about the future into a strait-jacket of prescriptions and guidelines.

Either one may not think about the future at all or — as is usually the case — one's thoughts must be in accordance with an orthodox, exclusively binding scientific code, i.e. cast in the mold of a compulsory prescribed model of the future. Of course it is true, as will automatically appear, that between an attitude of mind tending in principle towards dogmatism and the future-dogmatics specially elucidated here psychologically explicable links exist everywhere. In this sense, therefore, a separate analysis of future-dogmatics may, as an unsought-after incidental result, likewise make a contribution towards a greater appreciation of dogmatics pure and simple.

However, the primary aim is to show the close historical connection between the development of a future-dogmatics of this kind and a consequently one-sidedly limited prognostic vision. Then, by extending this line to our own period, it will be shown how this has led to a yawning intellectual gap, which has widened until now it is almost unbridgeable. An intellectual gap between a *future-dogmatics* that is the product of the past and has since then become rigid and a modern and flexible *prognostics* dissolving this future-dogmatics, wresting itself free with all its strength and penetrating much further, deeper and more widely into the future which it has breached.

In the second part, designated in particular as prognostics, are of course essentially concerned with this future now confronting us. It discusses the specific methods and prognostic techniques, which today, for the *first* time in the history of human civilization, are already available (or are in a more or less advanced stage) to provide a scientifically sound, analytical and synthetic vision of the future, and also for solving the present and coming problems of the future.

However, I have also given the title "Prognostics" to the work as a whole. For if prognostics is regarded not only in its modern form of development but, in the broader sense, as a general human datum from all times of the history of civilization, future-dogmatics forms an essential part of it. Viewed in this way, future-dogmatics often determined prognostics, with which it then practically coincided. But sometimes — as now — it blocks off an independent development of prognostics, whichs seeks individual, freer and better ways to achieve the aim set: the best possible insight into and outlook on the future.

Though future-dogmatics may be frozen and hypostatized, it is no less true to say that it incorporates one certain, indeed fixed prognostic view in respect of the future. For even the most rigid attitude of mind, according to which for instance the future is by definition unknowable and completely unforeseeable, nevertheless contains a future-prognosis, though in the prohibitive sense and moreover often an incorrect one. The violent opposition to all endeavors towards free anticipation of the future is itself based on one specific outlook on the future preferred as such, but generalizing and dogmatizing. In this process future and non-future are equated to each other as intellectual quantities, with only one single exception established a priori.

It is my point of view that free scientific development and appropriate application of the new *prognostics* techniques mentioned above are being seriously *hampered* today, and will continue to be, by the defense mechanisms proceeding from, and covered by, a *dogmatic* attitude of mind or by dogmatic habits of thought, conscious or unconscious, with regard to the future.

In a certain sense the historically developed, now prevailing future-dogmatics, with its strict rejection of any kind of reliable knowledge of the future other than the one modelled and limited by itself, thus forms a *negative* component of any free-thinking, progressively oriented prognostics. One can no longer control the problems of *tomorrow* looming up on all hands by the solutions of *yesterday* founded on an imperfect outlook from a distant past, and therefore defective.

That is why I decided, *after* the completion of the part on Prognostics, that I ought to write the study of Dogmatics now forming the first part and to allow it to precede the other part for a better understanding. I hope that the reader will accept that as a result repetition was not always avoidable. Indeed, notably where the deliberate ignorance of the social sciences with regard to the social form of the future is concerned, I have sometimes purposely used this repetition as a "frappez, frappez toujours", to attack the growing danger of this docta ignorantia on all fronts at once.

Of course, in a narrower sense prognostics proceeds from reality. From the reality that now exists in all kinds of new scientific development or applications. And likewise from the reality with regard to our definitely entirely different future which is now bearing down on us tempestuously. After all, the initial purpose of this work was to explain this *positive* component of the undogmatic prognostics now unfolding. This, of course, has *top priority*. Closely connected with this difference in rating of importance is a difference in approach.

The part entitled Dogmatics does not have the slightest pretension of being historically exhaustive or philosophically and scientifically complete. There could be no question of that, if only because, as explained above, only one aspect, the future-facet, has been detached from dogmatics as a whole. However, it will be self-evident that in reality this aspect is connected by all kinds of threads to the development of thought — religious, philosophical, scientific, epistemological or psychological — as such. Even that one future-facet will therefore be handled without any claim to a truly scientific completeness.

The set-up has a more limited scope, viz. to demonstrate more in particular how, in which respect and to what extent specific *socio-scientific* thought about the future has been and is still being most strongly influenced by future-dogmatics. In other words, how greatly this very socio-scientific thought has in many respects been constantly gagged and bound and, especially as regards its prognostic vision, directed one-sidedly or counter-directed with rebellious opposition. It is the intention to demonstrate by this at the same time, so to speak automatically, why precisely *this* intellectual freeze has exerted a tremendous and at the same time unfavorable influence at alle times, and therefore still does today: because the future repeatedly, and now more than ever before, makes itself felt precisely in that field of thought, that of *social reality*. The intellectual gap mentioned above has the most serious implications insofar as this gaping void manifests itself with steadily increasing severity between the practically stagnant course of a mainly *static* social science on the one hand and the vigorously pulsating development of social *dynamics* on the other.

Conversely — and I think it correct to postulate this with all due modesty — the part on prognostics, unlike the one on dogmatics, and precisely in connection with the last-mentioned phenomenon, does have at least some scientific pretension. For it is concerned with the emergence, probably confirmed by certain indications and symptoms, of the contours of a new *science in the making*, and is the *first* systematic contribution towards establishing a foundation for and elaborating this new science. So far this has been a field where angels fear to tread, and where consequently future-thinkers who are particularly progressive in themselves usually still prove to be highly hesitant and easily frightened off, and where they often seem to be overcome by ambivalence and, at the "moment suprême", by fear of their own daring. An antiquated future-dogmatics not infrequently seems to cast its dark shadow even over the creative and emancipated work of this forward-looking intellectual elite.

The situation is now such that in the firm belief of the present author such a new, developing scientific conception regarding the future will encounter many sorts of obstacles on its way to full development.

For every new scientific development and specialization opposition of this kind is, in itself, completely normal. If it possesses sufficient rational or functional strength of conviction for its raison d'être, it will without a doubt overcome this opposition or perhaps, precisely with respect to the future, step over it with sufficient elasticity. In that sense ever-further specialization and the scientific growth of new specialisms even form a characteristic of our modern age of science. It is not only usual that the new can develop only by fighting strenuous rearguard actions with the old but perhaps it is even as a rule desirable, so as to preserve a meaningful continuity. Moreover, contradiction forms the strongest mainspring in scientific progress.

For those to whose knowledge and social conscience the urgent call for the development of a scientific "prognostics" adequately appeals, the "dogmatics" may therefore be largely superfluous or further proof of their beliefs. For those whose opposition is aroused by this in their opinion pretentious and unrealistic prognostics, referring them back to the (i.e. their) dogmatics will probably simply incite them to intenser opposition.

Perhaps now my initial hesitation about whether it would be desirable to combine the two parts under one common denominator becomes more explicable, when it is seen that this is probably not necessary for the one and likely to have the opposite effect on the other. However, I finally decided, in view of the close connection existing between consciously pursued progress towards renewal of the framework of thought and obstinate adherence to the existing thought model, that I ought to maintain the bi-partite structure as a feedback that could not be disconnected. Above all because there is also a not inconsiderable intermediate category which perhaps sees something in the argument in favor of scientific change-over but which is equally susceptible to the attitude of mind still dominating and determining. I am therefore addressing myself in particular to this intermediate group, not yet definitely converted to a renewing exploration of the future but equally unconvinced about the absolute correctness of the negativistic ideas prevailing on this subject. It is to be hoped that this intermediate group contains a not inconsiderable section of the still flexible and progressive younger generation. Much would be gained if this "free-floating intelligentsia", to use Mannheim's expression, were to weigh the arguments contained in the two complementary parts as fairly and critically as possible and then consider their further position.

Partly for that purpose I should first like to state more precisely what exactly is meant by the two terms dogmatics and prognostics used in this work.

Introduction

CHAPTER 1

Definitions and thought models

Einer neuen Wahrheit ist nichts
schädlicher als ein alter Irrtum.

GOETHE

1. Dogmatics of the future as dogmatics

As already stated, this work refers more particularly to dogmatics of the future, and above all that of social science. However, for centuries social science was put on the same plan as philosophy and other sciences through its close ties with these. This may not be ignored in an analysis of dogmatics of the future. On the other hand, although I should like to concentrate in particular on this combined or separate dogmatics of the future, this does not entirely discharge me from the duty of making clear what should be understood by the composite term "dogmatics". However, it is especially difficult to indicate in a manner that is both clear and acceptable what precisely is meant by the general concepts dogmatic and dogmatics. These are greatly charged with emotional associations which usually testify to disapproval and are denigratory. There is always an inclination automatically to label an opinion we do not share as dogmatic, while on the other hand we are just as quickly convinced that having a differing opinion of our own testifies a priori to an undogmatic attitude of mind. Of course, things are not really as simple as that; if they were, the other person or the other idea of things would be dogmatic and our own opinion by definition undogmatic, which of course would be both an absurd and a dogmatic idea. However, without a personal value-judgment a valid criterion can hardly be given for the exact point at which a certain view or conviction becomes, or degenerates into, dogmatics. Drawing the right line between dogma and truth, if at all possible, is in any case a highly complicated and thus not infrequently disputable or disputed matter.

This is apparently somewhat more simple in the only field in which dogma and dogmatics thought that they had acquired a reasonably safe and permanent raison d'être: the field of religious and ecclesiastical dogmatics. And this occurred not only at an earlier date, but also much more strongly in Roman Catholicism — with its strict doctrines, its proclamation of dogmata and papal infallibility — than in Protestantism. Nevertheless, even in these fields dogmatics, viewed historically, has often not been able

3

to maintain or regain its position without shocks, fluctuations and violent discussions.

The dogmatism of the Catholic Church was not an independent thing. The Church was often obliged to adopt and confirm such a dogmatic point of view as a means of taking a firm stand and proclaiming the absolute authority of Biblical Revelation against what it regarded as heretical falsehood. Precisely what constituted heresy in this regard was of course determined by the Church itself and its own (and incidentally varying) historical interpretation. As long as the Church was victorious over heresy, falsehood continued to be falsehood. When in the Reformation sectarian heresy could no longer be overcome, its original falsehood was gradually confirmed as a new truth of its own and finally as dogmatics. The exclamation attributed to Pontius Pilate: "what is truth?" may also be interpreted as: what is falsehood, what is heresy? The relativizing wisdom from Pascal's Pensées: "Vérité au deçà des Pyrénées, erreur au delà" is still literally and figuratively true.

Above all because Protestantism in general had a less rigid and a freer attitude towards the authority of an ecclesiastical hierarchy, it was on the whole able to be less dogmatic in that respect, especially after the principles of the Reformation no longer needed to be quite as much on the defensive, which generated orthodoxy and fanaticism. Relatively speaking, Protestantism later received critico-historical and philological Biblical study somewhat more easily, relatively speaking. Liberal theological trends were able to gain support at an earlier date.

This does not alter the fact that precisely in the latter half of our century considerable influence has again been exerted on Protestant thought by the successive volumes of "Kirchliche Dogmatik" (the first appeared in 1932) by Karl Barth. However, as always, dogmatic action was followed by anti-dogmatic reaction. In our days this has doubtless reached a climax in a "God is dead theology", and "evangelical atheism" and a resurrection of the "secular city" (as opposed to Augustine's Civitas Dei). However, from the Catholic side, too, both the Vatican Councils and modern national movements (not least the Dutch) have entered into a highly dynamic period of accelerated development. This will in due course doubtless give rise to a modern dogmatics. At present the latest papal encyclical "Populorum Progressio" itself forms in a generally pleasing fashion a milestone of anti-dogmatic progressivity, although there would be no difficulty in quoting other recent papal pronouncements with a highly conservative trend to them.

But what now is dogma, or dogmatic thought, outside specific religious thought, or outside the still greatly varying religious beliefs of the various Christian denominations? The Greek word "dogma" is itself older than Christianity. At first it certainly did not have the dogmatic interpretation later given to it.

4

Initially dogma had a meaning almost the opposite of its current one, viz. little more than an opinion which could, however, consolidate into a conviction. Only later did it acquire the sense of a principle or even doctrine. In Roman Antiquity it was given in constitutional law the significance of *authority*: Senate decrees, imperial edicts ranked as legal dogmata after proclamation. From there it is only a step to dogma as God's law, although, especially in Protestantism, doubt and uncertainty will always persist regarding the share of human interpretation (or contribution), or even of human error, in the proclaimed divine truth, in other words a truth vested with unassailable authority. At regular intervals this doubt leads back from a historico-dogmatic, official theological proclamation to the original Christian evangelical preaching and the religious beliefs on that subject relativized for every temporal and spatial situation, i.e. demythologized and deideologized.

In other words, dogma and dogmatics themselves prove in the long run not to be susceptible to an unchanging, absolutized dogmatization, which could be invariably and universally valid for all times. They too are of only a relative historical importance, even in the light of the religious proclamation of eternal truths or of a creed regarded as orthodox, or of hierarchical authoritarian power exercised by one of Christ's deputies on earth with doctrinal infallibility. Dogmatics is anything but "saevis tranquillus in undis", peaceful amidst the turbulent waves, but is itself subject to constant change with the passage of time. The greater the acceleration of the rate, the greater the intensity and impact of social dynamics, the less the permanency and certainty of existing dogmatics.

The shift or elevation from dogma to norm is no more than a change of problem. Divine, moral or scientific norms can also lay claim to absolute validity but cannot substantiate it as unchangeable for all time.

The norm merges into the idea of normal and normality. What is regarded here and now as normal, or as abnormal, is of no greater authority than that of historico-relative morals and habits, including habits of thought. Human awareness of norms is likewise subject to permanent and fluid change, the more so according as the change in and of time itself is stronger in terms of rate, impulse, energy and intensity, and the prevailing staticism is replaced by a compelling, all-pervading dynamism. In this force field, with its high tension and heavy charge, the consequently changing awareness of norms in turn reinforces the temporal change in interaction. Firm definitions of the concepts norm and normal can no more be given than of dogma and dogmatic.

Even a critical, undogmatic thinker like Kant nevertheless tried to do this. As is known, ultimately only two things still made a deep and lasting impression on him: "the starry heavens above me and the moral law within me". As everyone knows, he endeavored to translate the latter into a humanistic and therefore nevertheless universal categorical imperative: "do not do unto others as you would they should not do unto you".

However, outside the specific fields of religion and morality there is above all a third area of particular interest to us here, where dogma and/ or norm have repeatedly settled and been preserved, viz. that of *philosophico-scientific* or *pure scientific attitudes of thought*. Repeatedly in the course of history we shall encounter a normative methodology laying claim to unassailable, absolute validity and autocratic authority. This validity and authority are proclaimed in the same doctrinaire, dogmatic and therefore both imperative and imperialistic manner as in religion and ethics, and are founded on equally axiomatic and thus invariable principles and universal prescriptions. Sometimes they are intermeshed with religious, religio-philosophical or more or less purely metaphysical ideas, and then again with ideas predominantly oriented towards the *natural* sciences and detached in appearance or reality from the former category. It is above all to this development that the explanation attempted here will relate for the purpose, as stated, of being able in particular to crystallize its effect on *socio*-scientific thought as exactly as possible.

It will become clear in the process that scientific dogmatics, where it lays claim to a timeless and absolutely immutable validity, is nevertheless also and equally bound at all times to a typically temporal and spatial situation or to a given pattern of culture. In other words, that this scientific dogmatics, like that of religion and morality, and often in conjunction with it, is repeatedly subject to historical change and fluctuation. This conjunction and change are studied above all by the history of science and the sociology of science. However, the remarkable fact occurs that this sociology of science searches its *own* heart too infrequently (or too superficially) and consequently proves hardly capable of exposing or at least continuing the line of its *own* socio-scientific dogmatics. An effort has been made in the dogmatics of the future below to analyse this socio-scientific intellectual process and its extremely great significance in a more lucid and critical manner.

Perhaps it is advisable beforehand to make some comments on the *aids* which, from of old, have been used by human anti-dogmatic thought — and are still used today — to unmask as such existing dogmatic thought and fossilized, distorted intellectual prejudices, deeply immured in embracing, rationalizing and generalizing thought models. In other words, auxiliary techniques for arriving at an undogmatic widening or progress of philosophico-scientific thought, or of thought regarded so far as being pure scientific. Beside and behind the history and the sociology of science there proves to lie a third field of thought of exceptional interest: that of philosophical self-reflection and philosophical fundamental research.

The most important intellectual instruments for overcoming dogmata include *sceptical* doubt and *critical* appraisal. Scepticism is one of the oldest philosophical touchstones. It was used systematically in particular by the Sophists, who became prominent in the fifth century B.C. Protagoras: "man is the measure of all things". Thus every opinion on Being or not-Being is at any moment relatively true for every man separately. Gorgias went a step further: everything is relative; no opinion on good or bad, true or false is itself absolutely true, because every opinion is comprised in the ever-changeable Being.

Socrates borrowed the ever-probing, sceptical and critical irony of the Sophists; for him, too, there are no fixed definitions absolutely valid for everyone. However, in the Socratic method an inner voice (cf. Kant's later moral law) tells everyone unmistakably what he should do. Moral duty is indicated not objectively and intellectually, but subjectively and intuitively. His scepticism with respect to the knowable and the known emerges from his famous saying: "all I know is that I know nothing".

The sceptical attitude of mind towards intellectual and moral sham certainties or dogmatically posited certainties reached a climax with Pyrrho. According to his teachings, sceptical wisdom leads to harmonious purification and redemption. This alone gives the true peace of mind (ataraxia). To achieve this, one should abstain ascetically at all times from any judgement (épochè).[1] Uncertainty and unknowability formed the props of this anti-dogmatic intellectual system. Of course, in its absolute and systematic negativism it led in turn to another dogmatism, viz. scepticism.

Sceptical and critical doubt later became a central starting-point for among others Descartes, Montaigne and Bayle, each in his own way. Intermingled with relativism this line of thought, which may be described as a French one, continues from Montesquieu to Voltaire. In England this sceptical and critical view was systematically employed by David Hume, who thus set about the concept of causality, together with other fundamental categories of knowledge, and rational religion. As philosophical criticism this new attitude of mind was to reach a climax in Germany in Kant, the "All-Zermalmer" hesitantly at first in his "Träume eines Geistersehers", then influenced by Hume and ultimately vigorously in the "Kritik der reinen Vernunft" (1781) and in his works for many years thereafter, until the beginning of the nineteenth century.

However, let us return for a moment to the dividing line of the ages formed by Kant. In his work "Was ist Aufklärung?" (1784) he characterized the era (the epoch!) of Enlightenment as that of man's final emergence from a period of tutelage which had been his own fault. In the Renaissance a first renewed humanistic attempt had already been made to restore the typically human dignity: the power to determine one's own future destiny. Now Kant advocated, precisely on the ground of this new coming-of-age of man, the combating of dogmatics and despotism, the acceptance of religious tolerance and, last but not least, freedom of research, combined with free expression of opinion. Religion and metaphysics became extra-rational or transcendental. According to Kant the critical capacity is diametrically opposed to the dogmatic attitude of mind that accepts traditional, religious, metaphysical, mythical, legendary, axiomatic and apodictic or doctrinaire habits of thought without further justification or verification, i.e. imposes them on itself and on others without the requisite criticism or self-criticism. Kant's theoretically rational criticism led in him too to a restoration of the primacy of practical reason, i.e. of volitional action, also for the future, in accordance with man's good will.

Rationalistic Enlightenment, with its criticism of dogmatic traditions and its plea for undogmatic freedom, ushered in a modern era, the era of the mainly scientific Encyclopédie and of a new enlightened philosophy, which was to prepare the ground for the French Revolution and the American War of Independence. Later ultra-rationalism and intellectualism were in turn to be exaggerated in dogmatic fashion into extreme isms and to have their repercussions in a converse dogmatics of reaction and irrationalism.

Nevertheless, at a still later date, extending deep into the present time, intellectual rationalism was to undergo a tremendous second growth in the form of logic, which likewise went back all the way to Antiquity. It is as if the same kind of film is run off every time: advent with critical doubt and verification, heyday, uncritical exaggeration of dogmatic certainty. Logic, too, initially formed a sharp-honed instrument for a cool, sober, unprejudiced opinion. The old Sophism (have you not lost your horns? If not, then you still have them!) was first refined into the logical paradox. Besides sceptical and critical doubt the paradox formed one of the most accurate weapons in the struggle against dogmatic opinions.

Modern forms of logic have been repeatedly worked out and enthusiastically welcomed as modern liberators from outmoded dogmatic habits of thought. For instance, Bertrand Russell (with Whitehead the founder of a new mathematical symbolic logic) calls logic "the great liberator of imagination".

Besides scepticism and critical, axiomatic and aphoristic philosophy I must first make separate mention here of an entirely individual kind of philosophy, which initially was also deliberately meant to be anti-dogmatic, that of Comte's *positivism*. It was directed against every form of theology and metaphysics and aimed at a purely factual science, from which a *new social science*, sociology, gifted with *special capacities in respect of the future*, had to be born. This vision of positivism as observation of the purely factual was later elaborated in two directions: philosophically by Husserl in a specific and subtle manner in phenomenology, and methodologically by finally developing it in its turn into an extremely overdrawn neo-positivism.

The positivism of Comte, who was associated with the Ecole Polytechnique, which had always been greatly oriented towards the natural sciences, was in essence an extension of pragmatic empiricism, as vigorously advocated for the first time, especially for the natural sciences, by Francis Bacon (in his work on "the advancement of learning") and applied with almost sensational, in any case literally spectacular (viz. telescopic), success by Galileo in particular. Empirical observation and experimental verification proved to be of tremendous value, as against speculatively dogmatic Scholasticism and Aristotelianism, to the progress by leaps and bounds of the natural sciences. It was self-evident that in due course they would be elevated to idols of *all* practice of science worthy of the name.

Thanks to the empirical positivism of Comte, at the same time building on Descartes' mathematical rationalism, it ought also to have been possible for the social and cultural sciences to become genuine modern sciences, freed from dogmatic assumptions and traditional prejudices. But things already started going wrong with Comte in later years, when positivism had literally to serve as a new religion. In the radical neo-positivism, developed above all by the Wiener Kreis of Carnap, Schlick, Neurath, Reichenbach et al., this doctrine also grew figuratively into the only true faith in the field of methodology.

It is in the latter strict methodology that practically all the former anti-dogmatic, again dogmatic lines of thought meet again. Not only does this demonstrate the effect, in science too, of action and reaction, the fluctuation of force and counter-force, but moreover this development again shows how a liberating, anti-dogmatic attitude of mind, by being exaggerated, becomes its own antithesis: a new formal and aggressive dogmatics. Again and again the *open* system, precisely through its over-strong and one-sided effect, becomes in turn almost automatically a *closed* system. The anti-schematic emancipation changes into another but equally dogmatic black-and-white scheme. Every anti-ism seems almost predestined, once it has made itself fully felt, to reveal itself as an equally suffocating ism, in an endless cycle.

It may then be asked whether a lasting anti-dogmatic attitude of mind is really possible. If I imagine that I am thinking anti-dogmatically, then surely in that very intellectual process I am almost automatically in the pupal stage of becoming dogmatic and intolerant.

Though the concepts tradition and authority form the two extreme boundary posts of the area covered by dogmatics, they do not go to the heart of it. If one seeks the essentials or the deeper roots of the concepts dogmatic and dogmatics, one soon comes into specific fields of sociology and social psychology, and also of depth psychology and clinical psychology. It can hardly be disputed that dogmatics and egocentric or ethnocentric isolation, coupled with intolerance, of a group regarding itself as the chosen one, far superior to all other peoples, minorities, formations or circles, are closely related, also outside religion. So closely related, in fact, that dogmatics, superior exclusivity and authoritarian intolerance are practically identical and interchangeable. This is most clearly apparent, apart from fanatical and murderous religious disputes, in dogmatic discrimination, aggressive contempt and persecution, or at least subordination, with respect to race, color, class, status, caste and descent. Much research has been performed into discriminatory prejudices against Jews, Negroes, and non-whites or non-Aryans. In this category also comes what is sometimes called "ticket" thinking: conforming partly voluntarily, partly compulsorily to the normal, the mass, the average man, the social group attachment, the other-directed human type (David Riesman), and so on. The latter is of course based on the rule of safety in numbers, which likewise ensures that "dogma rules", even though an occasional person can see through the paradox of the "lonely crowd". All these and similar studies have contributed a great deal to a greatly improved psychological insight into the essence and the effect of the authoritarian, intolerant structure of personality and character, into the typical aspects of dogmatic thought. But their definitions are usually in turn schematizing or tautological. In any case it becomes clear that the polar frames of reference of dogmatics are nevertheless formed as a rule, or at least most strongly influenced, by the two poles of tradition and authority connected as it were by an inner axis. But, as stated, these are not themselves "ruhende Pole in der Erscheinungen Flucht". The historical combination of tradition and authority does in fact tend at all times towards the narrowing or handicapping of a free process of thought.

As a rule tradition will relate more to blind faith in something that is true in itself and of itself, i.e. is regarded as dogma without further examination. Authority, however, is essential to the institution and lasting confirmation of such a faith, which therefore will usually also be partly founded on and maintained by an authority regarded as indisputable. But to some extent this is circular reasoning. For authority is regarded indisputably, on the strength of an identical faith, as the belief in certain ideas which are themselves automatically accepted as authoritative. In any case, however this may be, by virtue of this authority a further investigation of the content of truth, notably of the linked dogmatics, superiority and intolerance is not only *superfluous* but is also *forbidden* now in all severity as heresy, satanic temptation and intolerable dissension. It is therefore indissolubly bound up with excommunication, with rejection from the community in question and its inviolable supremacy.

The words authority and display of force are subject in our modern democratic society to a slow but sure depreciation and tarnishing. The adjective authoritarian has a doubtless antipathetic and almost equally unpleasant significance as for instance the pejorative expression totalitarian as against the completely innocent total or totality.

10

Doctrine and discipline are more or less acceptable, doctrinaire not at all, and disciplinary only half-heartedly. Come to that, the word discipline has already degenerated in meaning from a free science practised thanks to systematic teaching in the fundamentals, to a strictly bound form of control, also as discipline of thought. The word disciple, which at first was used in particular for the faithful followers of Christ, has acquired a bland and sometimes even slightly jesting meaning.

From the historical point of view, with respect to exercise of authority and discipline, the ruling regents do not have an overwhelmingly bad name, but in the modern Dutch view a "regent mentality" is anything but acceptable.

At present the expression "obedient to authority" sounds almost reactionary. In processions and otherwise the authority and political acts of authority of those in power are demonstrated against, or even rebelled against. Nobody in the Netherlands, let alone a political party, wants to be regarded as conservative today. But progressive is not always an ornament; often it is an insult.

Orthodox still compels respect in religion, but enjoys little appreciation outside it. The term "rectilinear" is not a pleasant-sounding one. Freethinking is permissible. But a freethinker was long regarded as a godless libertine.

Libertine, despite sharing the same Latin stem, has quite a different emotional content from liberal, which in general testifies to a wide outlook and broad, tolerant view. Once upon a time classical liberal was a prevailing, dogmatic-economic philosophy of life. But in Britain today "liberal" in the political sense means belonging to a small, shrinking middle group between the two big parties. In America a liberal is regarded as very progressive (sometimes falling victim to the witch hunts against Communism). In the Netherlands a liberal, according to public opinion, is — as the mouthpiece of the employers — more or less conservative, which will be fervently denied by the Young Liberals, since in this sense they are no longer liberal.

According to the critical older generation, the younger generation suffers too much from a lack of standards or an excess of the wrong ones. On the other hand, in the opinion of a critical younger generation (of "angry young men") the older generation displays evidence of obscurity, hypocrisy and abuse of power.

It is usually this sceptical younger generation which rejects the tradition and authority of an older generation and which sees in the prevailing mentality or habits of thought no more or anything else than a half-baked, purely formalized cliché, a practically endless repeating fraction of hollow phrases and empty terminology, in short fossilized ideology, dogmatics, prejudice.

It will now be clear, even from a highly superficial linguistic test, that the concepts tradition and authority, and also the word associations con-

11

nected with them, are too greatly subject to a process of attrition for it to be possible to use them as a sufficiently firm basis for useful research into the essence of dogmatics. Perhaps the term prejudice just introduced gives something more to go on.

Now what is the "precise" difference between opinion (the original meaning of dogma), interpretation, conviction, judgment and prejudice? Prejudice does not apply differentiating judgment and earmarks. The concept prejudice thus in any case contains the idea of an *un*founded "pre" (prejudice, preconception), i.e. like preceding, premature, prepossessed, predisposed. In American investigations the following comes to the fore as the second characteristic of these overhasty, immature attitudes: excessive generalization and simplification, plus a rigid and stereotype repetition, persisting and remaining constant despite all fundamental, structural and essential change. The essence of dogmatics, which moreover definitely comprises a systematic and reinforced *collection* of *prejudices* is now, I believe, most closely approximated by saying that hereby *the "normal" process of thought is largely eliminated*. It directs itself automatically towards the immovably firm data of an existing and evidently unassailable tradition and towards an axiomatically indisputable and thus permanent authority that is no longer susceptible to any kind of change. It may therefore help to clarify matters to state that tradition and authority really form the two sides of a mask evading and covering the truth. Unmasking this head of Janus then means reactivation of the process of thought concealed and ossified behind this mask. At first sight it seems irrelevant whether tradition and authority reside in religious revelation or proclamation, in political conviction or superior authority or in a scientific thought model. This is, however, of importance to the extent that dogmatics is encountered above all at a *higher* intellectual level. Prejudice is usually a general property of the public at large and of public opinion. Dogmatics, on the other hand, is mainly bound up with a higher (also regarding itself as higher) intellectual class of the representatives of religion, politics and science. There the elimination of the process of thought that is "normal" for *that* privileged intellectual milieu hits twice as hard and the distortion or obvious mental narrowing of this intellectual elite is multiplied many times in its effect.

This phenomenon is eminently relevant to the scientific thought model. A *static* scientific thought model in which and through which the intellectually circulated and *dynamically* fed process of thought is brought artificially to a state of paralysed and isolated standstill is a contradiction in terms. Science exists by the grace of endlessly progressive thought, freely propagating and renewing itself. *Scientific dogmatics is intolerable, since it precludes the true essence of science and makes a mockery of it.*

Nevertheless, this dogmatics repeatedly forms a characteristic and an almost inevitable concomitant phenomenon of science. The true practice of science therefore consists not least in the repeated aggressive liberation of science from the dead hand of dogmatics. That is why real scientific progress must so often occur suddenly and jerkily, presenting the unexpected appearance of a discontinuous and disparate happening. *The dogmatics of social science is at the same time the most persistent and the most dangerous of dogmatics.* It is the most dangerous because it always tends to keep social reality, i.e. the established order, immovably under the spell of its dominating theory, instead of following reality closely with its theory, indeed anticipating the *dynamics* of this reality and communicating the future social possibilities, chances, dangers or desiderata to the public at large trapped in prejudice. To my last breath I shall combat dogmatics in social science, possibly with a certain "déformation professionnelle" and, if it is the only way, even with apparent intolerance. If necessary I am prepared, like Don Quixote, to tilt at windmills of outmoded tradition and disputable authority, in the hope that others with greater discernment and a more accurate aim will lead to progress.

Social dogmatics, through its tendency to stand still in and with reference to time, and moreover accentuated into a fixed *dogmatics of the future* bound chiefly to the past, blocks our way to the future. It does so at the very time when, more than ever, the *future* is making an urgent call on all our abilities, and certainly not least on our socio-scientific knowledge, judgment and capacities. The ancient Chinese already had the proverb: "If people do not attend to the future, they will soon have to attend to the present"; how much more greatly and more strongly is that not true of our convulsive times of permanent revolution? The truth of a social reality evolving or even revolutionized at a high tempo cannot or at least can no longer be fixed. Moreover, we can gradually replace erratic and unexpected *inconstancy* by well-considered and purposive *changeableness*. In this way we ourselves create not only a new social reality but also a new social truth. Both can be approached by socio-scientific methods and techniques undogmatically renewed again and again. The history of science shows that scientific dogmatics is an eradicable evil, but socio-scientific dogmatics of the future may *now* be worse than sinful crime, viz. an irreparable error.

2. Prognostics as a science in the making

> I do not believe in a fate which strikes men *however* they act. But I do believe in a fate which strikes men *unless* they act.
>
> G.K. CHESTERTON

Here, to start with, I can be much briefer. For here hardly any criteriological, axiological or epistemological difficulties occur, at least in giving fairly exact definitions of the concepts used.

However, the fact that, as far as I am aware, the term *prognostics* is introduced as a new coining in this work for the *first* time is a different matter. This calls for a double explanation from me: A. to start with, *what* precisely I mean by the term prognostics, and B. why preference has been given to precisely *this* not yet existent name.

A. Quo vadis?

Let me start with a short and sweet statement: at present prognostics is *nothing*. The word has been introduced here to define a possible new science in the making which is now in its first vague initial phase. When it has reached maturity we might call it the *science of the future*.

As I have said, such a science does not yet exist. However, there are all kinds of trends pointing in that direction, especially in America, for instance the creation of separate university chairs or courses specially devoted to subjects relating to this. And nowadays research steadily growing both qualitatively and quantitatively, becoming increasingly specialized and sophisticated, is also being devoted at present to forecasting the future, with more and more effectiveness and looking ever further ahead. This is being done in many quarters (universities, government, military staffs, business, private institutes) and again America is in the forefront. In that country special future institutes with staffs of thousands (both generalists and specialists) are by no means uncommon today.

It is unfortunately true to say that the great majority of contemporary social scientists in Europe see very little indeed to be gained from a scientifically sound approach to problems of the future.

Against the prevailing opinion, I do not consider this view scientifically sound. However, it is often the case that when we have something which we hardly use, at least consciously, we are not particularly attached to it. But when there is a possibility of our losing it for good, that it could escape from its existing task, from its own special field, and possibly become part of a more progressive and dynamic approach, that is when the trouble really starts.

Such a short-circuit threatening from the outside would augur little good for the future of these social sciences, unless, at least, they adapt themselves in good time. Perhaps it would not be a bad idea if the concept prognostics were to assume in such circles the form of a cat among the pigeons. Possibly this would stir things up a little, if I may put it in so disrespectful a fashion (for I share some of the responsibility), in what is at present an almost stagnant, unruffled pool. This immobility tempts or obliges the practitioners of the social sciences to engage in the not very uplifting process of "muddling through" at a time when everything around them is on the

14

move. This process also leads to a kind of *double* standard, coupled with *half* solutions: the future, as long as it still is the future, is pushed on one side and declared inadmissible, but as soon as it has become the present it is treated with oily deference and servile obedience, a crablike retreat from "crucify it" today to "Hosanna" tomorrow, from breaking off diplomatic relations to jumping on the bandwagon.

In this sense prognostics may be interpreted in the context of challenge and response, as an answer to the very strong challenge of the future to our present time, already in existence and still to be expected. But also, conversely, as an intensified challenge to our social science, to which a suitable and timely answer, as is increasingly evident, has not been forthcoming for far too long, to our cost and its shame. For the future this could still lead in the final instance to an almost ideal cooperation, of actuality and perspective, of science of the present and science of the future.

B. *What's in a name?*

Of course the choice of a new name always rests on personal preference, if you like on a value-judgment. That is the case here too, but that is certainly not the whole story.

Anything but, in fact, since in the Anglo-Saxon countries and also in a number of European ones, including the Netherlands, *another* term for the same concept has in recent years begun to establish itself in the tentative manner peculiar to a vanguard and is now recognizable, if not yet recognized. I am referring here of course to the term "futurology" being used with gradually growing ease in certain circles. This term was coined several decades ago and defended in a number of articles in professional journals by Professor Ossip Flechtheim. At the time, shortly after the Second World War, it met with absolutely no response or rather, if it was not completely ignored, it then aroused, as was to be expected, an opposition operating rather in a negative sense.

Those who know me will admit that I would definitely not be put off in the slightest by that opposition in itself. After all, it is the inevitable fate of new ideas and of visionary thinkers first to arouse such opposition, sometimes violent and often personal. Nevertheless, a very long time elapsed before Flechtheim dared to take up his old idea again and to focus attention on it again in a book that was a collection of articles on rather scattered subjects. But possibly he had become too discouraged to attempt a more scientific foundation and systematic elaboration, although, even today, we certainly owe considerable gratitude to the spiritual father of "futurology".

The principal merit — and indeed no small one — of the term futurology is that the component or dimension of "future" finds particularly clear linguistic expression in it. However, in my opinion this advantage should be carefully weighed against other, possibly greater disadvantages.

Anyone who is realistic must be aware that in general the future is still regarded as the divine book with seven seals, the almost completely veiled mystery of Dame Fortune with her incalculable wheel of fortune, the by definition unknown (terra incognita), the riddle of the Sphinx, the ambiguity of an inextricable oracle or of the cryptic apocalypse or cabala. In this respect many adhere firmly and obstinately, with both feet on the ground, to the classic term "ignoramus et ignorabimus" — we do not know and we shall never know. Science above all should leave this field to tea leaf readers, crystal-gazers and fortune-tellers, to palmists and clairvoyants, to gypsies, spiritists, ecstatic poets or mystic muddle-heads.

Thus, according to that outlook, futurology in the sense of some kind of knowledge of the future or precognition is pretentious, reckless, misleading and unfounded. But, as a science of the future, it also runs the risk of exaggerating its own possibilities. C'est le ridicule qui tue, a highly undesirable, opposite effect. One is very quickly inclined to put it on a par with methods of foretelling the future used of old and established as unscientific, e.g. with fortune-telling or prophecy, which neither was nor is free from charlatanry, abuse and fraud. Or the very controversial matter of parapsychology and proscopy, i.e. really of what is regarded as abnormal or at least paranormal, is brought up. Finally, through a somewhat similar sound and sense a comparison with astrology, which usually still has a very bad name in scientific circles, is an obvious one to draw. Even the old linguistic suffix "logy", derived from or associated with the particularly unclear Greek Christian "logos", seems rather to work against the word. Are on the one hand theology and ontology, and on the other hand graphology and chirology, real sciences? Do neologisms like gerontology and pedology really have a chance? Indeed, is an introspective psychology entirely up to the mark?

And in addition there are not unimportant epistemological or even strictly logical objections. Futurology, as a science of the future, is said to be the only science that has no real subject, let alone a clearly defined one. The future does not exist — not yet. How could one conceive of a strict science with reference to something which does not yet exist as such, is neither observable nor verifiable? Would this not be at best comparable with a practically abandoned speculative metaphysics, and at worst hardly more than unbridled fantasy? How would an objectively establishable and universally acceptable science of the future be conceivable? True, in that case what is new is not assessed by means of individual, immanent criteria, but verified precisely by a historical scientific dogmatics, but nevertheless it is different to deny that the term futurology as such is more or less defenceless against sharp criticism, which cannot be entirely denied elements of logical correctness insofar as a contradiction in terms seems inherent in it at first sight.

Try the experiment of seeing how infrequently you can use the word futurology without evoking from the person you are talking to an at least

16

rather ironic smile or sardonic grin, or a disbelieving or disapproving frown or shrug of the shoulders, or without causing him to raise one or two hands in adjuration or to make other physical gestures of instinctive defense and aversion. A sensitive mind-reader could add quite a few other things along the same lines, because many people are too polite or uncertain to speak their mind when turning something down. After all, you never know with these modernists, and times change quickly. In itself, therefore, an inadequate reason for pertinent rejection.

As if this were not enough in itself, more and more popular American magazines have started to shorten "futurology" in otherwise serious studies to "futurism", perhaps because they find the former word too long or too naive. Apparently they do not know enough about the history of culture to realize its European meaning. It will be recalled that futurism began about 60 years ago in Italy as an anti-traditional renewal of painting, spreading to music and literature, and also to other European countries. In the minds of many it was closely related to, if not synonymous with, the somewhat later Swiss-French dadaism, which aroused feelings of considerable opposition and indignation among most people at a time when non-figurative art did not yet exist, although after the transition into surrealism it is now no longer so very remote from ultra-modern trends in art to which people today would like to give the name of gagaism or gogoism, or pop art and op art.

However this may be, the unfortunate reminiscences and emotionally charged associations with respect to the over fifty-year-old futurism would make the use of this term, at least in Europe, almost impossible, and certainly out of the question for a development into a new field of science coming forward with scientific intentions and pretentions.

I can consequently very well imagine that one of the first and most deserving European future thinkers, Bertrand de Jouvenel, emphatically rejects a term like futurology and rigorously refuses to use it for any purpose whatsoever. But what is his alternative? With typically French sophisticated esprit this erudite connoisseur of the classics merely speaks of "l'art de la conjecture".

De Jouvenel explicitly declares himself to be opposed to any true science or knowledge of the future. He is likewise against any pretensions to prediction, forecasting or prognosis, insofar as these could create the impression and suggestion of what is to him a fundamentally *unfulfillable* and *never achievable certainty*.

The furthest to which De Jouvenel is prepared to go, in deviation from and in contrast with a certain scientific knowledge, is a kind of art. This term was taken by De Jouvenel from the title of a work Ars Conjectandi, by the celebrated mathematician Jacques Bernoulli. The word "conjecture" means no more than a guess, and we are concerned here with the art of well-reasoned guessing which could lead to a responsible decision. De Jouvenel

17

tries to demonstrate that this usage also follows on that of the leading historian of Greek Antiquity, Thucydides, and on that of the crowned head of Scholasticism, Saint Thomas Aquinas.

In other words, De Jouvenel seeks the justification of his terminology not so much in the modern challenge of our near future as in the classical past. This terminology is not only highly modest, which is to its credit, but also, in the light of things to come, a little too conservative. One of the reasons for this, as I shall demonstrate in detail, is that during the writing of his work at the beginning of the 1960's De Jouvenel was evidently not yet aware of the latest forecasting techniques, which have a much greater "cleverness" and future range.

Quite apart from these drawbacks, which I definitely do not wish to worry about too much, although taken together they are not inconsiderable, I have an additional and decisive objection. As a true Frenchman De Jouvenel regards any usage of a word acceptable, provided that it is understandable in *his* language and derivable from a Latin stem. But in my opinion we definitely need a medium that can be used internationally. This would in itself have been complied with by the terms futurology and futurism which I rejected above. But if I take as my criterion Anglo-Saxon usage, then a translation of "l'art de la conjecture" could mean almost exactly the opposite of what De Jouvenel understands by it.[2] For, even though De Jouvenel does not wish to guarantee the slightest certainty, he does of course seek the greatest and if possible the exact degree of probability.

This untranslatability, or inevitable translation into an almost opposite idiom, in my opinion entirely excludes "l'art de la conjecture" as an international terminology easy to use and unambiguous. And in any case it complies just as little with another requirement of such a linguistic medium and vademecum: unambiguous briefness, indication of what is meant in one form of expression that is simple to use, i.e. consists of one word.

Similar but opposite difficulties would occur if we were to start from American usage, in which at present systematic exploration of the future has made the furthest progress. Usually the term "forecasting" is used there, as a rule decked out with an explanatory predicate or adjective, such as "long-range forecasting", "technological forecasting" or "economic forecasting". I fail to see — quite apart from the rather long-winded definition given by these terms too — how it could be possible to achieve an internationally standardized translation into other languages.

Moreover, "forecasting" describes a more or less technical process, viz. looking ahead with the aid of certain equipment and saying something about the future. But it would be wrong, and therefore not customary, to identify the technique used with the scientific view, basis or demarcation from which and for the practice of which certain instruments are used. In comparable fashion terms such as prognosis, provision or prediction — which

18

incidentally differ considerably from one another in meaning, as we shall see later — tend rather to indicate the aim pursued of exploration or forecasting, which after all may be applicable to *every* science but definitely not to the possible development of one given science, as stated or assumed above.

In addition there is another possibility propagated from certain quarters, partly to avoid the odium inevitably adhering to the term "futurology". Years before the pioneer De Jouvenel started his work — with the aid of the Ford Foundation — a French group had already been founded by the French philosopher Gaston Berger, with qualitatively very considerable support in leading circles. This group chose as its name "prospectivisme", which it also gave to a journal devoted to the subject. This name caught on here and there in other countries as well. Such a name is therefore in itself quite definitely most useful for an international linguistic code.

And yet, after ripe consideration, I am of the opinion that the term prospectivism could not render my meaning, or only very partially. This is quite apart from the fact, on which I do not wish to enlarge, that we are concerned here in the first place with an obviously antithetic contrast name. Prospectivism contrasts with historism or historicism. Research into the future is regarded as being of primary importance, as against and in preference to a study of the past (ending in the present). In principle this express orientation towards the future is of a particular attraction. Anyone who has read my "The Image of the Future" and my theory on the prospective picture of the future as a central category of socio-cultural dynamics will also hardly expect anything else from me.

Nevertheless, I have some quite considerable reservations. I regard historical knowledge as an indispensable aid to reliable knowledge of the future. I do not like the antithetic starting-point, the philosophical accentuation is perhaps overdrawn, the pendulum swings too far, too quickly or too strongly towards the other extreme. The dimension of the future does not stand alone as an absolutely autonomous, disparate and discontinuous quantity. The possibilities of influencing the future are always bound and limited to a certain extent. The forces from the past-present have their effect. Knowledge of the strength of these forces, of the desirabilities and possibilities of influencing them, i.e. of their possible changeability for creating another future in accordance with one's own responsible determination of one's destiny, ought precisely to form a very important part of a science of the future which has not only *philosophical* but also *scientific* claims and makes pronouncements accordingly.

Personally I am rather chary about any "ism" set up antithetically and taken to its ultimate consequence in all directions. Prospectivism, just like historicism, could develop into another dogmatism. Exploration of the future and control of the future must first prove themselves scientifically, substantiate themselves. They cannot present themselves a priori as the only true approaches. They must be able to show their positive results, achieved by their own efforts. The somewhat negative contradiction or reversal is without a doubt fruitful, but is in itself an insufficient condition of success.

What remains after this survey of existing possibilities and applications, at least those known to me? Only the introduction of a *new* term, answering as well as possible to the aim set, in other words a neologism to be invented (as once, not so long ago, economics and sociology were) seems to be indicated. A search could be made for certain compound words ending in "nomy" or "nomics" (such as astronomy or economics). Astronomy, detaching itself from astrology, the model of the first true science, independent of theology and metaphysics, is perhaps in itself attractive for a new science. But the suffix "nomy" points to a narrowly scientific type of thought model, connected with some natural law (nomos means law, natural law). The physical-nomothetic (lawgiving) knowledge ideal of the classical natural science is, however, seriously outmoded and has gradually been stored away in the museum lock, stock and barrel by modern science, as will be dealt with in detail below. If futurology is slightly ridiculous, futuronomy would be dangerously ambitious and self-destructive.

What about the suffix "metry" or "metrics", then? Geometry and econometrics are particularly successful, sociometry has been a complete failure and psychometrics seems to me at least to be extremely dubious in the general sense. However, quite apart from success or failure, I feel less than nothing for this connection with the concept of measurement. The implicit presumption here is always that what cannot be measured quantitatively must fall outside the practice of science. The tractability of measurability is decisive here for what can be studied scientifically or not. An all-embracing science of the future, however much it may and indeed must aim at the greatest possible exactitude, should never be coupled with such a dogmatic, literally exclusive and apodictic or aprioristic thought model. If it were, considerable parts, subjects, forms or forces of future-forming would in advance be stretched or cut as in a Procrustean bed, which would be quite wrong and would lead to malformation.

As a result, my ultimate choice fell at last on a theory of *prognostics*. This definitely does not shun exactitude, insofar as it links up with an older formation of concepts like that of logic, physics, mechanics and mathematics, or with a more modern one like cybernetics or biogenetics. However, nor does it disavow its partly qualitative directedness insofar as the latter leans on metaphysics, ethics or aesthetics, or on the still elusive or un-understood social dynamics. There cannot be the slightest doubt about its specific objective: work on scientifically sound forecasts. For international usage there is not the slightest problem: prognostics, prognostique,

Prognistik, etc., etc. However, prognostics is also more than prognostic work! For the time being I should like to define this prognostics as the science which, with advanced methods and instruments, aims at exploring the future and acquiring probable knowledge of the future. It is also the science which tries to control the future, based on this systematic anticipation, by purposively guiding the future by socio-dynamic techniques. It comprises those areas of prognostic reflection, viz. concerning the possible, ideally essential and actually achievable future developments, in economic, social, technological, political and cultural areas, and on both a national and a worldwide scale.

The greatest problem, and definitely no small one, is formed by the scientific foundation and demarcation of the specialized field developing as such. I have no illusions about the fact that I have not fully solved this problem in the present work. On the contrary, I am fully aware that for the time being this cannot be anything more than a first systematic contribution to further consideration, at most a provisional basis for discussion. Only critical reflection and examination can show whether and to what extent the path followed here will afterwards prove to be the right one. Nor, I believe, may one expect more from a broad-brush outline meant as pioneering work.

My sole pretension is thus the view that the first vague contours of a separate new science are beginning to form. I certainly do not presume to claim that this science is already springing up cut and dried, crystal clear and tangible, or even unassailable. We are only in the very first phase, which may or may not develop further. The possible future of a science of the future cannot yet be predicted with certainty or even with probability. There will consequently be no positive prognostication on my part with respect to prognostics itself. But on the other hand it is an empirical truth that "ce n'est que le premier pas qui coûte". This step *must* now be taken by someone in some fashion or the other, by someone who is prepared to function as a kind of try-your-strength machine. His consolation must be that, the harder they hit, the higher goes the heavy weight!

3. Exemplary American and free-floating European thought models

> Wer immer strebend sich bemüht,
> Den können wir erlösen.
> GOETHE, FAUST II, CONCLUSION

Before starting the work proper I believe that it is particularly desirable, indeed definitely necessary, to point clearly to and account for a paradox characterizing this work, a paradox which, I may say, is in some respects almost a tragic one.

If you peruse and study the first part on dogmatics, it becomes indisputably evident that thinking about the future is as such a European invention, if I may put it that way. However, on that continent it has repeatedly been choked or run to death, or at least calcified and mummified in dogmatic strait-jackets of thought models. Thought about the future is an idea and product of the European mind. It is also a brain-child that has been detained in a state of tutelage in Europe or has even been angrily shown the door as a stepchild, or so swaddled and corseted that it has grown crooked, suffers from rickets, anemia or hunger edema, or has come to a halt in its mental development. True, in the course of the centuries other and new ways of original thought about the future have been developed time after time, but ultimately the same fate awaited these products of the human mind almost without exception. They were all squeezed into certain molds, matrices or models, and bound to imperative prescriptions, dogmatic norms and methods which did not allow of any free life, any independent development.

In the America of the Founding Fathers, belief in the future, set in the American Creed, and propagated in the American Dream of the immigrants and the pioneers moving westward, was borrowed from the enlightened and revolutionary pictures presented by European thinkers about the future.[3] Come to that, the same applies — mutatis mutandis — to humanism and the Marxism of the leading Russian thinkers.

Now the tragic paradox is really a dual one. In the first place we in Europe discovered sociology as a social science and brought it to life as a specific science of the future (Comte), but it was in America that it was first unfolded in its true, full-blooded and vital form. It was there, too, that it first gradually bled almost to death. After the Second World War, and after five years of standstill, we have just chosen in Europe, and notably in the Netherlands too, to proclaim the models of this cold-blooded, almost dead American sociology, which has largely degenerated either into a timeless, completely abstract and empty formalization or into extremely fragmentary, disintegrated pieces of science of the present, as the only valid thought models. We have taken great pains to bow down to them in submissive worship, indeed as idolaters, to copy them exactly.

The other side of this dramatic event is, however, that in America itself they have not resigned themselves to this literally and figuratively bloodless revolution. In a certain sense they have ignored it, they have as it were simply stepped over it. This kind of social science proved entirely useless, especially with regard to future development, and certainly also for an attempted control of the future. Building on European ideas about the future, but giving them a completely American, i.e. purely pragmatic, twist or implementation, they have developed on the other side of the Atlantic all kinds of new, practically independent prognostic techniques and methods no longer strictly bound to any existing science.

22

That is why I described the paradoxical situation as a dual one, because it is precisely *these* American ideas and applied developments that were *not* taken over in Europe. This could hardly happen, because there was *no existing European science* that could borrow, imitate or critically correct these renovations. For in America it was not, or not yet, a science, but chiefly a development of technology, though also applicable as a *new social technique*. And in Europe we tend to observe a somewhat greater distance with regard to technology.

This places us before a dilemma, of both science and conscience, confronts us with an unavoidable ambivalence. I consider it only fair to say this at the outset, so that we bear it in mind thoroughly and continually and also, if possible, to nip in the bud what would otherwise probably have been a considerable degree of misunderstanding.

It will certainly not escape the reader that in the prognostics part repeated reference is made to the already highly advanced technical developments in this field in America. Nor shall I withhold from these developments the admiration which they deserve. If the reader gains the impression from this that we ourselves in Europe, with a few exceptions, have really become an *underdeveloped, backwards region,* this conclusion is, unfortunately, entirely true.

However, this in no way implies — and I should like to stress this point in advance — that this book is a paean of uncritical admiration and an appeal for indiscriminate imitation. The opposite is rather the case.

For the American development shows two sides of the coin which both equally deserve critical attention. On the *one* hand there is the development of fascinating new technical possibilities for reconnoitring and exploring the future as a probable shape of things to come. "Coming events cast their shadows before", and with projective techniques one can try to intercept these shadows and shafts of light or to convert them into recognizable images. But on the *other* hand, to at least the same extent, and often as a deliberate objective, the equally possible techniques can be developed which enable us ourselves to shape a future which we regard as desirable or optimal, or with which we can try to transform an expected future which we regard as unfavorable into a more suitable type of future.

We could distinguish between these two types of future techniques as *exploratory* and *normative* techniques. Now while what matters above all with the exploratory techniques is their operational usefulness, their plausibility, gradually increasing, maximizing and perfecting the force of their predictive capacity, we are in an entirely different world where the normative techniques are concerned. In a world where once again an ocean-wide distance could become a huge, perhaps almost unbridgeable intellectual gap between America and Europe.

I have deliberately spoken here of an *intellectual gap* and not a *techno-*

logical gap. In recent years enormous attention has been devoted to the technological gap that is said to exist between America and Europe. This has given rise to a great deal of discussion and has often caused alarm, especially when the phenomenon of the brain drain from Europe to America has been thrown in as well. Unfortunately, most of what has been said and written about this is not expert comment or relevant, or at least does not go to the heart of the matter.[4]

From the purely technical point of view we can do as much in Europe as in America, we ought not to lag behind; in fact, as is now the case, in certain fields we can perform better technical achievements than in America. As regards applied technology, various large European concerns definitely do not need to play second fiddle to their larger American brothers, and in fact have a temporary lead here and there.

But where there really is a difference, in fact already almost a world of difference, is in *mentality* and *thought patterns*, differences which come clearly to the fore not only in views on industrial management but also in those of the university world. This characteristic difference in way of thought naturally expresses itself in numerous respects, but nowadays it stands out perhaps furthest and precisely most significantly in an almost diametrically opposite *attitude of mind* with regard to the *future*. We therefore ought perhaps to speak of a "prognostic gap", which also has a deeper foundation and connection with a "socio-technical gap". Whilst America in practically all sections of the community is most characteristically and ultradynamically oriented towards the future, in Europe the mentality continues too greatly and in too many fields to be bogged down in a rather stationary, contorted *present-day position*.

It is *as a result of* this often awful and sometimes awe-inspiring difference in mentality and this almost 180-degree different attitude towards the future that the technological gap could in due course actually become a real danger. Because technical progress in America is to a much greater extent mentally and primarily purposive, and because this progressive urge towards the future is also given top priority there. In that respect intellectual and academic status has equally been impelled to such an extent to the highest peak of human ability and knowledge for future achievements to be attained or performed that, *for that reason* alone (and not only because of differences in remuneration), the brain drain will inevitably be intensified to a steady, ever-swelling stream. Anyone who brings with him new, daring ideas for the future and experimental future techniques or shows an inclination towards this renovating, penetrating intellectual habitat may be assured in advance of a cordial welcome in America and of a carefully tilled, fertile breeding ground for his ideas. The fanciful mind, and even the crackpot, the science fiction visionary, the speculative ideas man, possibly later unmasked, but not discouraged, as a phoney, but possibly also greatly esteemed afterwards for his correct and profitable anticipation[5], has in that country an undisputed reason and an established right to exist. He enjoys every possible facility for self-expression and also for the outspoken or even arrogant cultivation of intellectual fads and fashions. There, daring, readiness and the willingness of businessmen to take a chance are, in a much greater degree of mobility and elasticity, directed towards growth, expansion, change, renovation, revision and remodeling, precisely and above all where this leads to new figures, phenomena, shapes and kaleidoscopically shifting configurations of the *future*. A future which, already often referred to as "2000-plus", is moving ever further past the rapidly approaching year 2000.

In itself this real passion for the future fills me with admiration and even with a little envy. But on the other hand one must definitely not close one's eyes to possible consequences or unattractive, one-sidedly exaggerated implications which could very well be attached to this and in fact prove to be.

For it is always the question for *what purposes* this mental effort and the newly developed prognostic techniques are applied. What do people expect to achieve with them, what has in fact already been achieved? We can also turn these questions round: what *could* or *should* people have achieved with them, what has barely or not at all been achieved?

In the America of today the application of these prognostic techniques, which are as advanced as they are spectacular, is particularly concentrated in three strategic fields: *industrial, military* and *governmental*. Dr. Erich Jantsch has drawn up an extensive report on the subject for the OECD which, I trust, will be published in various languages. This report will be discussed in detail in the prognostics part. Here I shall just mention a few highlights, only insofar as this makes it possible broadly to visualize a black-and-white contrast with regard to the possible advantages and disadvantages of the use (or abuse) of these studies and analyses of the future.

Jantsch has analysed 500-600 large or medium-size American corporations with an annual turnover of as a rule more than $ 100 million. According to his estimate, these industrial majors are already investing about 1% of all their research funds in research into the future, and in some cases up to $5\text{-}10\%$. His broad survey indicates that expenditure on this research into the future has increased by leaps and bounds in recent years, and nowadays about $ 50-100 million a year is being spent by these firms' own internal industrial research departments and, in a proportion of about 10 : 1, an additional $ 10 million for specific external contracts for studies of the future concluded with separate think-factories or think-tanks, or specialized future research institutes.

Jantsch has also tried to arrive at a rough evaluation of the results achieved. By way of example he mentions extremely expansive growth firms like Texas Instruments and Xerox Corporation. According to his investigation, methodical technological forecasting definitely supplies about half of all ideas for new products. Sometimes a factor 4 applies to the increase thus obtained in the number of ideas for new profit-making products. The number of cases in which technological forecasting more than doubles the profit made on new products or the turnover of the latter is growing very rapidly. His simple conclusion is that as the ultimate result of this research into the future the profit on such investment rises in average about 50-fold.

At the present rate of dynamism the future picture of industrial developments also changes very rapidly. IBM, for instance, penetrated the computer market at the last minute by a resolute change of policy, afterwards acquiring some 70% of this market. European concerns in France, Britain and the Netherlands followed or are following considerably later. Purposive, systematic future market research and technological forecasting would certainly have had an accelerating effect on new European products in a number of European countries. In Europe not only the total expenditure on research and development (R. and D.) is considerably lower than in America, but so is the relative share of specific prognostic research in this expenditure. This industrial prognostics extends in America over a period in the future of at least 10-15 years, and indeed in a number of cases over a period of 25-50 years. On a rough estimate America, as regards purposive industrial dynamism, prognostics and the matching organization, is at present on average at least 10 years ahead of Europe.

In addition the new techniques and methods for forecasting the future have been tackled in America in a particularly intensive manner, in fact already since the last period of the Second World War, but in a much more extensive and systematic way from then onwards, by the Pentagon and by the highest military bodies. As in industry, the whiz kids and the brain boys have come very quickly to the fore here, in the organizations' own ranks or via big contracts signed with outsiders for research into the future. It is well known that for instance America's most celebrated long-term think-factory, the Rand Corporation, was initially financed almost exclusively by the USAF. The Army, the Navy and — last but not least — NASA likewise have their own extensive divisions for research into the future and generous budgets for meeting the costs of such investigations by separate semi-official or private future advisory institutes. It is a fact that a very large proportion of the new offensive and defensive weapons techniques and also of the ultramodern espionage equipment has resulted from this kind of research. The same is true of very many new ideas, technical apparatus and inventions which were required for the development of space travel. In addition new means and methods of air transport (the air lift to Berlin, the helicopter gunship war in Vietnam, the supersonic jumbo jets and air busses, the Mach 2 transports of the future) originated from this kind of research into the future[6], without mentioning such developments as early-warning radar, anti-missile missiles, artificial satellites or high-energy missile umbrellas with cosmic radiation.

A third area in which application of these sophisticated prognostic techniques is extending with ever-increasing speed along a steadily wider front in America is that of the central government economy. In more and more Federal executive departments use is being made of prognostic systems analysis and special purposive cost effectiveness methods to increase efficiency and yield and, above all, to obtain a result to be regarded as optimal for the future in terms of time, money, energy and clear *objectives* to be gained. Compared in that respect too European government policy may already seem rather archaic and parochial, and above all definitely not excelling in clarity or precise explanation of objectives whose achievement in a more distant period of time is aimed at.

However, in this very respect I should definitely not like to contribute to a possible misconception, viz. that everything is ideal in America, thanks to the application of modern prognostic techniques. That is anything but the case. Criticism from Europe, but equally inside America, is extremely outspoken on this very point. Foreign policy, the racial problem, the educational system and even the well-intentioned but partly unperformed, partly ineffective plans for "The Great Society" speak their own language, mixed with a satirical McBird, scandals extending to the highest regions of the Senate or White House, and a growing credibility gap between the top leadership and the country's intelligentsia.

But the weak point lies precisely in the definition of *objectives*. For the prognostic techniques serve not only to indicate as clearly as possible what *means* ought to be the most effective for a *given* end. They serve equally, if not more so, for acquiring a more correct insight into the *objectives* themselves or for showing whether, and if so how, other and better objectives ought to be selected and worked out for the future as a *task*. Or, to put it more formally, for the optimal transition from the status quo, which will have to disappear in any case through a radical process of transformation, to the terminus ad quem (the ideal final state). This refers to socio-political and socio-cultural objectives, and humanistic objectives regarding man's future and the future social system.

This certainly presents a not inconsiderable danger. Apprehension about the latter is definitely not removed by popular explanations of futurism or the futurists. Without any conscious or unconscious prejudice and detached from personal or political views of society, it seems to me that there is a fair risk of a development in a less desirable direction, even with an opposite effect. It would be nonsensical and petty to keep on regarding America with European arrogance and a sense of false superiority as a kind of wasteland of cultural barbarism. But it would be equally incorrect to romanticize the developments going on there. There is the unmistakable and real danger of

27

a tendency in America to direct these very objectives in accordance with vested professional interests, for the strengthening of the existing capitalist order, for opportunistic ends, in short principally to increase economic prosperity and to strengthen America's power in world politics and in what is to some extent undeniably neo-colonialism. That is even almost inherent in the applications mentioned above as coming most to the fore now: military, governmental, industrial.

It is by no means impossible that these progressive techniques, if reserved for and monopolized by a kind of parvenu but exclusive and esoteric priesthood, with almost unlimited funds available, would mainly benefit the forces of conformism and conservatism, forces administered and dominated by a relatively small technocratic elite, a new undemocratic oligarchy. In this way prognostics could become bogged down in a new dogmatics which no longer opens up a new future but closes the door to this all the more firmly, or distorts it in a prejudiced fashion. This new dogmatics would mainly serve the purposes of material prosperity and concentration of world-wide power, but certainly not those of spiritual well-being and the highest elevation of human values or goodness.

America must in any case always beware of the too easy identifications of "bigger and better": more technology = more dollars = more success = more good things = more progress. The advanced future-techniques, in themselves progressive and forward-looking, are in danger of being drawn over to that materialistic and opportunistic side. America leads in the field of industrial and military dynamics, but has contributed little to or does not amount to much in the field of socio-cultural dynamics. It has its industrial and its military technical think-factories, but knows hardly anything about civilian and cultural think-institutes. This threatens to lead to a distortion of normative prognostic techniques. As a rule the great fashion of American technological forecasting is at present still too purely technological. And therefore such exceptional importance attaches to the democratic and socio-culturally progressive manner in which the problems of the *objectives* for the future are incorporated in these techniques. Not just pragmatic but also and equally cultural objectives.

There is an additional and very important reason why there is a repeated danger of this less desirable development being reinforced and overdrawn. It is that in America too short-term thinking, especially as regards political policy, is still far from having been overcome. This short-term thinking automatically limits the objectives, too. For then the objectives remain on the whole limited to countering at the eleventh hour unfavorable developments that have already begun, sinister future possibilities which have finally become clearly visible. Erosion and the fatal consequences of the reckless use of pesticides, famine, bloody race riots, poverty, unemployment and disease, air and water pollution, slums, traffic jams and suffocation of

28

the cities, plagues of rats, smog, organized crime, intrusions on privacy, etc., etc., then successively attract attention after spectacular eruptions and explosions. Crisis, catastrophe and calamity ultimately compel pragmatic action time after time as "something inevitable".

This action serves largely as a reaction, i.e. the short-term averting or limiting of the most dangerous development trends that are expected to continue further. This intervention finally appearing necessary lies in the mainly *negative*, prognostic plane of "self-destroying prophecy". In many cases a challenge is not answered until after the event, after it has revealed itself in concreto with unmistakably destruction potency, and then the answer in those cases is in keeping: it is apt to be too simplistic, tending towards temporary relief, i.e. towards playing for time, deferment and a "with time comes counsel" attitude at variance with the essence of a truly progressive, comprehensive prognostics serving the public good.

The answer to the war in Vietnam then is: escalation; to the real threat of a civil war between black and white: pacification, compromise and of course a presidential committee; to a war breaking out in the Middle East: laissez-faire; to a feared Third World War: ABC-Z weapons; to automation: a presidential committee; to bureaucracy: automation; to China: no admission to the United Nations; to the developing countries: a peace corps; to world mortality from hunger: releasing stores of agricultural surpluses, and opposing the sacred cows; to capitalism: anti-trust legislation; to corruption: congressional hearings; to Communism: the CIA; to the assassination of President Kennedy: a presidential committee and the FBI; to the Kennedy Round: "you scratch my back and I'll scratch yours"; to the hippies of LSDisneyland: a hate-in and a teach-out; to space travel: "the first men on the moon"; to the endless spiral of world population growth: the free-of-charge inter-uterine loop; to the "other America"; essentially the same America, etc., etc.

In other words: the answer to the challenge of long-term prognostics usually comes too late at present, is too slight, too provisional, too fragmentary, in brief not visionary enough. Just as in the past, the Cassandras are hardly heeded if at all today. Rational action continues mainly to be defined as "wisdom after the event". Only when the crisis has set in in acute form are efforts made "to do something about it", and then mostly temporary palliatives.

Since the Civil War, now more than a century ago, relatively little has been done for the Negroes. The classic study by Gunnar Myrdal on the subject is already more than 20 years old. The civil rights program has got going too slowly, and real integration has been deliberately thwarted. Socioeconomic and educational discrimination against colored people in America is appalling; if anything it has become worse. *After* the Black Power movement has almost inevitably gained in power and suggestive influence, any-

29

thing which may still be extorted by force will always and largely again be *within* the framework of the existing political and capitalist structure. This will be imputable to both a faulty long-term outlook and the lack of a volitional attitude towards the requisite fundamental change and a preconceived changeableness of the existing social pattern, in accordance with objectives laid down beforehand. In other words, this is due to neglect of a utopian-normative and idealistic directedness, which ought to reach its completion and have its effect in the eminently *positive* self-fulfilling prophecy, methodically setting its sights further ahead to a dissection of "the American Dream"!

As regards the objectives, the highest priority will always have to be given at the top of the hierarchy of values to the creative, imaginative effect of desirable and achievable projections of the future, not so much for "the great society" as in anticipation of and leading to "the good society" inspired by the dream to be realized one day of the other and better society on earth gradually to be approached, which will soon already be widening, indeed growing in all directions to cosmic scope, including the planetary and extra-planetary, oceanic and galactic worlds.

Now in Europe, latterly not least under heavy pressure from modern American sociology in particular, we have unfortunately sadly defaulted almost completely both in theory and in practice in this thorny field of humanistic values and objectives for future human society. Serious thought has been given to these matters almost exclusively in the field of economic policy, where, broadly speaking, a pleasing degree of agreement has been arrived at on the objectives to be pursued. In social and cultural areas there is an enormous lack of anything of the kind; our ascetic, unworldly attitude of mind is, like one of the 28 dominoes, still double blank. Our dominant social science is, in the field of objectives, methodically absent and deliberately abstinent, rigid and frigid.

However, this does not detract from the fact that, when we are able to think our way out of this rather miserable and sterile intermediate stage and, in particular, when we think back to the highspots of the European spirit, which after all has left its permanent monuments and milestones "aere perennius" precisely in this enlightened humanistic, socio-ethical, progressive revolutionary and idealistic utopian field, we may no longer avoid this task bequeathed us. There will have to be sufficient self-confidence that, even today, a valuable contribution can be made by Europe, precisely with relation to these *normative* problems in which individual human happiness, well-being and dignity, the pursuit of the highest universal values of collective human existence and social life are at stake.

The future of man and of human society are involved in our times — still mainly subject as yet to the whimsical and dangerous interplay of free forces. The survival of a flourishing Western culture is in the balance.

30

We are concerned among other things with maintaining and evolving a democratic social order, with man continuing to grow above himself in the direction of the "summum bonum" forming the most exalted ideal. And with the question of how the ultra-dynamic development processes now rushing on their way, which without any doubt will result in one way or the other in radical social transformations and fundamental structural shifts, can best be controlled, where necessary and attainable corrected and where desirable and possible guided in our favor. It is definitely not just a matter of the problems — however important they are in themselves — of how we could build up a kind of early-warning system in the socio-cultural field as well, aimed against the harmful risks, possible crises or even nihilistic consequences of the in themselves equally probable chances of the future as undesirable forms of the future. Our task is more comprehensive and above all constructive, namely how we can exercise in optimal fashion our function of *responsibly determining our own destiny* in our present situation with regard to a future dawning tempestuously and radically upsetting the established order.

We may and must study the new American thought techniques and thought models, for the time being without engagement. After that we shall have to take a stand ourselves. We shall have to choose and on the strength of this choice decide whether and how we can apply it in reforming and improving our existing social order, against the background of our prevailing values of freedom and democracy, and also in the light of a perhaps necessary renovation of the values themselves, which might need to be regarded as being of higher value or deeper content for a future, different and better society. Freedom and democracy are of course eminently current concepts also or precisely in America. However, there the interpretation, indeed the philosophical reflection, seems polarized between the extremes of dogmatic and pragmatic.

In conclusion I should like to add a few short notes for the concrete elaboration of the European point of view outlined here.

(1) In the first place Europe already has at its disposal a number of institutional agencies which could very well be put to work on this task in a more specific or methodical way: EEC, Euratom, ECSC, OECD and the Council of Europe.

I have already mentioned the expected publication of the OECD's extremely interesting report on the new prognostic techniques now in full development.

I know that the Council of Europe is studying a plan for the creation of a "look-out institution", a permanent forum in which problems of the future (or matters with a future-aspect) can be thoroughly discussed by intellectual leaders, managers, prognosticians and politicians, thanks in part to compact institutionalized and specialized machinery. They would thus form a Council of Wise Men for tackling in good time and thinking out the key problems of the future, long before these are ripe enough to be submitted to the national parliaments or political parties for a final decision.

(2) The establishment of an international future-research institute in Europe is highly desirable for the coordination of the work which is now both scattered among various countries and divided into different sectors. It is to be hoped that European *and* American philanthropic foundations or modern Maecenases will also be prepared jointly to further the creation of such a body.

(3) What *can* Europe's own contribution be? I am firmly convinced that a forward-looking attitude of mind oriented more strongly towards the future could lead to a particularly rich harvest in very many fields:

(a) a highly important contribution could of course be made by social science. However, this would first have to renovate itself thoroughly, revise its fossilized methods. Entirely new information and communication techniques are awaiting application. Soon, perhaps, social data banks will become available. However, these ultra-modern techniques need not be awaited, although here too computers can be of great use for improved and accelerated data processing. We shall not have to be afraid to extend social dynamics to form a dimension of the future. The idea of a science of the future should no longer be ridiculous or contemptible; it must not in itself be inferior to a historical study or to knowledge of present-day reality. We shall have to learn to work with propositions and hypotheses on various possible alternative forms of the future. Social science will also have to seek a future truth, but at the same time must sacrifice its most beloved and venerated value: certainty. For all possible futures contain by definition elements of uncertainty.

It is clear that increasing fear through uncertainty about the future also forms to a proportionately increasing extent a neuroticizing factor of pressure and depression in present-day human society. Social science could contribute towards reducing this anxiety by providing more future certainty. But first it must overcome its own inhibitions and will have to be prepared to shoulder some uncertainty itself.

Only on this unstable basis of uncertainty, intangibility and insecurity, of risk, adventure, ignorance and misjudgment can it begin to build again. This will be its service and at the same time its principal merit.

(b) European philosophy will have to undergo a similar metamorphosis. So far it has been hesitating between three possible directions.

First a continuation of the endeavors of the classical Stoa, later to be found in Spinoza, among others. This trend would like to banish completely both feelings of hope and fear. For both relate to an *uncertain* future. They lead to inner doubt and disquiet, to a life oscillating between hope and fear, without peace of mind. Poetic echoes are to be found above all in Goethe, Schiller and Rilke, without their entirely mastering this ambivalence.

Secondly existentialism, prepared by Pascal, Kierkegaard and Nietzsche and continued by Heidegger and, above all, Sartre. The choice now falls on the positive reconciliation with the negative fear of living and dying, the revulsion, the despair, the evil, the death that leads to nothing and the unchanging hopelessness from now to all eternity. Literary interpretation of Nothingness may be found in particular in Camus, and in music, but with a much stronger ambivalence and a change of general tone, by Gustav Mahler.

Thirdly the retreat from all philosophy and metaphysics into an absolutely peaceful timeless symbolic logic, into semantics and significs, into syntactical and grammatical linguistics, into analytical tautology, which as of today and for all the future is meaningless, even dead, frozen or in hibernation.

Philosophy, too, will have to muster the courage to face the unknown and frightening future again. An all-embracing future, or different conceivable futures, which in all cases call for an outlook on totality, i.e. a synthetic judgment.

We no longer live in a messianic world of prophets, saviors and redeemers. We live in a world of "Entzauberung" and debunking of myths. For us there is no longer a prestabilized harmony, no theodicy, no automatic, irresistible progress, no historical predestination towards the millennium. We must think out our own future, think in advance by thinking *back*. Change too is changeable. Where are we going, and why?

This is a new task for deep-digging philosophical reflection; thinkers such as Heidegger, Bollnow, Bloch, Marcel, Buber, Berdyaev, Mounier, Jaspers, Merleau-Ponty and Guardini have made cautious, tentative approaches towards solving it. And not in the last place Teilhard de Chardin, however impenetrable his views may perhaps be. All these are European thinkers of a breadth and a stature which, generally speaking, barely appear or flourish in the more pragmatic America.

Pragmatism, coupled with philosophical exploration of the objectives on the intellectual horizon and the aim that man shall be allowed to determine his own destiny, can have a particularly salutary effect; on the other hand, operating alone it may become almost disastrous. It is still true for America too — indeed precisely for America — that "there are more things in heaven and earth than are dreamt of in your philosophy". Horatio is too predominantly operational there.

(c) Most closely related to the field of philosophy proper is that of values, norms, ideals and criteria for a future society, a borderland of social ethics, religion and humanism. From these quarters, too, a renewed effort is required for the further and also concretized definition of objectives. The tentative start that has been made with the discussion on a "responsible society" ought in fact to be converted into and widened to a discussion on a mankind responsible for the *future* society.

33

(d) There still remains the urgent rehabilitation of what once formed one of the principal intellectual driving forces behind socio-cultural dynamics, a typical intellectual product of European soil: the utopia. There is the greatest need for new, inspired and inspiring, positive and motoric visions of the future. Methodical, instructive and idealistic visions of the future, which can take over from the counter-utopias that have prevailed too long and which, instead of the horrible nightmare of a "Brave New World" or of the despotic terror of "1984", can project an attractive and meaningful picture of the years 2000, 2100 and 2500, which would be more than worth aiming at with all our enthusiasm and our spiritual capabilities, and also with the aid of all our prognostic techniques.

This is primarily a task for those whom Karl Mannheim once christened the "free-floating intelligentsia", and Arnold Toynbee the "creative minority", in brief of a cultural and intellectual minority, responsible for answers, suitable and timely answers.

(e) Finally, when I speak above about Europe, I do in fact mean Europe. Confronted with such a great, comprehensive and constructive task, an intellectual separation between Western and Eastern Europe is senseless. It ought to be possible for joint study groups to exist for mutual consultation on these social and cultural problems of the future which affect the future existence of all mankind.

(f) In this advocated East-West collaboration it is in essence a matter of overcoming and then bridging two kinds of mistrust, each of which is in itself not entirely unfounded. In the Communist countries there is a somewhat understandable suspicious inclination to regard the gigantic American research into the future as a diabolical new and perfected invention or Machiavellian conspiracy of capitalist and imperialistic making. In the West, on the other hand, one is conversely inclined to disqualify methodical studies of the future by Soviet Russia and the Eastern European satellite countries in advance as serving for the expansion and consolidation of preconceived Marxist positions. In my view, for the sake of an open future we shall have to put aside any dogmatic ideology as much as possible, irrespective of whether capitalist or Marxist dogmatics is concerned. I am convinced — and there are more than enough facts to support my belief — that progressive thinkers about the future in every country of the world are very willing to meet one another on what is fortunately still largely free ground from the intellectual point of view — that of the future — and jointly to consider in undogmatic fashion how the best possible socio-cultural and socio-political realization of an ideal picture of the future could be effected for the *whole* of mankind.

Both dogmatics of the future rooted in the past are outmoded, and for that very reason useless as dogmatics for the new, the other future. The future encompasses the whole earth; it decides the fate of mankind. Socio-humanistic study of the future is *planetary* or it does not exist. As soon as the dogmatics on both sides — or the mutual accusation of a dogmatic attitude — no longer cling desperately to their own former basic tenets, a forward-looking prognostics can have shining results: "forever . . . the twain shall meet". There is also a very close link between prognostics, the future of the world and future world peace!

(4) In my words of conclusion for this first, exploratory chapter, I should first like to ask for recognition of the paradoxical situation in which we find ourselves at present. For in my opinion there is no getting away from the last conclusion that we are obliged — perhaps in spite of ourselves, possibly grumpily and sulkily, but without a doubt simply *compelled* by force majeure — to make a complete change of front out of inexorable and irrevocable necessity. We must moderate our undirected freedom and curb the completely free interplay of forces, precisely for the sake and the preservation of our freedom. Enforced freedom. Enforced change of front with regard to the future, the future which we have not dared to look straight in the eye, as if it were a Medusa's head, the sight of which would turn us to stone. But the exact opposite is true, it is when we anxiously avert our gaze and our interest in that future, when we pretend, as we have done so far, to be blind to the future, and when our consciousness of the future gradually atrophies through disuse, it is precisely then that our fate runs the danger of becoming an unhappy one. It is urgently necessary to get to know the future as well as possible, in order that we can still direct or drive our destiny in an optimal direction as much and as far as is possible ourselves.

In our day we should give a new and thus a different answer to the three essential questions already raised by Kant: what can I know? what may I expect? and what must I do? And this must be a particularly clear, unambiguous and urgent answer.

What can I know? If we really want to, we can now also know about the future. Certainly not everything, nor with complete certainty. But doubtless much more than has been assumed up to now by too many people, including those who could have known and should have known better. And we can do so with what is in many respects a degree of probability that should definitely not be underestimated.

What may I expect? We may believe in a future, even in one which is not only different, but also *better*. We may also cherish that expectation, partly through a renewed and confirmed self-confidence in *human power*. With sufficiently developed scientific skills and purposeful, i.e. future-directed activism of the will, we can determine our own destiny better and more strongly than at any other time in the history of human civilization. Never have we had at our disposal so many sophisticated techniques still susceptible to further perfection than is at present already the case, for application to a development of the future that can be controlled and dominated.

What must I do? We must now use the powers and possibilities given us, which form the essence of our human dignity, in the fullest possible measure and to the furthest possible limits. In our human activity this determination of our own destiny should again move up with irresistible force to the top of our hierarchy of values. This zenith has already been achieved once before, in the renewed humanistic outlook of the Renaissance. This was followed by a development which first declined into an overtrained rationalism, next veered round to an equally overdrawn irrationalism, then resulted in an impotent fatalism, combining despair and fear, ending in complete passivity and in feelings of predominant impotence and hopelessness.

We must combine our intellectual forces. The future is neither determined nor closed. To a considerable extent it is still open; within certain limits it can still be determined by us. The future is not a completely unknown thing; we can explore it, learn quite a lot from it, also let it make our acquaintance. We ourselves can now largely *make* the future of our future.

The future is no longer for us an *order* to be awaited as given, that is to say in resigned surrender, whether a divine or a natural order, but it is a human order. More than that, in fact, it is a *plan* to be created and recreated by purposive mankind.

The future is neither a delusion nor an illusion which is absolutely unavoidable and must always lead to disillusionment.

The future may also be a truth, but not a "vérité faite" fixed in advance and to be accepted willy-nilly, but both a "vérité en marche" and a "vérité à faire". Man's most difficult and highest — but fulfillable — task is to *prove* this future truth to the best of his ability. He is now helped in this by the new, nascent, two-sided prognostics: exploratory and normative, speculative and active, rational and moral, knowing and striving, open and breaking open, future-directed and purposive, unprejudiced and with discernment, especially between good and bad.

It is we ourselves, those living today, who can write the history of the future now. Let us hope that it will be greeted with a more favorable judgment by those who will be living shortly than, with the best will in the world, we can now apply to our forefathers. What they left us includes war, overpopulation, lack of food, air and water, underdeveloped peoples, the overdeveloped megalopolis, an urbanized Lumpenproletariat, the eradication of nature and living space, pauperization, juvenile delinquency, class education, mass neurosis, synthetic leisure, racism and genocide, alcoholism, drug addiction and suicide, materialism and degeneration — and unrealized slogans of liberty, equality and fraternity, of humanitarian progress and of Christian salvation. Anyone who wants to work to improve this legacy, to rehabilitate a more distinguished intellectual patrimony, is by definition a man spurred on by the future. However, for the first time in human memory the contemporary *idealist* can at the same time also be par excellence a *realist*, by thoroughly studying and where necessary perfecting extremely desirable application of the new prognostic and supervisory techniques.

For the *first time*, too, man need no longer automatically be taken by surprise by the overpowering future challenge of technology, in particular that of the applied natural sciences and of the revolution of automation. He will be able to answer this challenge using the *same* intellectually sharpened weapons of modern technology.[7] For with the aid of prognostics socio-cultural and socio-humanistic technology can now be placed on the same plane, given the same impulse and impact, in order ultimately to establish a new comprehensive equilibrium all along the line at a *higher* level than achieved or achievable before, though with trial and error and also of course with ups and downs. Even now we can still seize these new chances for the future before they are already choked in the oppressive grasp of the future and mankind is hurled back into even greater impotence. The moment of truth and of the *decisive choice* has dawned. Anyone who is not for the future is against it. If we are activated at the right time and in the correct manner, the future will unmistakably be *for* us and for *us*. If we continue in our attitude of neglect and abstention, we shall in due course find the future turned directly against us, with immense dangers and serious threatening possibilities of evil probably vastly, almost conceivably, exceeding the troubles of today. These two opposite forecasts can now be given with absolute *certainty*. The real choice is therefore by no means one between optimism or pessimism, but one between activity and passivity, between purposive human power and resigned fatalism. If we consent to the future, then the following step is also inevitable: we must at the same time accept in the positive sense a technology of the future which outstrips in the socio-scientific field the present limited scientific practice and which, in our highly technical days, is the only way of arriving at effective solutions.

However, this has already taken us much too far much too quickly. At the end of this chapter the beginning looms up for us again like an almost impregnable bulwark. For now we are confronted with all those dogmatic attitudes of mind that repeatedly implant themselves against the future, also in the form of supreme scientific models of the future fixed in advance. With combined energy and with the greatest ingenuity these attitudes of mind try to frustrate — or at least discredit as much as possible — any new systematic approach, as advocated above, on the strength of their vested authority and conservative tradition. The occasional future-directed endeavor is summarily condemned as such, without any knowledge of the subject, as an offence against decency and as being in conflict with scientific integrity. Without a better insight into the immobility of this closed dogmatics of the future an open scientific view of the future will not be able to develop vigorously enough.

PART ONE

Dogmatics

The sad story of the coercive mutilation of thinking about the future

Der Mensch kann was er soll;
und wenn er sagt: "Ich kann nicht",
so will er nicht.

J.G. FICHTE

CHAPTER 2

Prenatalia: broken love-affairs between the past and the future

1. The vicious spiral of the prevailing attitudes of mind towards the future as a subject of study of the sociology of knowledge.

It is extremely difficult to find a reliable path or guide, preferably a thread of Ariadne, through the confused and confusing maze of historical attitudes towards the future. In this introduction to the subject-matter I should therefore first like to apologize for the initial caution, perhaps even apparently unnecessary circumlocutions, with which I am feeling my way. Even then it is impossible to make matters clear enough as long as the problem proper is only touched on.

Attitudes of mind towards the future are, together with this future in the making, themselves subject to a constant process of subtle change, so that they are difficult to grasp or understand when viewed in the form of a random cross-section or snapshot from the course of time. However, a study of these inconstant attitudes towards the future and of their intellectual development processes, in their interrelation to the course of cultural history, is particularly fascinating. It might even be said that these evolving attitudes towards the future are characteristic of the evolution of the history of human civilization as such and vice versa. For this history of civilization only really begins when and through the fact that man starts to be clearly distinguishable from animals in particular. Such an essential difference — man really becoming human — is especially marked by the fact that he commences to think about time and future.

In the same way, biologically speaking, man's liberation from the animal state is characterized by his purposefully forward-groping hand with the opposed thumb, his upright and forward-striding locomotion, his perspective vision enabling him to view the world to the horizon, his growing brainpower and shape of the skull, due in part to a gradually included future dimension. And probably a further characteristic was the possession for a sufficient length of time of an intuitively developed "sixth sense" of future dangers lurking in the inimical nature all around man and also in the eternal return of the barren autumn and the severe winter. In brief, the never-ceasing struggle for daily existence called for never-slackening vigilance in respect of tomorrow, extending and intensifying itself into a purposive foresight on behalf of the survival of the species as such. For the fact that man has on earth climbed to the summit of evolution is due above all to his own guiding of that process of evolution by an ever-improved, ever-extended existential orientation towards the future.

The great thinkers, the founders of our Western civilization, from Plato to Augustine, understood this very well. Consequently, as is known, both Plato and Augustine reflected most profoundly on the concept of time. It is definitely not a coincidence that both of them bequeathed to us classical pictures of the future, philosophical and religious respectively: Plato the completed Politeia and, in his Critias, his unfinished sketch of the arcadian Atlantis, Augustine the "De Civitate Dei". In those striking heydays of Western civilization, the Renaissance and the Enlightenment (if I may be permitted to lead you in seven-league boots through history for a very broad preliminary survey), i.e. from about the 15th to far into the 18th century, human thinking about the future reached new intellectual heights via different routes. In the 18th and 19th century Kant, Hegel and Marx were in succession totally different titans among such thinkers. Philosophical reflection on time was continued in the first half of our century by, among others, Husserl and Bergson, and in our present day by — to mention only a few — Jaspers, Heidegger and Teilhard. I need hardly say that these philosophical time analyses were performed by the thinkers mentioned and by others in rather divergent ways and fashions.

Personally I should like to give my point of view here for the present with a variant of a statement by Buber: In the world now known to us there is only one being that knows a future as a future and knows itself to be the one aware of that knowledge.

On too many important points we still know very little indeed about the nature and the operation of thinking about the future in the oldest and not even so very old history of human civilization. The same may be said about the more earth-directed speculation about the future, and with respect to the supermundane, transcendental, metaphysical or mystic-magical thought about the future going far beyond the former category. What we do know is in our eyes sometimes surprising, and mostly singular. A small example which I believe is little known but is nonetheless a striking one, may be given of almost inextricably tangled, purely worldly and at the same time supermundane thinking about the future which may have been of considerable influence on the historical development of mankind, though this is something which we can no longer exactly establish. We know from the correspondence that Columbus conducted with the Portuguese and Spanish royal households to beg a sufficient sum of money for his costly maritime expeditions that a certain religio-eschatological picture of the future is a recurrent theme in that correspondence. It was argued that, since the end of the world was in sight, it would be of overwhelming importance before that event to convert as many heathen peoples as possible, so that they too could enter new heaven and earth at the right time. Now in this connection it is not of the slightest importance whether Columbus was the first man to set foot in the "New World". Nor does it matter to us here whether this argument really formed his genuine motive or was merely the perhaps rather hypocritical mask that had to be donned in his capacity as a "fund raiser" by the adventurous explorer who was convinced that he could sail round the globe. All that is important to us here is that evidently this argument was regarded as indubitably effective for the aristocratic elite in those days, in that mental climate and on the strength of a religious conviction anchored in the latter. Again of secondary importance, though significant, was Columbus' fate; twice falsely accused between his voyages of discovery, ultimately not rehabilitated, and dying in poverty and oblivion. The discovery of America has been taken from him.[1] An attempt to have him beatified was turned down by the Vatican in 1873. After the eclipse of his feats by space travel, we may have almost forgotten his achievements by 1973. Except for the reminder of Columbus Day.

It is important to return for a moment to the main theme of religious conviction applied to the future. Fanatical religious zeal was largely a zeal with reference to the future marked in one certain way. For instance, the Conquistadores were animated against the Incas, who, on account of their other-directed belief in the future, did not defend themselves against their downfall through systematic genocide. The same was true of the active participants elsewhere in the world in the Inquisition, heresy-hunting, witch-burning, the religious wars, the extermination of apostatical or rebellious sects, etc., etc. At the bottom of all this was their unshakable belief in their present and future election and their consequent exclusive, strictly delineated possession of the only true doctrine of future salvation. Despite its initial protests against this, the Reformation ultimately was also to proclaim and to defend at any price its own, sometimes equally implacable doctrines of future salvation, though these did branch off in a number of directions.

For this reason I should already like to state once and for all, in a very provisional form as yet, that, even for a convinced thinker about the future, enthusiasm is not enough; one also needs a reasonable dose of scepticism and to preserve a certain distance. Thinking about the future is not just by definition and thus automatically salutary, true and good, let alone, forbearing fine. Once again each individual case depends on: *what, how, where* and *whither?* In addition there is the decisive matter of conscience: how much freedom is left to people who think differently, after this has hardened into a strict *dogmatics of the future?*

Thinking about the future will as a rule *include* something definite, but it is inclined to *exclude* all the rest and anything that differs from it. All speculation on the future calls for a critical judgment on what it *contains* but also on what it may *forbid.* If application of the free process of thought is formally forbidden, thought about the future is transformed into material dogmatics of the future. With regard to this thought content the clear difference between a free "may" and a compulsory "must" has therefore to be more closely examined. Finally, the "must" breaks down in turn into an authoritative prescription and a scrupulous sense of the fitness of things, the difference between "must" and "should".

The motto from Fichte that heads this introduction, "der Mensch kann was er soll", is therefore correct in itself, and certainly the same is true of the conclusion drawn from it, which designates the inability to do something as the rationalization covering the desire not to do something. However, this once again covers and immures something else, namely that we usually do not know of man "was er soll", or in other words what he ought to do, how and whither he should proceed. To this extent, therefore, Kant's celebrated three-forked question: "Was kann ich wissen, was darf ich hoffen, was soll ich tun?" digs deeper. The Kantian "do" comprises a voluntarism and activism in the ethical humanistic sense.

Nevertheless, in conclusion, the historian and the sociologist will have to dig yet another layer deeper that the philosopher to find out *why* (or at least to understand *that*) these three questions have been answered in the course of the history of human civilization not only in a manner which has repeatedly *varied* considerably, but moreover in a closely entangled, practically inextricable relation between *knowledge, belief* and *willing* or *assiduous action*, or conversely in a systematic *abstention* from or *neglect* of *action*.

It would require a very extensive study to elucidate these relations adequately, going far beyond the scope of this explanation of dogmatics of the future. For these relations are much more complicated than might be derived from the single illustrative example given above of the religious conviction determining future action or awaiting what the future brings. And yet I should like to explain them to the extent that something of an elucidation is given of how much attitudes of mind towards the future are neither fixed for ever nor ever exist in their own right. Not only do they change according to place and time, but they are also attached by countless threads to a temporal and spatial network of complicated, ever-shifting relations of belief, knowledge and volition, of morals, customs and habits, of thought, commission and omission. They form part of an in turn variable, complex totality of ideas, attitudes of mind, starting-points, prevailing conceptions, codes and norms, patterns of behavior, ways of life and styles of culture. These again could be labelled as for instance resulting in, reflecting by or crystallized into a certain view of *God* and *man*, and also a view of the *world* and *society*, which in turn are recognizable by or expressed in the matrices or mythology, ideology, habitus of thought, social mentality or also in all four: dogmatics. However, this classification barely offers a firm grasp, since these four ways of thinking form the field of operations of more than four philosophic-scientific approaches, each of which illuminates different aspects of them. But on the other hand another, more differentiated approach comes up against the difficulty that only one aspect is illuminated at a time.

To give an example of the latter, it is obvious — although far too little specific research has been done up to now on this very point — that one should start from a plausible working hypothesis, viz. the assumption that the special nature of attitudes towards the future must be in particularly close relation to certain other characteristic facets of time. For instance, the characteristics of certain historical periods (e.g. more static or more dynamic), of certain peoples (e.g. more contemplative, i.e. devoted to theory and reflection, or more expansive and therefore more practical and pragmatic), of a given social situation (e.g. a relatively stable established order as against a revolutionary, entirely newly constructed social organization). Likewise it is almost a truism (though not yet demonstrated as such) that the historical fluctuation of attitudes towards the future must be closely connected with the change characteristic of that time in religious, philosophical, cultural, ethical, scientific and social ideas or psychological ways of thought which are themselves influenced by the changes in thought about the future and, in turn fructify, transform or temporarily fix this thoughts.

The reason why research into this is relatively scarce and in my opinion is still very incomplete is doubtless the fact that this material is so comprehensive and is so widespread. Upon closer consideration this spread proves to relate to at least *six* main fields which, though closely connected in this matter, are usually trodden separately. Each of these is in addition often subdivided into countless separate specialisms and generally isolated (not to say sealed off) from the others in a practically watertight, airtight and lighttight compartment.

These main fields are: 1. *theology* in the widest sense of the word (notably here the comparative history of religion, the philosophy of religion, religious phenomenology and religious psychology); 2. *philosophy* (in particular the history of philosophy, and also cultural philosophy); 3. the *science of history* (in particular the history of culture, social history, including secularized projections, and the history of science); 4. the *natural sciences* (notably the successive revolutions of the prevailing cosmographies and of scientific methods brought about by these sciences); 5. *sociology* (in particular the sociology of knowledge or science, the sociology of religion, philosophical sociology and cultural sociology, which has hardly got off the ground or been recognized); 6. *psychology* (besides religious and social psychology, above all the psychology of thought and the too little developed psychology of science).

Now that I have tried to make it clear in broad outline what I shall *not* or cannot do, either because it would take us much too far or, an even more likely reason, because I do not have a sufficient knowledge of this comprehensive material, I have now at last advanced at any rate to such a point in this virgin forest that I can state which way I could, I trust, hack through it.

In the following Chapters 3 to 7, and also Chapter 9, I shall try to show in somewhat more concrete terms the interaction of the intellectual trends in the six above fields in general and attitudes towards the future in particular.

Besides these interrelations, with their many sides and their many threads, the historical changes in or even complete reversals of prevailing attitudes towards the future touched on above will automatically come more clearly to the fore. However, I must first add a few comments to this last point, which is by far the most important for the essence of my argument.

2. Certainty-seeking attitudes towards the future as a cause of the coercive thought models of human bondage

In his imagination man hovers between hope and fear. Hope and fear both relate to the future. Hope of future salvation, fear of future disaster. Man is obliged to live between the two poles of hope for and fear of the future. Man lives by hope, but fear is ever-present in the background. Where does the stress lie for the future?

The resultant ambivalent attitude to life, the constant oscillation between these extremes, cannot ultimately be borne by everyone. Then in turn extreme tendencies are born, either to flee or to want to know for certain. Flight from the future, certainly about the future. It is not difficult to summarize a number of typical attitudes of flight — I shall do so very briefly — but my principal attention will be devoted to the second type of reaction, the *longing for certainty*. For it is due above all to this that thought models of certainty (mostly with the pretention of *the* truth, but often revealing themselves as pseudo-truth, or at least proving invalid as exclusive truth) will try to claim to their coercive sole right — in each case until the moment when their apparent certainty is unmasked as an untenable monopoly on too shaky a basis.

Mental attitudes of flight may of course end in mental disease. For Freud, for instance (if I may generalize in that way) the twin concepts of hope and fear were in themselves really rather suspect with regard to the individual (patient): hope as concealed fear, and on the other hand fear as a supplanted wish. Since then we have learnt with increasing skill to see through the increasing uncertainty characteristic of our present consciousness of time and of the future ("the age of anxiety") as one of the strongest driving forces in the continued neuroticization of contemporary man ("the neurotic personality of our time").

A very common attitude of flight is of course the return to and entrenchment in the present. There, from moment to moment, one can find certainty and also enjoy the fulfilment in pleasure (carpe diem). The future (hoped for or feared) does not enter into consideration; it is eliminated with a stroke of the pen.

In a related manner, but not entirely equivalent, since the future is admitted in principle, one can try to find in the present an equanimous equilibrium between all possible futures: both the favorable (hoped for) and the unfavorable (feared), or, to put it differently, by eliminating both hope for and fear of the future in commensurate fashion and with complete peace of mind, as it were allowing them fully to compensate one another. This has been aimed at in various ways in philosophical views or systems, going from the Stoa to Spinoza, if I may forgo further gradations here (i.e. of differences between these philosophical schools and both those that followed them and those that preceded them). Without hope and without fear — or letting these cancel each other out — one can set aside the future as aproblematic or await it in impassive, calm piety and trust in God as soon as it becomes the present ("let us cross our bridges when we come to them").

Both more paradoxical and more cogent is a third attitude, to be found for instance among French atheistic existentialists like Sartre, Camus and Simone de Beauvoir. There is no God and there is neither prospect nor hope in man's earthly life; nor is there anything after death. There is only despair and fear. But precisely in that man ought to find happiness. The endless struggle of Sisyphus is for ever in vain. He will never succeed in rolling the stone to the top of the hill and keeping it there. Repeatedly rejected, he must taste the sweetness of precisely this bitter misfortune. Consequently, he may not withdraw from the desperate, revolting struggle for daily existence by committing suicide. The futureless, existential today is — here too — the last line. Eternal despair is by definition and par excellence the only hope; in the dignified and voluntary acceptance of fate in its absurdity, approaching that of the Attic, heroic tragedy in respect of the curse of the gods, once pronounced, lies man's allotted happiness.

However, there is also an entirely different attitude of flight, which brings us much closer to the subject of this section. For the attitudes of mind outlined above still have in them elements of freedom, or at least of a reaction in freedom, with a free choice, in an area which has admittedly very narrow limits (the present, destiny, death, etc.), coinciding with the extreme limits of bondage, which are after all given.

But now we come to two thought models, quite different in themselves, which in fact — though with certain historical gradations — may proceed to assume an equally coercive and absolutistic character.

One of them is the product of philosophical meditation. Neither the present nor the future is in itself interesting and relevant there. Only the permanent timelessness and timeless, universal validity are of value. The first beginnings are already to be found in the universally and eternally applicable Platonic theory of ideas or forms. Not the here and now, nor a certain time, i.e. the future coming in human history, can be "apprehended", but the true, the good, the beautiful and the just in an absolute sense. This implies serenity and also to a certain extent (in respect of both the concrete present and the unfolding future) resignation or an "amor fati", a loving attitude of mind towards every possible determination of one's destiny, an attitude which, following these lines, can also come close to the Spinozistic view of life.

However, this idea of timelessness can assume an entirely different function or play a completely divergent role as soon as it also penetrates science and, on the promise of lasting certainty, encloses it as it were in this strait-jacket, so that the practitioner of science also falls under the spell of this magic circle — or if necessary is banished via the judgment of science. Of particular danger is the escapism bound up with this fixation or absolutization, if it infiltrates into the practice of social science, which then misleads itself and others under false pretences, while nothing is so temporary and changeable, especially in the future, as socio-dynamic reality.

A second form develops again as a separate variation on the same theme, since it likewise originally proceeds from or is related to the same idea of timelessness or eternity. However, in this form hope and fear are both fixed and reduced to one single point of view. For then in certain circumstances a religious expectation for the future, or rather a promise for the future, guarantees one absolute certainty for all eternity. Either in the form of eternally blessed (or damned) life after this earthly life or in the form of one elect future on earth for the people of good will, designated by selective criteria.

In the case referred to here the future is no longer *open* but *closed*; mankind is in principle no longer free to determine his own destiny but broadly subject to an unchangeable predestination. Human endeavour may no longer be volitionally active, but is in essence powerless and largely passive. Rebellious human might must give way to divine supremacy and to God's all-wise dispensation. However, the latter is apparently always known to a number of wise men to the extent that on the strength of it they feel obliged to impose in all ways and at all times their imperative commandments and ordinances on mankind for ever — without tolerating any departure or exception. These commandments and prohibitions are now coded and compulsorily prescribed as eternal, invariable thought models. But, and this is the point, the future itself, and the only way to that future, are likewise compulsorily prescribed in that manner.

We then have a law of the Medes and Persians, an iron law which cannot be altered by anyone. Those who obey it to the letter may hope with a clear conscience; those who do not must fear with great trembling. The present and death are transcended along fixed lines. There is a future, true, but it is subjected and subordinated to a coercive thought model. The attitude of flight has been replaced here by a *confrontation with the future* in the *certainty of faith* or of *knowing for certain*. Here, then, our study proper begins. For science had its schooling from religious belief, became just rigid in its faith, just as *dogmatic* in its attitude towards the *future*, where it is a matter of gaining and retaining that most valuable and purest of all jewels: *certainty*. Here too on payment of the same particularly high price: *bondage*.

47

CHAPTER 3

Theological models of the future

Religious images of the future, once embodied in theological systems, often acquire an imperative nature. Come to that, religion in the sense of service of God is predominantly service directed towards the future. Gods or God and future are complementary; they condition one another. The living and active God or Deity manifests himself par excellence in the forward motion from today to tomorrow, in the future determination of the destiny of the individual and of mankind. The extended and shifted projection from today to an initially extremely uncertain future bears an all-embracing and numinous name, a hallowed one giving absolute certainty: God. God as the citadel of trust is a citadel of the future, a guarantee of the future, faith in the future, in short a permanent source of never-failing confidence, of assurance and conviction regarding the future. The future is in God's hands, the future is God's Plan, is the same as God. The future and God form an indissoluble duality. God without future-directedness or without an image of the future is inconceivable.

The oldest law was likewise religious, the legislation given by the gods or God. It was applied by the king (ruling by the grace of God) and, in many cases, by priests.

It is therefore not at all surprising that, from of old, a connection had existed between the recognized religious writings and their content which also preserved the terminology of the law or legislation. It is true that elements of secularization had already penetrated the old legislations of Hammurabi (1700 B.C.) and, still more, of Solon (600 B.C.). Nevertheless, one spoke — and still speaks — of the Jewish or Mosaic law (the Torah or Pentateuch: the first five books of the Old Testament), and also of the Old Law (the Old Testament) and the New Law (the New Testament), while one sometimes hears the combination "under the law and the Gospel" used.

The Jewish scribes have also been designated since time immemorial as jurists. At the same time this gave rise to a conflict, with lengthy fluctuating and often far-reaching consequences. At the centre of this conflict were precisely the legal character and the legal interpretation of a thought model regarded as legally imperative or of a code of behavior which distinguishes exactly between what in broad outline or even down to the smallest detail is or is not permitted, absolutely commanded or, conversely, strictly forbidden.

The common Old Testament and later too New Testament expression "this is the law and the prophets" thus already contains, seen in this light, a contradiction in terms testifying to that conflict. A double one, in fact. First of all the law was directed towards exact maintenance of the status quo, whilst it was precisely the prophets who opposed fossilization and too literal an interpretation of the cult. In the second place, of essential importance here, the interpretation and practical application of the law became increasingly directed towards and confined to the daily life of here and now, while the prophets, naturally qualitate qua, above all fastened their wide gaze on a possibly close-by but more often distant future, not regulated down to the smallest detail or established with elaborate precision, but fixed only in its embracing totality. Of course efforts were made to solve this antithesis by as it were bringing prophecy in spite of itself in line with the law: "this is the law and the prophets". This is a stereotype procedure which, besides always being applied by a religion which gradually widens in the course of time, on pain of disappearance has likewise been employed with success in a secular, especially political respect, through the centuries and throughout the world.

It was particularly these practical prescriptions of the Torah that were later to form a very important part of the Talmud, increasingly refined by shrewd scribes and erudite rabbis. Although the famous Jewish philosopher Maimonides already systematized the strongly developed casuistry (comparable to the medieval Christian scholasticism) in the 12th century, the term "Talmudism" ultimately acquired and has even retained in usage, rightly or wrongly, associations with hair-splitting, or more elegantly with "legalism".

This was inevitable, too, because, again in emulation of the prophets opposition could not but repeatedly arise of old against the narrow, coercive and dogmatic interpretation of the religious thought model, which after all also completely controlled social and civil life. When Jesus appears with a new gospel, he must come into conflict with those who demand strict observance of the law. That is why we now put Pharisees on a par with hypocrites, thus obscuring the actual event rather hypocritically ourselves. For the conflict proper is still the same dual conflict: on the one hand between the existing and the renewing, on the other hand between the present and the future or between two different possible futures. In this case for Israel the Messiah, who will still come in due course as soon as Yahweh wants him to, and on the other hand for Christianity, according to which God has already sent His only Son to earth, the redemption of mankind that has already begun, leading to the future glory of the Kingdom of God.

In the interim I may point out that Judaism, against or beside the orthodox observance of the law, and also since the prophets running from Elijah and Elisha, Isaiah, Jeremiah and Daniel up to Jesus, has always in principle been strongly susceptible and open to renovating intellectual trends with respect to the future. As an instance I shall mention only the ideas about the future crystallized in three separate movements: the apocalypse (awe-inspiring disaster, necessarily preceding with hard strife the ultimately triumphant salvation), the cabala (a mystic, visionary theory of the future, connected — even then — with a cosmic speculation on numbers or gematria) and Hasidism (legendary expectations for the future, communicated in anecdotal imagery, handed down to us above all thanks to Baalshem Tov and Martin Buber). All this, again in various mixed forms, was transposed into Zionism (Herzl and Weizmann). Once the State of Israel had been established, the conflict between strict orthodoxy of the law (the famous ghetto of Jerusalem, Mea Shearim) and the liberal pursuit of emancipation was to break out again. The Mizrachi (also called the modern zealotry) demands the absolute unity of Church, Jewish "law" and State.

Christian theology — and its thought models — set its stamp on thinking about the future until far into the last century. Sometimes it did so in extremely scholarly forms, e.g. in the doctrine of predestination or of transsubstantiation, or in literally dead simple ones: "Are not two sparrows sold for a farthing? And one of them shall not fall on the ground without your Father". Sometimes it was mysteriously formulated: Jesus as the immortal Son of God and as the mortal Son of Men. And then again in universally understandable language: the crucifixion of Jesus as a purifying, expiatory sacrifice for original sin damning every man since Adam. Sometimes it evaporated into transcendental concepts like those of eternity, grace, infinity, regeneration and omnipresence. Or it offered a mainstay, depending on the religious denomination, in baptism, prayer, the sacrament and the altar, the preaching and liturgy of the church a tangible cross, the image of a saint or a rosary, confession, catechism or the benediction and above all the text or letter of Scripture, the canonical books of the Bible which, however, in the course of time were again to lend themselves to many kinds of interpretation and just as many different thought models, including thought models as models of the future. This transition from the present to the future culminates in the predominating function and special qualification of the almighty God, more in particular as omniscient and merciful *Providence*. With regard to the future one could attach all kinds of reflections to the idea alone of a divine "Providence" active at all times.

The same is true of the strange contradiction between the conviction that the future was completely subject to God's almighty all-good and all-wise, but inscrutable Dispensation and the repeated claim that God definitely wanted this and just as definitely did not want that. Further, that once again, in His name and in that of Christ, a great deal of blood had to flow again, also in endless wars of religion and crusades, in inquisition and heresy inspired by piety, and, above all, in the relentness suppression of other-directed visions of the future, even if they were just as pious and visionary. The extreme antithesis between canonized eschatology and outlawed utopia, or between the one theological eschatology and any other eschatology equally based on the Bible (e.g. the chiliastic movements for the establishment of the millennium,

50

or for the Third Testament and the like) was completely irreconcilable for centuries. While on the one hand the future was surrendered and abolished, lip service being paid to the complete confidence in God's hand, on the other hand efforts were made at the same time to form this future at any price in accordance with one's own anthropomorphic representation of God, peculiar only to the time in which one lived. It was not God who formed the future in reality in His image; it was man who transformed or deformed this future in accordance with the human, all too human, image of God everywhere evoked in those days by theology and the church, and thus all-prevailing. Whilst constant reference was made to God's omnipotence, it was par excellence *human power* which, with religious inspiration, on the strength of authoritative human interpretations, answered for the future and asserted itself in historical events.

Perhaps I must even say that this thought model has prevailed until far into our time. For, to choose a striking example, how else can one solve the completely logical contradiction between the historian Toynbee, who first "proves" in a number of volumes that man may determine the fate of his civilization himself in accordance with the system of "challenge and response", and the Christian theologian Toynbee, who thinks quite differently. After all, in the concluding volumes he "proves" that the fate of our Western culture, already in decline after a breakdown, now depends solely on a possible divine miracle. Only a universal Christian conversion of mankind, who must then await events calmly but pray fervently to God and serenely await His decision, could perhaps help at all. In fact the human power of response has in that case shrunk again to zero, or become fossilized in one exclusive thought and future model.

For the common man, who does not immerse himself daily in theology, religious philosophy, poetry or belles-lettres, or in theological analysis of history, a simple, easy-to-use recipe has often been prepared beforehand, which contains a translation for daily use of the Christian thought model. This recipe is usually cast in the form of a rationalization after the event.

Man — according to a doctrine simplified for the common man — simply *cannot* know the divinely determined future, and so much the *better* too. It is preferable to live in daily uncertainty, but then to trust exclusively to the one absolute certainty of faith, than to want to or be able to know in advance about for instance future disaster on earth and personal misery. With time comes counsel. Such a life, oscillating between fear and hope, despairing between punishment and grace, deeply longing for happiness, but at the same time possessed by fear of a possible fateful misfortune, is normally speaking unlivable. It is in essence waveringly negative, while the positive surrender to restful religious conviction is open to all and can offer complete relief — it alone. Thus once again the two poles of fear and of hope are eliminated again — except for deserved fear of hell after a sinful life and just hope of a place in heaven after a good or at least really contrite life. Loving forgiveness,

51

to be gained either by confession to and absolution from a priest, or by personal communication with God, preferably under the auspices of the Church.

Later opposition was to arise against this "sop" from the most varied quarters, such as the socialist circle of Bebel and Marx (as Lenin was later to say, "religion is the opium of the people"), from theological circles themselves via Kierkegaard (the inescapable "disease of deadly despair, seized with trembling"), from philosophical circles via Nietzsche (a "superman" must in the future replace that unsuccessful creature man) and from Sartre (the "revulsion" of human life, petering out in "Nothingness"). Modern theology has not yet been able to recover from this succession of traumatic shocks systematically administered in the last century with universally accepted thought models which are now current again. To some extent dogmatic thought has gone adrift, seized by the violent wash of the turbulent dynamism of today. However, I am anticipating myself here. Let us return — to remain in style — to the theological shepherds of the flocks of sheep entrusted to them.

Needless to say, the rule of life described above applied very definitely to the "common man". But for centuries popes, pious rulers and God-fearing statesmen, before taking any decisions which might be decisive for the future, sought the advice of astrologers, soothsayers, seers, wise men and of course also professional charlatans, who formed the opposite numbers of court jesters and equally honored fools. Nevertheless, offenders against the commandments and prohibitions concerning the acquisition of knowledge of the future were for centuries very severely punished — both the consumers and the suppliers. Such penalties are for instance still in force with regard to fortune-telling in the predominantly Catholic France, though they are seldom applied.

The original reason for such penalties was at the time not far removed from the celebrated cynical maxim of "keeping the people stupid" — also by withholding good training and general education. With of course the hypocritical addition that, as always, this was truly being done for the good of the people, to protect them against themselves. It was really by far the best thing for everyone not to know about the future. After all, it was surely not for nothing that the seer Teiresias was struck blind by Hera, or that, though Apollo presented Cassandra with the gift of accurately predicting the future, he attached to it the property that nobody would believe her? No, the Greek gods too wanted to keep the future to themselves, although they in turn had to give way as regards domination over life and death to the three Fates to whom the thread of life had been entrusted. But this was at Olympian level, beyond the mental grasp of the pedestrian, tragic human being.

And yet other sounds were heard from religious and religio-philosophical quarters even in the first half and above all in the second half of the 19th century, though at first these lonely voices in the wilderness did not carry far. Or rather we must perhaps first go back to a period from 1780 to 1788, the period of the main works by Kant, the founder of a new metaphysics and theory of science, and also of a non-rational religion and ethical system. It was only afterwards that the "All-Zermalmer" was perceived in Kant; it took half a century before Heinrich Heine established that Kant had killed God, although some German ecclesiastics had at an earlier date, whilst Kant was still alive, christened their dogs "Immanuel Kant" by way of furious protest and reprisal, rather a long name to give a dog, and probably no longer used by theologians for that purpose.

Then, among others Dostoevski followed, together with Kierkegaard and Nietzsche. It was Nietzsche who — unlike Kant — himself posits "Gott ist tot" as a thesis. Not, for instance, as is often wrongly assumed, in one of his later works, perhaps also already touched by madness, like "Also sprach Zarathustra", "Antichrist" or "Ecce Homo" — in which among other things the idea of the superman to be created or re-created by his own hand appears — nor in his earliest works, from the beginning of the 1870's, such as the "Unzeitgemässe Betrachtungen" (an appropriate title, since this book was definitely already directed towards the future). No, the statement is to be found in a seriously intended scientific work, to which he gave the critical-satirical title of "Fröhliche Wissenschaft" (1882).

Kant was about two centuries ahead of his time, and Nietzsche about a hundred years.

This does not imply that in the 19th century the strict theology thought model — with the exception of for instance Kierkegaard and Dostoevski — remained entirely unimpaired. Among the non-theological religious thinkers and writers one can find pronouncements enough which again went in the direction of a human, hopeful expectation for the future. Instances are Goethe, Schiller, Hölderlin, Rilke and many others, although in these authors one can also find contradictory statements, the product of a change of mood.

But it was not until our time that a new version appeared, provided in particular by French atheistic existentialism, building on the ideas of Heidegger. In a different context I have already mentioned this intellectual trend several times. In view of its tremendous influence on our contemporary thought, this repetition — I shall later return to it in more detail, in fact — is not, I think, uncalled-for. What is new about this humanistic intellectual trend is that for the first time it tries to combine the loss of belief in God of "God is absent" or "God is dead" constructively as a pertinent but negative pronouncement with a pronouncement which is just as harsh but is meant positively. The latter is that the complex of fear, despair, and complete hopelessness for man — who has no say about his coming into this world — will be for once and for all the fate thrust upon him, his lot for all eternity. Literary "translations" of this theme may be found for instance in Albert Camus, Dylan Thomas, Beckett, a number of "angry young men" and, in part, in Graham Greene.

53

There are then only two theological answers possible: either essentially unchanged retention of the thought model existing for centuries or the devising of new thought models which are still sound and conclusive. Both answers have been and are being attempted. Great objections adhere to both attempts, at least from our undogmatized point of view.

The celebrated dogmatics of Barth is probably the most gigantic attempt at a synthesis of preservation and (the least possible) renovation. The question remains whether such a dogmatics, taken to all its logical conclusions, must not of necessity ultimately lead back again for our time to the historically notorious and not very elevated system of "double truth", e.g. of religious truths and scientific truths, while it is precisely the fundamental compatibility that is always so greatly desired.

However, Bultmann and his pupils took the path of demythologization and existentialism. It was predictable that logically speaking this path, once trodden, could not but end at an ultra-radical "God is dead" theology. Heroic theologians now drain this goblet themselves to the last bitter drop. The then visible bottom of the goblet looks deceptively like Nothingness, but they keep on looking hard for the false bottom that must be there somewhere. Why shouldn't the paradox and the absurd bring relief here too? Or should, in the future, a Percival discover the Holy Grail again?

Finally, some seek the most difficult theological way of all, viz. that of combination with the atheistic humanism of Sartre, which more or less closes the circle, if indeed we might not have to speak of squaring the circle. Nevertheless, should it prove possible — though it is hardly to be expected — to jump over one's own shadow, how particularly attractive such an eminently humanistic theology would be! But let us not rejoice too soon: the shapes of the future also cast their shadows before. And the latter foreshadowing now forms the most essential and vital problem for mankind today.

This assiduous theological industry, although definitely of absolute integrity, sometimes creates the impression of an almost panicky, "every man for himself" search for passable and acceptable ways of escape, or if possible for a return to the abandoned heavenly throne of God and to healing of the deep wounds made. Of course I am not stating this here for its own sake, quite apart from the fact that both my competence and my reading fall far too short in this respect. What prompts me is solely the end-result of these attempts at recovery, insofar as they relate in particular to a by no means impossible and indeed rather self-evident resurrection of the coercive thought models, like old wine in new bottles.

In fact a feverish search is being made on all sides — though in an extremely vague and often illogical manner — for a *new future for God*. And also, if I may say so with all due respect, for a modern task and a new field of work for God. It almost seems as if the tempestuous forward rush of automation not only will increasingly and within the foreseeable future replace the work of man, but likewise threatens in addition to make superfluous the work of God.[1] What can God do on earth for the coming new type of man from the age of automation? What can man, in a time when robots will occupy a dominant position and exert by far the strongest influence on the fortunes of mankind, still expect from a God who, according to rapidly growing views, is absent, or at least elusive, or do for Him as an evaporating abstraction? If God is truly dethroned as the undisputed ruler of a divine order and if man has produced robots of his own accord, he will at the same time have to create for himself, entirely on his own responsibility, a new, robotized but viable order.

To put it differently, one is not only seeking a new future for *God* from the theological side; we have at the same time to seek, with the full deployment of our efforts, a new future for *man*.

A new *image of God* and a new *image of man* must be sought. New values for the future, both religious and humanistic, are urgently required.

Getrennt marschieren, vereint schlagen? Or, starting from totally different beginnings, will the paths cross each other again, will the socio-cultural dialogue and communication pass each other by, precisely at the decisive point? Is a theological or religious model of the future directed specifically towards the future progress of human society in accordance with socio-scientific criteria conceivable in theory? I believe that it is, but I do not know whether it will happen: this future is still "in the lap of the gods". But one day a real peace with clear demarcations will have to be concluded, if only for the sake of everyone's self-preservation and self-respect. And if we turn a blind eye to the potential sources of conflict, which unfortunately are still abundantly present, our prospects for the future in that respect do not appear very hopeful. In my view three things will have to become absolutely clear to Christian theology and be accepted by it unconditionally: that the future of the earth is still largely open (insofar as it is not historically determined and limited) that this historical future of the earth from of old to the present day is not God's work but purely the work of man and, finally, that the hour of collective, purposive and scientifically re-creative human power, free and volitional, to affect socio-historical events has at long last irrevocably struck, almost at the twenty-fifth hour.

The real dilemma lies in the fact that man has ultimately gained powers equal to those of God for the independent creation of his society and possibly soon for the re-creation of himself. He can no longer withdraw from the responsible use of this human power nor can he continue to pass it, or its consequences, on to a higher, superhuman power. On the other hand theology, which has always stated that man is created in God's image, cannot in principle deny or thwart the use of these powers by and for man without contradicting itself. But conversely it cannot fully recognize this far-reaching process of human evolution without reducing the divine share in it to an abstract minimum or even completely disavowing it.

Let both sides, denominational and humanistic, do their very best to avoid as far as possible all intolerant arrogance and, above all, *apartheid*. Each in its own way, they will have to try in the best of team spirit to arrive not only at peaceful coexistence but also at fruitful collaboration. I might almost venture to put it this way: united in a partly secularized but nevertheless sacred duty! Their efforts must be directed towards the urgently necessary "populorum progressio". Directed from the theological side, with recognition of the present socio-scientific capabilities, towards the future *progress* of the peoples, of *all* peoples. However, for the theological models of the future that will obtain in many cases this means nothing less than a Copernican change of front!

Philosophical models of the future

As the reader is aware, at the cradle of our learning stood the philosophy of Asia Minor and Greece, itself influenced in turn by Indian and Oriental philosophical and religious conceptions. It is the tragedy of this philosophy that, although it was traditionally directed towards the undogmatic acquisition of wisdom and virtue, always regarding the freedom of human rational thought in visionary fashion as the highest good, it nevertheless inevitably led to a *mental* hardening of the arteries into coercive thought models. However, this repeatedly met with philosophical opposition from a renewed urge for liberty, which tried to break though this mental strait-jacket. The history of philosophy reflects this alternating and largely repetitive movement: gradually developing intellectual freedom — imposed intellectual restraint — provocative protest — revival of independent research and so on. Here, in the special context of models of the future, as far as my knowledge extends, are a few random instances.

For a historically sound understanding of Greek philosophy one will in my opinion in any case have to go back to Pythagoras (6th century B.C.) and his school, i.e. to the founder of mathematics, of the theory of music and the theory of motion, to the religious reformer and architect of one of the first scientific associations. To his thought models: the arithmetical number, the geometric shape, the cycle and the circle with centre (symbol of the divine circle without beginning and end, but with central emanations). To his ideas concerning harmony (of music, of the spheres, of motion, of opposites), the multiplicity-in-unity and the unity-in-multiplicity, the essence of things and the natural order of the universe: the well-ordered cosmos and nature (physis). Here we already clearly find an incentive to thought = reckoning and thought = knowledge of the natural, cosmic laws or necessities.

Even before Pythagoras Ionic natural philosophy had in any case already begun to seek a rational explanation of the opposites and contradictions that confused thought. Thales of Miletus, one of the seven wise men (born ca. 625 B.C.), is commonly considered as the first representative of this awakening and wondering thought. The wonder always concentrated on understanding the contradictions, of the polarity or contradiction between light and dark, male and female (Chinese yin and yang), lasting and transitory, unlimited and limited, unity and multiplicity, thesis and antithesis. This led to two types of thought model; either a model in which the contradiction was reconciled or a model in which one of the two sides was clearly chosen as the essential and thus the true one.

This then, was the origin of a philosophical parting of the ways, which for centuries was to lead to diametrically opposed thought and future models. On the one hand there was the crowning of the Ionic trend with the two most powerful, progressive new thinkers, Xenophanes and Heraclitus. On the other hand there were the two top figures, likewise head and shoulders above all the others, of the Eleatic school, which had developed from the Ionic one but was in essence more conservative, Parmenides and Zeno.

Xenophanes, one of the greatest and thus least known, was at the same time a transitional figure between Ionic and Eleatic philosophy in the 6th century B.C. He was a religiously inspired philosopher, a poetic prophet, the opponent of polytheism and anthropomorphism, the founder of monotheism who may perhaps himself be described as pantheistic. God is absolute Being: unique, eternal, unbecome, imperishable. Oneness implies impassivity and essential immutability. God needs no treacherous sensory perception, nor movement from here to there. His whole being is all-embracing Sight, Mind and Ear. What is essential is the combining All-One (hen kai pan), the all-embracing One is the Perfect One, the Wise One is the almighty, all-seeing, all-hearing and all-knowing God (for the first time, as opposed to the Greek gods, in the singular). Opposition to the ancient, traditional Greek cosmology and the Homeric, heroic mythology (from about the 9th century B.C.). Despite his auditive, visual and cognitive powers, which are infinitely superior to those of man, God does not have a human shape, but plastically or optically that of the completely true and absolutely perfect globe (sphairos). Motion and change (the very things that were usual among and characteristic of the mythological and Homeric deities) are, according to Xenophanes, at variance with God's dignity and immutable perfection.

However, the very special thing about this new religious view in Xenophanes is that it is in no way contradictory to an equally grandiose prophetic *image of the future* of human progress. On the contrary, whilst he (as the first philosopher to do so) recognizes that human philosophical knowledge can never penetrate completely to the frontier, let alone the centre, of the all-dominating *divine* perfection and comprehensiveness, on the other hand he expressly states (likewise as the first one, and even as far as is known the only one to do so), his belief in possible *human progress*. To mortal man — so his pronouncement runs — all that is divine has certainly not been revealed from the beginning, but by searching of time. According to Xenophanes, man himself creates both his religion and the rest of his civilization. Here in fact, more than twenty centuries beforehand, the Age of Enlightenment is already dawning, together with that of man's determination of his future destiny by his own volitionally active endeavors.

However, the first very tight turn of the philosophical screw is applied in the 6th century B.C. by Parmenides, the recognized founder and leader of the Eleatic school. In his own way he continues the ideas of both the Pythagoreans and Xenophanes. However, the results are almost totally different, and often completely opposed. The contrasts detached from the preceding philosophical study, and only partly bridged, between Being and Becoming, remaining and changing, between the extremes of Being and Non-Being, of divine and human, or those between eternity and temporality, are revived. Such contrasts, with which are also connected those between cosmos and chaos, truth and pretence, idea and reality, or between objective and subjective, theoretical and practical, absolute and relative, universal and historical, abstract and concrete (to reproduce ancient concepts in modern terms), are for Parmenides insupportable, intolerable and therefore impossible. For him and his followers all that exists is Being, unchangeable and imperishable for once and for all. Non-Being, negation, is illogical, inconceivable, unimaginable and unreal. This view — which of course has been given here in an extremely simplified form, reduced to its purest nucleus — recognizes exclusively as essentially true and positively existing only the eternally unchangeable, immovable Here and Now. This way of thought automatically and radically closes the door to a changeable Future that might ever be different. The one Being is all the Being and at the same time in advance all the Beings.

Parmenides no longer recognizes, in the slightest respect, a polarity of pairs of concepts. In his philosophy the One is literally absolutized, i.e. at the same time banishes the Other, the opposite. The One is now the same as the absolute, the total, the infinite and unbounded and — also or precisely — as the naturally necessary. This is the beginning of all ontology and metaphysics — but unfortunately it is equally the forerunner of dogmatism and exclusive orthodoxy. The extreme antipole is this essential Oneness of existentialist Nothingness. The latter is the purely antipodal but equally apodictic premise of the absolute negation of all essence (except one's own) about 25 centuries later by Sartre, thus demonstrating that extremes meet. In its poetic form Parmenides' philosophy is a religious doctrine of salvation — borrowed from the Orphic mysteries and Indian mysticism — but in its essence and content it is a strictly logical path — i.e. a path made obligatory as the only true one — to the sole and sole existing Kingdom of Truth, Light and Justice.

Parmenides — recognized by Plato as the "father of philosophy" — states most definitely that Nothingness or Non-Being cannot be. And he therefore speaks scornfully of the "double heads" who believe this to be possible. Being resides in itself as unchanging, continuous unity and is kept by strict necessity within the narrow bounds of a divine circle. Rational thought and this unchanging Being are identical. And therefore, logically and consistently, neither Being nor the Thought coinciding or consonant with it are subject to time and place, to a multiplicity of forms, to a change of place, to external or internal transformation. In this way becoming and passing away, i.e. by definition all future changes, phenomena and metamorphoses, are excluded from Thought as irrelevant or non-existent, or are denied by it.

For centuries this thought model was to hold good as a coercive *model of the future without a future*. But first it was to be further intensified, extended beyond itself and oddly transformed, though without its essence being affected.

The most celebrated pupil of Parmenides, Zeno the Eleatic, tried to prove his master's doctrine as undeniably true by explicitly developing its extreme logical implications. Down to our day his indirect demonstrations and in particular the aporias have preserved an indestructible vitality. In particular Zeno extends precisely those lines directed towards the complete exclusion of motion and future change. "The arrow in flight stands still" and "The fleet-footed Achilles can never catch up the provocatively slow tortoise" are the classical aphoristic illustrations of his argument.

To be fair, this struggle to eliminate the contradiction (in itself really a contradiction in terms) should be viewed in the light of what was at stake and in the background for these logical thinkers. For if changing Becoming and a possibly different future ought to be regarded as part of the essence of things, how was one to arrive at a fixed, thinking order of things? How could one penetrate to a systematic, creative examination of the deepest essence of Being, of matter, nature and the cosmos, of eternity or of divine, indeed of rational wisdom itself? There had to be unchangeable basic principles, essentials and constants, magnitudes of order offering something to go by and laws providing absolute *certainty*, i.e. operating and recognizable in accordance with strict necessity, which, if comprehended, would lead man to exalted virtue and supreme happiness. It was therefore anything but stubborn "Rechthaberei" but a pursuit, as profound as it was spiritually ennobled, of what was thought to be the only passable way to banishing from thought illogical multiplicity and inexplicable change. But at the same time it was believed that this would lead to the elevation of man, with heart, soul and mind, to the highest peaks of this Being to be discovered, the only true and eternal lasting one. However, this penetration to the very heart of truth was possible only after elimination of all contradiction, change and decay, of every aberration and denaturization, of false appearance and (as we would say today) of optical illusion, but equally of evolution, illusions about the future and delusions about progress.

Nevertheless, there was one who spoke out against this firmly anchored and unshakable doctrinal structure. This was possibly one of the greatest — and again least understood — thinkers of all times, Heraclitus of Ephesus (ca. 540-480 B.C.). Even Socrates did not entirely understand him, and hence he acquired the nickname of "the dark philosopher". Indeed he compared himself to "the sibyl oracling in ecstasy who, possessed by God, proclaims the hard, unadorned truth". He was a champion of free philosophical thought, the forerunner of the later critical Sophists, Cynics and Sceptics, the inspirer of the Socratic, dialogical method of thought, a grand master of the paradox, the founder of the philosophical dialectics of motion, the inventor of the logos — later borrowed by Christian theology and, after a flood of conflicting commentary, still extremely complicated.

60

Some of his celebrated pronouncements, recorded in preserved fragments of the oldest known Greek philosophy, this time in prose form, have been handed down to our day. "Everything flows" (panta rhei), "one does not bathe twice in the same stream", "struggle is the father of all things", "nothing is permanent except change", "day and night, youth and age, waking and sleeping are the same", "unity through conflicting endeavor" and "discord produces the greatest harmony" are among his most celebrated aphorisms. They re-establish the reconciled unity of opposites (coincidentia oppositorum), the union of each thing with its own counter-thing, stress with counter-stress, efforts pro with efforts con, action with reaction, recognition with denial, by elevating them jointly and upholding them as a high, comprehensive order of nature or the universe. The eternal struggle of things, the constant changing Becoming and the lasting transciency are not the product of chance but in turn themselves obey the eternal basic law of the true and essential supreme harmony.

To quote another of his finest paradoxes, "the finest cosmos is like a dung heap thrown up by chance". For, though pure beauty and justice prevail in a universe governed by divine reason, in our earthly human reflection of this ordered scheme of the universe beautiful and ugly, good and evil, justice and injustice, Being and Becoming are de facto interwoven. The wise, infinitely deep reason of the human soul can and must try to follow and to grasp the eternally existing, unearthly reality, and thus try to substantiate it ultimately as alikewise earthly harmony. This is, at the same time, one of the oldest and most elevated attempts to reconcile *divine* and *human power*.

Heraclitus uses in his *aphorisms* "die Magie des Extrems", to borrow a description which his fellow spirit Nietzsche applied to his own philosophy. In this way he links in concentrated fashion the rational and the irrational, the logical and the illogical, the capricious fluctuations of reality with the laws or rules which in turn apply to these fluctuations too. He effortlessly combines the "from everything one" with the "one from everything". The whole and the parts, Being and Non-Being form one homogeneous, all-embracing totality. In brief, Heraclitus sets against the *static* world of Parmenides and Zeno *dynamic* reality. Thanks to a synthesis of opposed predicates he creates the dynamics which, in his own words, is an "eternally living reality, which at once embraces birth and death, Being and Becoming, and the perfection of God". It is this synthetic view of "Ganzheit" that contains "satiation and hunger", "war and peace" and welds these, just like other antipoles, into a significant twofold unity. Also or precisely to the extent that war and hunger in themselves are entirely pointless and therefore ought to be abolished in the future.

However, Heraclitus knew in advance that he would not be heeded as a philosopher. His work begins with the sad but wise words: "This logos exists for all eternity — but people are not prepared to follow it, neither before nor after they have once listened to it". People, he argues, must listen and understand what they hear, but they willfully avoid doing so. In this way Heraclitus posits indirectly both the dogmatic attitude of mind and the fundamental freedom of man, and he appeals to the task which they are obliged to fulfil as a result of the latter intellectual freedom, which has repeatedly to be regained. This is an ethical task, above all in respect of the other and better human existence on earth to be aimed at in the future, which he reliberated philosophically from the stifling strait-jacket all around it.

There are three reasons why I went somewhat more deeply into this philosophical prehistory. The first is because it is perhaps the most instructive and the least known. Secondly, because the principal philosophical contrasts that come to the fore in it have dominated thinking, but then mainly in the Eleatic direction of Parmenides and Zeno, which was deliberately preferred to that of Xenophanes and Heraclitus.

But there is a third reason which I personally consider so important that it will repeatedly thrust itself into the foreground in this work in changing contexts. Why was there, from of old, this repeated return to, and then election of, the unchangeable, immobile Eleatism? The principal explanation lies in the insatiable, uncheckable human urge for philosophical and scientific *certainty*. Certainty is ultimately preferred to and more highly valued than the truth. The longing for indubitable certainty is always at the bottom of every dogmatics. The fear of uncertainty forms its strongest protestation, lack of intellectual courage its cover, inner weakness its fortress.

Fortunately, in the course of history critical judgment could not be silenced always or for good. After the Sophists had initially continued or exaggerated the theories of Heraclitus to such an extent that everything flowed and not the slightest certain knowledge or fixed moral standard remained, Socrates went back to the beginning to seek a refoundation for the lastingly good, just and true human values to be realized in liberty. As is well known, he paid for this freedom with his life by draining the cup of hemlock. Plato carried on the work. He included elements from his predecessors, from Parmenides, Heraclitus, the Pythagoreans (Timaeus) and from Socrates, in his mathematical, scientific and philosophical system. He also, as he admitted, committed "parricide" with respect to Parmenides by at the same time incorporating Non-Being. However, Plato too was obsessed by the Eleatic hunt for the essentially permanent and the absolutely constant. It was from this source, among others, that his eternally valid ideas and his doctrine of the universalia sprang.

In his turn Aristotle again rebelled against his teacher Plato. But he too ultimately adopted, in somewhat amended form, precisely what he had initially attacked most fiercely. I mean his doctrine of eternal substance, of fixed categories and of immovable syllogisms — in short his entire doctrinal system. For centuries this was to have both a vigorously stimulating effect on continued philosophical thought and an equally vigorous inhibiting influence — through his coercive thought models — on free scientific thought. Intertwined with older theological thought models, such as Augustine's, it dominated the religious thought systems evolved in particular from the 12th to the 14th century, culminating in Thomas Aquinas. The essential Being and the divine norm, the true and perfect, Sein und Sollen, Christianized philosophy and Christian revelation coincide in these for over three centuries.

However, to win new freedom of philosophical thought, new blood had to flow. Three main streams of development were finally to intersect and meet in the person of the Dominican Giordano Bruno, who was burnt at the stake in Rome in 1600. One of these streams began with a revival of natural philosophy in Paracelsus, at the same time a start of a renovation of medical science and chemistry, among other things. A second stream began with a renewed mysticism, especially in Meister Eckhart, who in turn exerted considerable influence on Nicholas Cusanus. A third commenced with free empirical research, continued against tremendous opposition by Copernicus, Kepler and Galileo, vigorously advocated by Baco and crowned with success by Newton's synthesis.

Their repercussion on current philosophy too reflected the enormous influence of these new ideas. For Descartes freedom to indulge in critically thinking doubt was basic. Cusanus was to emanate his emancipated and liberating spirit to deep into the Renaissance, especially with his work "De docta ignorantia" (1440) ("Of learned ignorance"), in part indirectly via Bruno, and his influence was still to be felt two centuries later by Spinoza (who in 1656 was condemned in his own circle and banished from Amsterdam). Many lines finally met in the universal genius of Leibnitz, who simultaneously embodies much of Aristotle as well as more modern religious, philosophical and scientific insights.

Even in Kant, the All-Zermalmer in the field of religious dogma, the idea of divine laws of nature still lived on more or less unimpaired. However, this did not prevent him from, ethically speaking, drawing up a categorical imperative — recalling Heraclitus — and thinking ahead in daring fashion to a future of eternal peace attainable by man.

But it was not until Hegel that there was a real recovery or rather breakthrough of the dynamic-dialectical movement in philosophy. In him the rational world spirit traversed world history in spiral form, sometimes descending, then rising, via the repeated triad thesis-antithesis-synthesis. In his theory this spirit, ultimately striving heavenwards, left its marks in that history in dual, interconnected fashion. Firstly, in accordance with the law discovered by Hegel (in aphoristic form): "die Weltgeschichte ist das Weltgericht". That is to say, as the stairway still ascending from the past, despite — or thanks to — punished irrationally, nonsense and immorality, leaving this past permanently behind it. Secondly, as the gradual climb to an ever-higher level of mankind, by means of a rational self-awareness developing, with dialectical countermovements, towards the future. Unfortunately Hegel himself put an abrupt stop to that historically progressing idealism, proclaiming that the highest plane of perfection of this rising and falling process of intellectual evolution had been or would soon be reached in his own time in his native Prussia, as the completion of metaphysics. With him and through him, still during his lifetime, this grandiose, rational course of development would, Hegel asserted, have broken through to the final state of complete fulfilment and immutable perfection and would then be brought to a final halt.

As is known, Marx adopted dialectics, merely reversing the philosophical signs and converting it into a historical materialism active in the successive economic systems of production. I shall return separately to this in a later chapter.[1] What is principally of importance here is the much cited pronouncement by Marx (in one of his propositions on Feuerbach's work): "Die Philosophen haben die Welt nur verschieden interpretiert; es kommt darauf an, sie zu verändern". Philosophy must therefore, in his view, not only examine, but also create and re-create.[2] Nobody will deny today Marx has in fact changed the world. And yet in his system of strictly natural laws of motion, operating with necessary dialectics, a principle of immobility and fossilization was also inherent. I shall leave open the question whether Marx intended this himself, or whether interpretation of his theory as a realization and thus termination of philosophy could not but lead to this. After the complete fulfilment of the law, i.e. after the expropriation of the expropriators, after the assumption of power by the formerly exploited proletariat, after the introduction of the classless society and after the abolition of the State, and also of capitalism, private property and the profit motive — what motion could then still be initiated by what law? Marx himself did not wish to fill in this future.

Such contradictions were equally contained, and found increasing expression, in the great philosophical system of Comte. Once again his great merit is that, beside and against the artificially fixed statics, he devoted very great attention to a theory for building up *social dynamics*, for which he had in particular predestined the brand-new *sociology* that was to be created. However, to put it briefly, he halted between two main lines of thought, which were irreconcilable with each other. On the one hand for this dynamics he gave a central place to a tripartite law of development ("loi des trois états"), which in his view developed from the past to the future in accordance with the triptych theology — metaphysics — positivism. However, this in itself eminently progressive positivism (which after all deliberately wrested itself free from all former dogmatic prescriptions of theology and metaphysics choking off free science) ultimately — and indeed inevitably — entailed a new, coercive theory of science. A renewed scientific theory, according to which the practice of science, as is known, was from then on permitted to be founded only on the processing of experimentally verifiable empirical facts. On the other hand his own (and in actual fact his only) main law of such as three-stage development could not possibly be derived from experience; it was and remained mainly speculative, in fact even dogmatic. No wonder that Comte, initially going ahead with great intellectual power, finally himself became the conservative founder of a new metaphysics and even religion. With this reversion to the two theological and metaphysical scientific stages, which he initially overcame and eliminated respectively, he too largely closed the door again on free thinking for the future.

It proves particularly problematical to draw up new thought and future models which are not later reconverted into coercive formulas. A further typical instance of this may be found in Nietzsche, a rebellious spirit and a nihilistic break-through specialist. And yet even he throws speculation about the future into irons again, notably by his invention, which he himself so boundlessly admired, of the "ewige Wiederkehr des Gleichen", which repeatedly thrusts the future back into the past.

Another example. In his "Evolution Créatrice" Bergson gives an iron-clad refutation of Zeno and his Eleatic school. With his "élan vital" he breaks through the absolutization of the eternal present and again gives priority to the motion of fluid Becoming. He absorbs the latter in duration ("durée"). However, it almost seems as if the future as a separate entity nevertheless sinks like a stone in this infinitely progressing duration. Indeed, Bergson says in so many words that the future of mankind is not determined but dependent on itself, and also that mankind needs a "supplément d'âme" for the favorable development of that future. However, it cannot be said that in this philosophy the future acquires as such a clear shape, let alone a dimension of its own.

In Teilhard de Chardin, on the other hand, the primary orientation towards the future is very much in the forefront. But this fascinating view is so intermingled with a specifically Catholic, partly mystical and perhaps even, for the outsider, deliberately dogmatic metaphysics and theology (philosophy of history and salvation theology respectively), that as a result the pure philosophical and scientific intentions are rather pushed into second place or even obscured.

Meanwhile the systems of Heidegger and Teilhard themselves are in danger of contributing building blocks to new, compulsory thought models. A complicating factor here is the break-up of existentialist or related philosophy into entirely different trends (Heidegger, Jaspers, Sartre, Marchel, Le Senne, Merleau-Ponty, and others).

My own philosophical position, if I may put it that way, is very briefly as follows[3]:

(1) I think about the future, therefore I am and can be a human being;

(2) The future is partly knowable for man: thinking back = thinking forward;

(3) Anyone who ponders the future will learn that this is still open to a

considerable extent that can be further determined from case to case, and that consequently man can determine his own future destiny to a considerable extent and in collective fashion. He can do so by appropriate control and if necessary redirection or even purposeful re-creation of the future;

(4) Determining one's own destiny implies two things: ready acceptance of a stewardship for the future and of the duty to make a choice;

(5) Everyone must therefore be able to have access, as soon and as completely as possible, to all available data for, and possible consequences of, this choice to be made. This must include its most probable favorable and unfavorable possibilities, its good chances, its threatening danger, its adventurous results and inevitable risks;

(6) For this purpose everyone, choosing in complete freedom and on his own responsibility, must be able and permitted to utilize all the philosophical and scientific thought models useful for this vital choice;

(7) Thought models, or models of the future, are useful insofar as they can reasonably contribute towards the optimum realization of man's future-directed wishes and actions in a given situation or period;

(8) Optimum realization aims at a harmonious synthesis of *effectiveness* and *justice* in the furthest possible surveyable part of future time;

(9) The effectiveness to be aimed at calls for the application and refinement of all conceivable prognostic techniques for adding to knowledge of the future, including those which can be effectively developed over an ever-wider time scale. The justice to be sought calls for constant reflection on the desirable, realistic objectives that are capable of realization in any given temporal and spatial force field. However, this reflection cannot be dissociated from simultaneous research into the highest objectives planned long-term and for the time being completely unrealistic;

(10) All objectives meet in the endlessly continued approach to and progress towards the ideal "summum bonum", though this, the most valuable humanistic good of a full human society, may perhaps never be capable of realization in total perfection.

CHAPTER 5

Historico-philosophical and historico-scientific models of the future

L'histoire n'est pas utile parce qu'on y
lit le passé, mais parce qu'on y lit
l'avenir.

J. B. SAY

1. From the Third Testament from the 12th century to the testament of the 18th century

Once again about halfway along and like a crowbar thrust into the historical axis extending from Augustine to Bossuet, the theological dynamization of temporal events on earth was to lead to a violent eruption. Towards the end of the 12th century the prophetic and visionary abbot of Calabria, St. Joachim of Floris, predicted in a book on the Apocalypse as his renewed gospel an imminent breach in time. What he himself designated as a new phase in the world, beginning with a Third Testament, was to remain famous under the name given to it by one of his pupils: the "eternal Gospel". Joachim linked the three main ages which he had discovered (viz. those of the Old Testament, the New Testament and the Third Testament) with the Holy Trinity of the Father, the Son and the Holy Ghost. His theory was that this third and last historical age of the Holy Ghost was then imminent, in accordance with the will of Providence, and was accordingly to usher in the historical last stage of perfect freedom. In that final phase the ecclesiastical hierarchy and the dogmatic theology adhered to so far, preaching and the sacrament could be abolished as completely superfluous. All that would still hold good would be the rules of the order of St. Francis: poverty, humility, love, charity, piety and truth.

During the first half of the succeeding 13th century this revolutionary movement of the Spirituals acquired a tremendous following, until it was forcibly eradicated from Rome. However, first in the Renaissance, then later in 18th century Germany (above all thanks to Lessing), great interest in the works of Joachim and his fellow-spirits was again to develop. Lessing in his turn proceeded to exercise a particularly strong influence on the French Saint-Simonians in this direction. Joachim's theory of the three ages was also to continue to occupy a dominant position in the philosophy of history in different forms for many centuries to come.[1] I shall return below to the prognostic strain in this conception.

The 14th century was largely a quiet one, viewed in our historical context, but towards its end, and especially in the 15th and 16th centuries, the break-through from the medieval cosmography to that of the Renaissance became increasingly perceptible precisely in this respect. Logically speaking, it was simply inevitable that the newly flourishing belief in human dignity and in the closely related human task and power of determining one's own destiny would collide with the equally firm belief in a predestined higher guidance of human fortunes. The new impact manifested itself everywhere in a gradual extrication from the static immobilization and absolutization of a theocratic thought model. A dynamization of history both created and encouraged by mankind itself could not but explode this coercive religiophilosophical model of the future at a given moment. At a given moment: in reality this process took some 350 years, from about 1500 to 1850, in a large part of which period the crowning work of the theological philosophy of history of Bossuet (the end of the 17th century) could still continue to exert a dominating influence.

This was notwithstanding a series of powerful injections, which could not but gradually cast increasing doubt on the contemplative, deterministic interpretation of history as the effect and fulfilment of God's Plan for and with, through and against man predestined since the Creation. These doubts were originally refuted partly by means of doubt itself, as the basis of the Cartesian *deductive* method of reasoning, which placed only God beyond any doubt. But increasing opposition grew to this very method of reasoning too through the development and ultimately the prevalence of new empirical and *inductive* methods of thought for establishing fixed causal relations in reality, also in that of history. The thinkers and devisers or investigators of these new scientific methods were not always aware — any more than many of their contemporaries — of the radical and revolutionary character inherent in them, also in respect of the omnipotent direction and working of God's will. On the contrary, not infrequently they were deeply religious themselves and regarded their scientific work as still being entirely in accordance with the doctrine and law of Providence, indeed even as an irrefutable proof of it. In many cases it was only after their death, sometimes centuries later, that the true, the deeper-rooted essential conflict between the *sacral* historiography applicable so far and a consistently extended *profane* version was discovered. After the intellectual threads had been taken up again, this transition to new thought and future models was finally to be completed quite deliberately.

One of the predecessors, and at the same time one of the greatest, whose true significance is really only beginning to be properly understood in our day, is doubtless Niccolo Machiavelli. As a rule he is known only as the author of "Il Principe", i.e. as the founder of the later "Machiavellian" fascism, but not as the philosopher and historian, the connoisseur of Antiquity, as evidenced by his work on the historiography of Titus Livy (written in 1519 after his dismissal as secretary of the Florentine Council and for that reason published posthumously). Exactly a century before Francis Bacon was to formulate this new method of scientific research in his "Novum Organum" (1620) in classic fashion, it was already being fully applied by Machiavelli: not a religio-theological interpretation of history on the basis of Revelation, but in accordance with strictly empirical and objective observation, incorporated in a strictly rational consideration of the facts. Thanks to the historical, cyclical identities which he found, from which a natural law or at least regularity imperatively applicable everywhere and always could be derived, according to Machiavelli the *future* could be predicted with ease and precision in every historical situation on the strength of accurate research and also in view of the fact that human nature never changes.

The second great pioneer of genius was another Italian, Giambattista Vico, who published his "Scienza Nuova" in Naples in 1725 for the first time and, during the decades that followed, worked on improved editions (the last one dates from 1744). However, the book passed almost completely unnoticed at the time, and it was not until no less that two centuries later that its fundamentally renovatory significance for the philosophy of history was comprehended as a basis for a modern philosophy, viz. in 1927 by a third great Italian philosopher, Benedetto Croce. It was indeed a "new science", so new, so far ahead of its time, that Vico himself, as a pious and faithful Catholic, was hardly aware of the fact that his work dealt a death-blow to Catholic theological philosophy of history.

Indeed, how could he be aware of that? For he himself characterized his new science — without, I assume, meaning this as a concession to the Church — in a seemingly rather prolix but revealing definition as first and foremost a "rational theology of divine Providence in particular for the mondo civile, i.e. for historical world events".[2] However, he too, as an enthusiastic admirer of Baco, tried to follow a purely empirical procedure. On the strength of this he wrote an eternal "ideal history", according to which the history of all peoples proceeds in characteristic schematic form. As he endeavors to demonstrate, history proves to be subject to immutable laws which must evidently have been instituted by divine Providence as lawmaker.[3] In actual fact two schemata are concerned: one is the repeatedly attempted historical tripartition, now called a divine, a heroic and a human period of history. The other again relates to a chiefly bipartite cycle of "corso" and "ricorso", of rise and fall. In this eternal cycle, however, besides pure repetition, there also occur — and this is a new idea — historical renewals, as a result of which the cycles assume a spiral form. There is thus neither steady progress nor a return of exactly the same, but only consequently a *partially possible prognosis*. It *is* possible to forecast an upward endeavor which inevitably ultimately changes into and recedes to a downward movement, but impossible to predict how far this will fall back or when, or therefore how and in what direction a historical recovery will set in again. On the other hand there is nevertheless such a broad planning scheme of so wide an effect and so great a flexibility, in which upon closer examination immanent motive powers within the force field of history literally "in fact" eliminate a preordained and transcendental fixed plan of movement of Providence.

Only a few years after the completion of Vico's work in its final form (1744), "De l'Esprit des Lois" by Montesquieu was published in 1748. He too discovers, empirically and rationally, the fixed laws which he believes rule "les histoires de toutes les nations" in binding fashion. These causal and constant relations revealed by him could be regarded as the Newtonian laws of nature for history. Montesquieu too ascribes these invariable laws to the fact that God so willed them, for the preservation of the world — but now this is already by way of defence and sounds more like lip service. It is clear that, at least implicitly, the power of prediction had to be inherent in such historical laws of nature. Montesquieu consequently himself attempted various predictions on the strength of them, some correct, others incorrect.

Again a few years later, in 1750, a couple of Turgot's speeches were published: one on the merits of Christianity, the other a "Discours sur l'Histoire Universelle". Turgot, belonging to the school of Physiocracy — according to which there was an "ordre providentiel" for social and economic life that was the product of natural law (or natural right) — was a great mind, also great in his ambivalence that was still typical of that age. On the one hand he still leans firmly on Bossuet's theocratic view of history, and on the other hand he forces one of the first break-throughs towards the secularization of history. For here is the first dawning of the explicit belief in the *progress* of history, achieved by the development of the human spirit, and expressed in corresponding human action. This progress is clearly visible in the law of development in three stages which he was the first to apply purposively to it. However, it is equally apparent from the law which he was again the first to formulate regarding the *acceleration* of progress — which is again in the foreground of historical development for the first time in 200 years.

Once again nearly half a century was to pass before this thread of Ariadne through the historical labyrinth was taken up again. Condorcet, mathematician, universally enlightened spirit, one of the authors of the Encyclopédie (among the subjects which he championed were rights for women and birth control), wrote his "Esquisse d'un tableau des progrès de l'esprit humain" in 1793. He did so as a refugee, shortly before his imprisonment and his suicide as a sacrifice to the Revolution which he had

70

served so well. In this "testament of the 18th century" he describes the essence of human history. This is by now a completely secularized history, in which the Christian faith plays a part only as superstition.

This history is subject to fixed laws of nature to be discovered by empirical research. According to Condorcet, these prove two things. On the one hand, his optimistic thesis on lasting progress through a possible "perfectabilité" or future perfection of mankind. On the other hand, when, thanks to a Newton of history, the science of history has one day developed into a perfectly rational and exact science, his corresponding conviction concerning the possibility of replacing *prophecy* by *prognosis*, of *divine Providence* by *human vision*. However, in a later age these two undogmatic future-expectations, which completely revolutionized existing thought, were to be rejected on the grounds that they were as naive, utopian, dogmatic and absolute as the Christian expectation for the future which, for these very reasons, they had to replace. But at first this new *image of the future* had an overwhelming effect.

In the half-century that followed, the stage of the philosophy of history was, however, first still dominated by the powerfully creative spirit of Hegel, inspired by the same idealism. I believe that he may be regarded as the last of a series of thinkers who, intentionally or unintentionally, were to give the final shove that overturned the theology of history. To the present day it is still uncertain whether Hegel assigned himself this role. Many thought themselves justified in automatically identifying his "Weltgericht" (which Hegel combined with "Weltgeschichte") with a Christian judgment of God which he evidently meant at the same time. Others argued — and still argue — most strongly against this, backed by other quotations from his extensive work. Both Hegel himself and the countless commentaries in their authoritative interpretations of his theory, fluctuate in ambivalent fashion between two contradictory views.

Did Hegel deliberately try to fuse the still extant theology of history with, or replace it by, a philosophy of history that was completely independent of it? Was the World Reason just another word for God and was the Weltgeist in its dialectical-dynamic progress through history bound to or even the incorporation of the development of the Christian idea? Or, conversely, was the Hegelian Weltgeist precisely the progressive rational (and moral) development of awareness of the human self, that is to say of the above all free and freedom-seeking human spirit? But precisely because these are and will doubtless remain questions, and perhaps because all the answers in that respect are both true and false, for these very reasons Hegel is in any case a typical and certainly no longer completely dogmatic transitional figure.

2. From sacral to profane historiography: from divine to human power

The answer to the doubt contained in the above question (for an identical ambivalence was characteristic of the majority of his predecessors in thought mentioned above) is perhaps less important if we confine ourselves to the historical effect of this reasoning on the further history of history. For there is not the slightest doubt that after Hegel's death (1831) the most influential effect came to lie among the group of younger left-wing Hegelians, above all in a period concentrated in the following decades, but with emanations over more than half a century. Members of this group — leaving aside Marx, who will be dealt with separately — included in the first place D. F. Strauss, Feuerbach, Stirner and, in a somewhat later period, Engels as well (who published on this subject after the death of his friend Marx). Now their purpose was a particularly explicit one: the historical uprooting of Christian dogma, as a rule partly to free the future development so that human freedom could change it as thought fit and, without interference from outside, reshape it for the best.

I have already stated that, starting from about 1500, it was to take nearly 400 years before sacral historiography gave way almost completely to profane historiography. The latter was a liberated historiography which could afford to replace the one final objective of the history of salvation fixed for the future by other, actual, historical trends, and also by other possible objectives pursued in reality or considered probable, possible or desirable. Orthodox theological historiography put up a stubborn resistance for a very long time, although its original tenets could not be fully maintained and it had to fall back on lines erected and reinforced behind it.

The first and principal shift lay in the fact that it was gradually obliged to share the theocentric supremacy that it had exercised for centuries with other, newly discovered powers and forces, and had likewise to try to embrace these in attempts at synthesis. The world-conquering forward march of modern science, at first mainly the trio mathematics — physics — astronomy, was one of the forces forming a particular threat to orthodox historiography. True, at first the greatest scientists of the 17th and 18th centuries, mostly still sincere believers, who also introduced the term laws of nature for their successive discoveries, such as Descartes, Huygens, Newton and Leibnitz, saw these very laws of nature as evident proof of the existence of God, to whom these laws in their opinion owed their existence without any doubt. Descartes ascribed the invariable constancy of the laws of nature to the immutable nature of God. Newton did not only base the exactly prognostic capacity of such mechanistic laws on this, he also wrote — something that is less well known — an interesting work in particular on the prophetic predictions of Daniel.

Perhaps even more important in this respect is Leibnitz, who, besides being a celebrated mathematician, physicist and philosopher, was an equally famous historian. It is fascinating to see how even he already had to wrestle with the subject-matter so as to be able to preserve in essence the theology of history. Of course it would take us too far to describe this intellectual process here in detail. I shall simply mention two aspects that are particularly appropriate here. In the first place he could not succeed in his intention of tying up the loose ends without employing a massive artifice, viz. the requisite "wonder" of a prestabilized (fixed and postulated as permanent) harmony deliberately introduced by God. Positing this cosmic harmony introduced in advance into world history in accordance with God's Plan compelled him, however, to draw a second logical consequence. This was to demonstrate how the evidently conflicting, complete disharmony (of evil, immorality, misery, chaos and absurdity, discord, injustice and unhappiness, in brief the suffering of men — even the pious and devout — on earth) could be reconciled with the first assumption. As a result he was forced step by step to devise the most celebrated theodicy in history. This was an answer to the age-old question of the justification of evil in a divinely created world and furthermore an attempt to find by verification in that very situation proof of almighty God as the perfect, just, holy, merciful and loving ruler vis-à-vis His faithful subjects, sinners and otherwise. However, others were driven by the same problem to insubordinate refutation.

But the first artifice of preordained harmony, too, proved to have other consequences for theological-philosophical historical models. For it is known that in the 17th century deism acquired increasing strength. According to this rational religion, though God originally created the laws of nature with which He set the world in motion, He withdrew from "day-to-day management", leaving them to go their own way in dominating world history without further intervention from His side. In essence this view is already contained in Leibnitz' theory of harmony, for which he repeatedly uses the image of two clocks synchronized in accordance with God's original instructions, with which process of synchronization He, as the creative clockmaker, has no longer to concern Himself thereafter. His pupil Christian Wolff continues this line still further: the world is a machine, faultlessly constructed by God and functioning automatically, which He leaves in peace to function further, without having to intervene personally.

This view has two implications: firstly, God's creation is good, evil is simply the imperfect work of man (an argument to support the theodicy). Secondly (an unintentional undermining of the theology of history), the laws of nature are given autonomy within the framework of a natural order instituted by God for that purpose. However, men can dominate that natural order by discovering its laws and then learning to use these for *their own power* (according to Baco's motto). However, via the techniques of science this will ultimately mean the end of both the theology of history and the theodicy connected with this. For once again there rises here, against an originally *divine* power, a power which, though derived from the former one, is nevertheless very individually *human*.

Things had not yet quite reached that stage. In the same 17th century Spinoza devised his deeply religious and profoundly philosophical ethical system for good and loving human life. This ethic was "more geometrico", i.e. built up on the principles of geometry. In Spinoza's opinion this mathematical-intellectual synthesis led to the purest and most blessed love of man for God (amor Dei). However, for him the Bible was a book like any other historical work. Neither religious worship nor theological history could retain their conventional meaning vis-à-vis his critico-historical and anti-dogmatic attitude, either as religious or as philosophical thought models, coercive or otherwise. On the contrary, his work formed a daring impetus, and this time a deliberate one. Revealed faith remains, but only so far as it is locked in the heart of man, that is to say, in Spinoza's view, as a natural and rational morality. He was firmly convinced that the State should serve not in the last place to ensure spiritual freedom, including freedom of thought and opinion. Socrates redivivus!

Come to that, theology itself did not ultimately succeed either in escaping the triumphant successes of modern science. What one could not permanently banish, on God's supposed authority, one could better build in lastingly, to the greater glory of God. A certain John Craig won for himself in 1699 a (viewed in retrospect rather ridiculous) place among the immortals as one of the leading representatives of the "physico-theological" school.

En passant I can only mention here the intermediate position of so complicated a figure as Kant. Inspired by a work from 1784 by his former pupil Herder, of which he incidentally wrote a rather sour review, he — the philosopher, and among other things physicist and astronomer — also engrossed himself in the science of history and in history (a subject in which he was otherwise not greatly interested). His essay, from that same year 1784, was called: "Idee zu einer allgemeinen Geschichte in weltbürgerlicher Absicht". Even the formidable All-Zermalmer proves here to be a child of his age after all. According to Kant history is determined by something like laws, comparable to the discovered laws of nature, and in accordance with a "Plan of Nature". In his view this was the only way to explain how it is possible that stupid people (even philosophers, he states, are not wise in everyday life), without knowing these laws or this plan, let alone understanding them, were led to progress in spite of themselves. Kant stated that the revelation of such a teleological plan of nature, unfolding itself in history, would be the task of a new Kepler, while further establishing the necessity of the laws contained therein would call for a second Newton. True, according to Kant himself, this idea of a teleological plan of nature cannot be proved, but unless we operate with it we cannot understand history.

In Kant's opinion progress in history comes about in spite of man and his unknowing, irrational actions. But, according to plan, this process gradually leads to a type of man acting more rationally, gifted with greater intelligence and more moral freedom. Only two remarks will be made on this: Kant does not designate all-wise Providence, and even less so innately good man, as Rousseau does, as the potential prime mover of this law of development — on the contrary, bad, imperfect, wordly man is instrumental. But, and that is my second remark, Kant nevertheless concludes on the strength of his argument that an optimistic prognosis is called for. And despite a fundamental difference of argumentation, this prognosis still displays considerable internal resemblance to the eschatological history of salvation, progressing towards the future. When all is said and done, his natural order and a divine order are not "poles apart", and the difference between a Plan of Nature and a theological Plan of God seems perhaps little more than a difference in terminology (which had already entirely disappeared with Spinoza's "deus sive natura", God, that is Nature). Which of course in no way detracts from the fact that Kant too must definitely be regarded as one of the transitional figures from sacral to profane philosophy of history.

Somewhat arbitrarily I should like to conclude this series (which is definitely not meant to be exhaustive) of these transitional figures from a still prevalent to a newly dawning thought model, whom I regard as the most important ones in this context, with an author of quite a different kind, a historian by profession, Alexis de Tocqueville. His two-volume main work, "De la Démocratie en Amérique" (1835-40) is of importance here for several reasons. In the first place, as a modern work, still highly readable, which also introduces the New World as a phenomenon into history. In the second place, to show that far into the first half of the 19th century the spirit of Bossuet was still extremely alive after more than 150 years in a leading writer who now gives the central position precisely to democracy (following on the historical periods of Enlightenment, Revolution and Progress). According to Tocqueville the stepwise development of the equality of conditions of life is a matter of Providence and possesses all the characteristics of a divine dispensation: it is universal, it is lasting and it frustrates all human opposition; every event and every person serves its progress. Consequently, to him every attempt to hold back democracy and its steadily continuing development means fighting against Providence and "against God Himself".

However, there is a third aspect that attaches to this proposition that seems significant in this connection. Given the starting-point that the development of democracy cannot be halted on account of its providential necessity, the possibility of *forecasting* the coming historical development in this respect also follows explicitly in Tocqueville. Admittedly, like so many theologians before him, he trips up over the old question of how this providential necessity determined as fate can be reconciled with the free will of men who either want to hinder democracy or want to foster its cause (precisely because Tocqueville, to avoid a fatal outcome, vigorously advocates the latter). However, greater minds have racked their brains on this to no avail. For this very reason, too, Tocqueville is a transitional figure, because he is very well aware of this ambivalence, or rather contradiction. Nor is it material here whether this or other prognoses of Tocqueville proved right or wrong in the event. What seems to me of importance is that Tocqueville proves to be a great advocate of historical *prognostics*.

3. From the atheist Proudhon († 1865) to the Christian Proudhon (resurrectus 1965)

Like Montesquieu and Turgot, Voltaire helped to write the Encyclopédie, the great pacemaker of the scientific (D'Alembert), anti-orthodox (Diderot) and rationalistic philosophy of history, and therefore repeatedly banned. This philosophy of history came into being during the 18th century in Germany too. One of the most advanced figures in this direction was Wilhelm von Humboldt. A pregnant quotation from one of his works, testifying to his advanced historico-prognostic attitude of mind, runs as follows: "Von dieser Seite betrachtet, liesse sich die ganze Weltgeschichte in der Vergangenheit und Zukunft gewissermassen mathematisch berechnen . . ."

Of course Voltaire, but also Vico and Comte, and finally Hegel in particular, find a very important continuation in Proudhon. I have deliberately used the word "important", because this author is usually viewed either within the limited bonds of the history of development of socio-economic doctrines, or as the man who was the subject of annihilating criticism by Marx (although strongly influenced by him), viz. as socialist avant-la-lettre (i.e. before Marx' message). But Proudhon means much more than is suggested by just about his only aphorism that has come down to us: "la propriété, c'est le vol". As evidenced by his principal economic work and his many other writings (collected in 26 volumes!), he is one of the most important thinkers in the context envisaged here. As such he also forms an essential link in the development of the philosophy of history. While for instance both Jaspers and Collingwood make no mention at all of Proudhon, Löwith has — in my opinion quite rightly — devoted a separate and fascinating section to him among the thirteen persons whom he discusses individually.[4] I shall borrow some of the information that follows from this section, giving it my own interpretation.

Proudhon's express intention was the systematic, *complete* replacement of divine Providence by *human forethought* and *foresight*. Instead of the ultimate end of history revealed by God and of the theological progression of history towards that predetermined completion, Proudhon wanted to give the central place to man himself and make him entirely independent. In his view man himself had been elected to set objectives for the movement of history towards the realization of progress.[5] On the basis of these causal objectives impelling history onward, the *desirable* development could be *determined* independently, and moreover the *probable* development can (and must) be *predicted*.

What means were required for this process of intellectual transformation? As in Voltaire, but now more sharply formulated, a total conversion of theological into absolutely secular historiography, i.e. also including man's *influence* on history. However, while for instance a Condorcet and a Voltaire, although radically anti-clerical, are usually still regarded as deists, Proudhon tends to be classified as a pronounced "atheist" and even specifically as a revolutionary, anti-theistic fighter. Judging by the letter of his pronouncements this is certainly not surprising — and yet not the final truth.

God is Evil — according to Proudhon in another aphorism — and Lucifer is Good. For, the explanation runs, the Christian God robs man (we would today perhaps say Promethean and Faustian man) of his own free will, active creativity and liberated, theologically unburdened foresight. Lucifer is Good, as the good genius of rebellion and revolution. Proudhon regards revolution as the indispensable medium in the centuries-long struggle of human power against divine supremacy. According to Proudhon the Christian faith has merely replaced pagan Fatum by Providence, which determines human destiny (and fate) just as completely and arbitrarily. The time of total and final emancipating "défatalisation" which is unavoidably revolutionary on account of theological and reactionary resistance, Proudhon preaches, has now dawned as a milestone of history, is ready at hand.

Deliberately and vehemently anti-Christian, that was how this charged call to general bourgeois resistance in various works was interpreted by his contemporaries. Persecuted on account of it, he had to flee to Belgium (just as Voltaire, banished from France, lived in England and Prussia before settling in Switzerland). Many of the free thinkers and freethinkers mentioned in the preceding pages as opposing coercive thought and future models suffered this fate in their day, while if they were rehabilitated at all, this happened one or more centuries later. This is interesting from the point of view of both psychology and the sociology of knowledge, because with these coercive thought models too there is evidently an almost natural cycle of action, reaction and renewed action, which is greatly reminiscent of a Hegelian-Marxian dialectic. The anti-dogmatist should always be on his guard too, lest he fall into dogmatics or tempt his possible successors to do so. This applies a fortiori when, as has happened with Proudhon, the rehabilitation goes so far that the atheists are restored to respectability and neatly incorporated in a highly modernized but nevertheless not de-dogmatized Christian theology. For instance Joachim became a recognized precursor of the Reformation, whilst Hegel, as we have already seen, became a proclaimer of Christian doctrine. And in the same manner Copernicus and Galileo were finally restored to grace, though attempts at having them canonized have not (yet) succeeded. Later we shall see how Christian theology eagerly pounced on atheistic existentialism and on the God-is-dead proclamation, likewise appropriating these two contrary intellectual trends to its own use. In the long run, strangely enough, nothing attracts dogmatism like anti-dogmatism. Evidently in a number of cases this anti-dogmatism forms the best springboard for renewed dogmatism!

It cannot be denied that in the Proudhon "affair" points of contact for this attempt at religious synthesis can be found. In essence his attacks are in particular anti-theological (i.e. against his own contemporary theology), notably against the current theological philosophy of history. His attack on God too, if I may put it this way, is almost impersonal and specifically aimed at one given image of God, the image of God ruling everything and His attributes of almighty, omniscient and all-wise Providence in that function. This is, in Proudhon's opinion, a caricature of humanity and human dignity. It is completely irreconcilable with his image of man. Human beings are equal to one another and, precisely in this respect, at least *equal to God*. Man is lord and master of his own fate, entitled and obliged to *determine his own free destiny*. Man is called upon to make a free choice concerning his future, and he is capable of doing so. He himself possesses the power of prognostic foresight and of directing this future that still lies open before him.

Nowadays, perhaps, this is a view which, at least for most progressively minded persons, is gradually and increasingly becoming almost self-evident, but in Proudhon's time it was an almost entirely revolutionary one, which did not begin its gradual and cautious development until the course of the 17th and above all the 18th century. Even the revolutionary, radical Proudhon still observed this caution. He could not do without the hypothesis of God, he says (cf. Voltaire's "if God did not exist, he would have to be invented"). But Proudhon goes further; he compares himself with the ancient Christians, and is therefore really a deeply religious man. If one peels away the rhetoric, one finds behind the philosopher Proudhon a moving and passionate theologian, in fact in the deeper and certainly in the modern sense a Christian theologian.

The *"Christian robbery of man"*, viz. the theft of his pre-eminently human determination of his own destiny, Proudhon argues, can certainly not be blamed on God. On the contrary — still according to Proudhon — God presents to man the figure of Job as a most pitiful and significant example of absolute passivity and of human tragedy resulting from inconceivable, unacceptable and intolerable ignorance. This reprehensible tragedy is recognizable by a completely needless, irrational and senseless suffering. It is not due to God's will or intervention, Proudhon goes on, that mankind is confined to a passive wait-and-see attitude and serene resignation with regard to historical dynamism.

It is, I think, fair to say, as did in fact happen afterwards, that the torch of Christian eschatology of salvation was possibly handed on precisely and in particular by atheists like Proudhon, Marx and Nietzsche, or at least the flame was kept alive or a dying spark revived. What Proudhon aimed at in so many words was the founding of a "foi nouvelle", of a new, if one likes pseudo-theological *doctrine of salvation* which would later be elevated to the optimistic philosophy and religion of progress.

4. From the left wing Hegelian critics of religion (N.T.) and the Messianic Marxists (O.T.) to the God-is-dead gospel of Nietzsche (Third Testament)

From Proudhon and Hegel historical lines of thought of contradiction, conversion and identity run to Marx. Such a tremendous amount has been rightly written about Marx that it seems to me quite superfluous to enlarge on this central figure. The laws of dynamic-dialectic development formulated by Marx, applicable with the strict necessity of nature to history, are well known, as are the two mainstays of this argument, on the one hand that the Being of men determines their consciousness and on the other hand that men make their own history. It follows from the first that improvement of the social situation and the environment, or improved education, will improve human thought. From the second it follows that it is not an abstract God — or any other providential mythical power — that predetermines human destiny but that in concrete reality men themselves fully determine this, where necessary with the aid of revolution.

As far as is known from his extensive work Marx — like Comte — never really accounted for the epistemological and also strictly logical collision between a rigidly deterministic conformity to natural law and the freedom of man to determine his destiny, which is therefore open and still undetermined. Whether or not deliberately, he flung this as a "polyinterpretable" (Jan Romein) and eagerly picked bone to his executors, as befits an obscure, New-Old Testament prophet. Marx also deliberately avoided a more precise delineation of the image of the future that he evoked, which many regard as his strongest point and others as his Achilles' heel. However this may be, a forecast broadly based on his laws of economic and technical development, and applicable to at least the near future, was definitely present. Rightly in my opinion, he has been described in this respect as proclaiming a *secularized prophecy* or a *profane Messianic gospel*. Indeed it cannot be denied that the theocentric and sacral philosophy of history is for the first time replaced by a new anthropocentric philosophy of history with its own doctrine of salvation worthy of human beings. Such a profane, humanistic doctrine of salvation is characteristic of the views of the younger Comte and of Proudhon, and also of those of historical materialistic Marxism and of evolutionistic idealism of progress. The *future* is now the exclusive product of *human manufacture*.

From Hegel and Marx, and also from the Young Hegelian critics of religion, clear trend lines run to the intellectual giant in whom practically all that had gone before culminated for the time being and from whom practically all that follows seems to flow back: Nietzsche. Without any understanding of Nietzsche the contemporary philosophy of history and of culture is entirely incomprehensible. What lies at the heart of the new ideas that he propagated, what is the cause of his influence and of his failure? Is it perhaps one and the same cause, operating in opposite directions? As we approach the present day, in which Nietzsche's tremendous influence is still active, I must go somewhat more deeply into this, although I shall of course confine myself as much as possible to the connection with thought and future models. For Nietzsche fundamentally and consistently rejects all thought and future models that were or had been applied to human history.

In their place he offers us what he is firmly convinced are other, better and literally soul-saving attitudes of mind, though, as we shall see, once again the only true ones. This was a reason for inflated veneration or humiliating vilification, in the polarity that seems inevitably to fit prophets like a cloak that can be turned inside out. And it was also a cause of tragedy, for him personally as a renewing philosopher and Messianic proclaimer of glad tidings, but also for the whole of mankind, in the sense that the newly opened access to an eagerly awaited future proved to make this future (as the result of an impenetrable and insurmountable vacuum at the same time introduced behind it) as elusive and incomprehensible as the ever-unattainable horizon, or a fata morgana evidently reflecting nothing whatsoever of coming events.

No philosophy of history dealt with so far found favour in Nietzsche's eyes, not even the philosophy that formed the avant-garde in this respect. But least of all could he accept the Christian philosophy of history. In a number of works he tries his best to demonstrate that Christianity has slowly but surely been eroded and devalued to what is only a weak and hollow moral theology, an emptied Christian ethic of which both the moral and the theological value, which in any case have no historical effect or emulation, are also completely unacceptable. Nietzsche, in his "Fröhliche Wissenschaft", is the first to state that God is dead. There never was a creation, and there will never be a completion. The *eschaton*, the Christian hope of ultimately redeeming salvation, is nothing but a treacherous *myth*. History has no beginning and no end, no sense and no purpose, no significant, purposive, surveyable connection. A finalistic, teleological movement of history, running according to a preconceived plan, is nonsense, nonexistent.

But equally so the *secular* expectation of a historical development in the direction of a natural or other evolution is, in his opinion, nothing more than a dreamy utopia and complete illusion. He rejects both *idealistic* progress and *fatalistic* ruin. There are no values or norms applicable in advance[6] to which history conforms, there is not a single *real* or *ideal* prospect. This is the beginning of nihilism, usually misunderstood or deliberately abused.

In other words there is nothing, no value, salvation or ideal. Nothing that sets the trend, improves, elevates, redeems. And yet throughout his life Nietzsche was obsessed by the problem that shattered the peace of his soul (a problem in origin both religious and humanistic), namely whether man could arrive at another and better future, how, despite everything, he could re-create this future for his salvation. Nietzsche, a passionate opponent of strict logic, which he saw as choking all original thought, aesthetic beauty and Dionysian poetry, could not of course, as we shall see, avoid a logical contradiction that nevertheless equally dissolved his own system. This was the inescapable, uprooting contradiction caused by his first demonstrating in great detail, with an accumulation of reasonable arguments, that any future salvation that may be expected is fundamentally unthinkable and, viewed philosophically, is entirely pointless, and then, after this complete demolition, showing precisely the — in his opinion — only possible and accessible way to such an essentially identical and equally ideal construction.

Nietzsche's sharp mind was not unaware of this antinomy, but he believed that he had found a sound solution for it. This may be reconstruction in the main by combining in particular the main themes from "Also sprach Zarathustra" (1883-85) and his last major philosophical work, "Der Wille zur Macht" (1888).

Man must first wrest himself completely free by the action of his own will from all dogmatism and fanatical prejudice, from all despotic, coercive ideas and tyrannical, sacral or profane ideas of the future. In an unsparing iconoclasm he must demolish all these, eradicate them root and branch. Only then will he be truly free, will the true future be open to him. In itself and to this extent this approach is highly conceivable. A clean sweep is made. But to what end? Nietzsche too, after Marx, also says: "You have nothing to lose but your chains". Marx needed as midwife for the birth and growth of his natural law of development only some material aid to start: class struggle, revolution and dictatorship. Nietzsche in his turn required only enough spiritual insight to reject both the existing God and the existing man. The human will to power, brought to a historical climax, is, by a fantastic manoeuvre, replaced by a complaisance that emasculates itself in heroic fashion, the pure negation precisely of the ultradynamic, hyper-sensual and evil lust for power which he first designated as essential. Free will is suddenly and exclusively instituted and converted by a wave of his magic wand into the absolute passivity of a "yes and amen" pronounced in mass obedience.

Now, if once the process of evolution follows this twisting path precisely set out by Nietzsche, he, like Joachim, then introduces a *third* historical phase. When for that purpose he causes the password to fall from a clear blue sky and resound for man, both the reprehensible Biblical "thou shalt" and the contemptible pagan "I will" will, he prophetically assures us, ulti-mately be permanently succeeded by a ravishing cosmic "I am". True man, Superman, has then been born, been created by Nietzsche. However, this future salvation depends on man first making a spontaneous-forced journey to Canossa. To that extent this new metaphysics and new gospel also form a new utopia which, however, as he himself says, always amounts to a fatal illusion.

His pseudo-Greek solution limps, for the same reasons as the Greek god Hephaistos, cast out of Olympus by the wrathful Zeus on account of an "aberration". Just like Hephaistos, Nietzsche then builds an unbreakable metal cage and places in it the man first liberated by him, and liberated for that pur-pose. He has this man, imprisoned and sunk in the deepest vale, addressed and admonished by Zarathustra from the infinite heights of his oriental mountain-top. But the ultimate future resulting from this preaching, and designated as manifest for man, seems at all times untimely.

For, when all is said and done, Nietzsche simply replaces the *one* coercive model for a religious doctrine of salvation by *another* which, completely un-realistically and illogically, offers neither freedom and redemption nor de-liverance and future. Like so many philosophers before him, Nietzsche is prepared to *make* the way free but on no account to *keep* it free. Man may only want what Nietzsche wants. "La critique est aisée, l'art est difficile" is a pronouncement which is by no means always true as far as the first part is concerned. However, the art of the second part would be a good deal less difficult if one did not repeatedly commit the same fault (it almost seems to be a law of the psychology of thought or the sociology of knowl-edge) which one has previously criticized — often rightly — most strongly: a *dogmatic attitude of mind*. That Nietzsche, like many whom he attacked, not without cause, failed after drastic demolition in a constructive approach, can only be regretted, but it continues to be highly instructive and fascinating. But it is a decidedly tragic fact that in so doing he too, the great liberator, like so many predecessors and followers, completely immobolizes men again, or at least tries to tame and train them with cracks of the whip like wild circus animals and having done so, again lays down the law to them in dictatorial fashion.

5. *From law of nature to diametrically opposed socio-natural evolutionary tenets*

It may be useful to pause here and consider the idea of the "law" just mentioned. This concept of law has itself evolved through the ages with the course of history and with the development of successive thought models. It is immediately clear that the stupendous development of modern science, and in particular its discovery of the classical laws of nature, could not but exert a tremendous influence on all other fields of science. Its nomothetic-physical thought model everywhere became *the* thought model pure and simple. Now as these classical laws of nature were above all characteristic laws of motion, it is equally evident that attempts were made to use these Copernican, Keplerian and Newtonian laws of motion to find historical laws of motion and development for the dynamic force field of history which, if not identical with the former group, then, insofar as already sui generis, were at least comparable with these exemplary laws of nature.

That is to say, laws of the same universal validity, strictness, absolutely without exceptions and of inescapable necessity. Only in that case could one, as in science, use such a thought model at the same time as a *model of the future*, thanks to the strictly determining causal conformity with natural law. For then the historical laws of motion and development found in that way would, as fixed laws of historical dynamics, have the same certain predictive or prognostic power. *Thought* models can in themselves already become coercive forms of thought within their relative frame of reference when they, as the best possible, are compulsorily imposed for the optimum practice of science. However, they also become coercive models in the absolute sense as soon as they begin to apply as pertinent models of the *future* too. Their character of as it were natural, absolute inescapability and necessity, sparing nothing and nobody, traps all future events in an iron net of cause and effect, in a frozen fixation from earlier to later.

We already found such strict historical necessity in the 16th century in a predecessor like Machiavelli, then more generally in the 18th century in Montesquieu, Turgot and Condorcet, and afterwards especially in Comte, Hegel and Marx, culminating as a cosmic natural law in Nietzsche. True, the *after the event* always proves to be a historical creed, or even simply wishful thinking, wrapped to greater glory and authority in the scientific cloak of a natural law inevitably unfolding in future events and thus foreseeable and predictable in its panoramic development. If the prediction

83

proves incorrect a posteriori, then the natural law claimed a priori also loses all foundation. The soufflé served collapses into an indigestible mess.

But now we must go a step further back. Scientific study in the wider sense did not confine itself to the cosmological motion of the heavenly bodies or of the earth around the sun. Explorers went round the earth too. They brought into being geography, ethnology, and later anthropology. Moreover, they gave birth to systematic research into the historical movement and development of all life on earth: natural history, geology, biology and genetics were added to the sciences. As a result of this manifold development the names of Linnaeus, Mendel and Darwin, among others, entered history. But they too fructified historical thought with new thought models. For they led to a further dynamization and historicization of the world-picture. In particular Darwin's theory of evolution had an effect on historico-philosophical thought that it would be difficult to overestimate.

This almost overwhelming influence extended in quite different and in some cases entirely opposite directions. To mention two extremes: Spengler versus Spencer. Oswald Spengler, by origin a mathematician, greatly influenced in his philosophy by Nietzsche, transplanted biology into the history of human civilization. Its expression in cultures was therefore irrevocably bound up with the law of life and death, or origin and decay. This, thought Spengler, occurred with an "eternally returning sameness" and accordingly a "simultaneousness" comparable throughout all history of certain congruent stages of development of cultural rise and inevitable fall, all entirely in accordance with the biological life-cycle. Perhaps the work would never have left scholars' studies if there had not automatically been an inherent part of this strict natural law and necessity which was of an unassailable prognostic nature and which therefore logically and consistently extended to our own Western culture too ("Der Untergang des Abendlandes").

In direct opposition to this fatalistic pessimism, Spencer had already extended the biological theory of evolution to a socio-historical Darwinism which, however, preached an equally fatalistic but for that very reason irrepressible optimism. If nobody at all were to interfere with the process of social development (no State intervention and certainly no philanthropy, let alone social legislation on behalf of the under-privileged or any kind of protection of or aid to the socially weak), the optimum and maximum development of history would automatically begin. For the progress of human society and of national and international historico-political events would spontaneously bring into action, under the relentless pressure of the merciless struggle for life, a natural selection in the general interest, i.e. also in everyone's interest, with as tempting fruit the extremely desirable survival of the fittest. The supposed do-gooders were therefore in actual fact evil-doers!

The theory of evolution induced renewed philosophical reflection on the problem of a possibly preconceived or inherent end (telos) as a (teleological) creatively active driving force for *progress* in the continuing history of mankind. The adoption of this, in origin, biological thought model by the vitalism or neo-vitalism of for instance Dilthey, Driesch and Bergson ("elan vital") will not be dealt with here, since it forms a sideline in respect of the philosophy of history.

6. *From rationalistic optimism of progress to existentialistic pessimism of Being or from human supremacy to complete impotence*

It is in the philosophy of history that one finds the most important reflection of biological Darwinism, namely in the form of a marriage between this evolutionism and rationalism, which had developed strongly in the 17th and 18th centuries. This was indeed a "mariage de raison". The intellectual child of this union which, rapidly reaching adulthood, was to reign almost supreme in the 18th and still in much of the 19th century was, as is generally known, christened at the time as the doctrine (or the idea) of historical *Progress*. It was also designated as the immanent idealism of progress, though afterwards it came to be deprecatingly characterized as naive optimism of progress. As I have dealt with this new thought model and, at the same time, dominating philosophy of life elsewhere at length and may refer the reader to that work, I should merely like to add here what stamps this thought model as a specific model of the future too.

I shall thus not concern myself with the question of birthright, viz. whether we ought to assign this to for instance the Abbé St. Pierre, to Jonathan Swift or to Fontenelle. The last-mentioned certainly has a claim, because (in the celebrated "quérelle des anciens et des modernes") he exerted a decisive influence on the conclusion reached in those days that, in respect of Antiquity, progress had in fact been made (a balance that was not to tip in the other direction until about two centuries later, with Nietzsche). As we have seen, this trend was resolutely continued towards the future in France by Turgot, Condorcet and Proudhon.

What they added forms the very essence of the crystallizing new *model of the future*, viz. the changing of the guard at the gate to the future. It was no longer divine, ruling Providence that formed the sole guarantee and also, thank God, was exclusively responsible for the other and better future. Human forethought and foresight now proceeded to take over this task entirely independently. Progress, since then written with a capital P, now was conversely no longer God's work but, equally exclusively, *man's work*. This Progress was no longer *transcendental*, operated as it were from above and almost inscrutably in favor of historical events. Progress, as an *im-*

manent force in the dynamics of history, was as autonomous as it was manifestly active. It was the force incarnate of a mankind that had reached adulthood, had become increasingly more rational, knew what it wanted in a progressive direction, what one could and therefore must do on a rational basis.

It is perhaps as well to warn at this point against two possible misunderstandings. One could be engendered by the impression that the final victory of profane over sacral historiography had been won, the other by the belief that the historical philosophy of human rational progress is accepted as such without reservation by all professional historians. Neither view is correct.

Even after Bossuet, whose theological historiography concluded and crowned the 17th century, sacral historiography never completely abandoned its point of view. It is true that the sober, extremely influential historian Leopold von Ranke, whose influence emanated in the 19th century and later, abandoned the theocratic, purposive movement of history with the admonition that the historian's task is simply to investigate objectively and factually "wie es eigentlich gewesen sei", without pronouncing on the deeper significance of the event, let alone on any kind of progress measured by human standards. On the other hand, his personal Christian philosophy of life is evident from his equally celebrated pronouncement made qualitate qua: "jede Epoche ist unmittelbar zu Gott". Even in our day this found an echo in Herbert Butterfield, with his historic statement on history: "every instant is eschatological". Finally, Toynbee's ten-volume "A Study of History", dating from the twenty-year period from 1934 to 1954, like his other work, is again pre-eminently Christian-sacral historiography, to which I shall return separately.

As regards the other point, that of profane historiography viewed in the light of rational progress, for instance Jacob Burckhardt was already strongly opposed in the 19th century not only to the concepts meaning and progress but also to a continuation of the historical lines from the past to any future, whether or not intended for eternity, but in any case unknowable. In our day K. R. Popper, for example, has opposed even more sharply and most disapprovingly the historical idea of a future, continued progress as such. On the other hand the British historian E. H. Carr, though particularly sceptical with regard to naive optimism of progress, is very positive in his attitude towards the historical dimension of the future as such.

It is of course easy after the event to amuse ourselves with the group of professional historians who firmly believed in a historical progress-directedness. For instance, there is the witty quotation from Carr, who in one sentence ironically reprimands sacral and profane historiography — insofar as the latter also admits to an ever-progressive movement — prevailing in the 19th century: "This was the age of innocence, and historians walked in the Garden of Eden, without a scrap of philosophy to cover them, naked and unashamed before the god of history". Carr himself regards history as an attempt at synthesis between past and future. It is certainly not the future-directedness as such that arouses his displeasure, but the idea of progression that this contains in advance. And indeed there was ever-increasing exaggeration in that very respect.

For some went considerably further with regard to the active process of progress than the generally accepted view, with a reasoning that was decidedly most attractive in its simplicity and effectiveness. In this view the inherent force of Progress, which pushes and pulls the Past towards the Future, was not only of unparalleled strength but was moreover entirely independent. Independent of a sovereign God and of rational man, if necessary going *against* unwise decisions or actions by man forming impediments. In this way the idea of Progress was absolutized. It was believed to work in a manner which was almost mystical but which, viewed matter-of-factly and realistically, was incessant and irresistible, operating through, for and, where necessary *in spite of* irrational and obstructive men, without there being in theory any kind of bounds for this in the future, or any which could in practice be set for this Progress, marching inexorably forward despite everything. A new, *coercive, dominant and determinant model of the future* had been born.

Even today it is often not sufficiently appreciated just how great the significance and the reach were of what was in fact no less than the almost overwhelming intellectual *transition* from a religious eschatology that had prevailed almost undisputedly for nearly twenty centuries to a new, soon all-prevailing pseudo-religious eschatology. The Land of Promise and the future final fulfilment were transposed to earth again and into the historical course of time with a tremendous, no less than revolutionary change of spirit. Perhaps this change of spirit was the only possible one at that time. People had become so used and attached to a divine doctrine of salvation that when the predicate divine was replaced by human they did not dare at the same time to interfere with the datum of the doctrine of salvation as such. Taking *two* new steps would evidently in those days have been one too many, more than could have been tolerated then. Indeed, the dogma of the historical doctrine of salvation in its new secularized version had even to be radically sharpened and exaggerated to enable it to continue successfully during this transitional phase. The comparative analogy seemed good, the superlative still better!

According to the view of the theology of history, Jesus' appearance meant that the final state had already begun in essence. Viewed precisely from the historical standpoint, this became increasingly difficult to accept. How did the historical fall of Jerusalem, Athens and Rome tally with this Christian view? And what about the disastrous history of the world in the historical age, pre-eminently a Christian one, before and after the Reformation, and the ever-increasing worldly, predatory pursuit of money and power? How could the spreading technical materialism and comfort, the capitalistic craving for wealth, acquired by robbery, exploitation, abuse of power, plundering and injustice, be reconciled with the suffering, the asceticism, the poverty and self-deceit of the early Christian preaching, with the attitude of mind of the catacombs, the martyrs and the Franciscan principles? In that way doubt even grew about the "historical" Jesus as the Son of God, while on the other hand the historical image, and at the same time pre-eminent example, of the rational and moral Socrates as a milestone of continued progress of Western civilization continued to stand firm against the wild waves of history.

Accordingly, as against the claimed progress and predestined final fulfilment of religious Revelation, via Enlightenment and Rationalism, it was now possible to draw up a synchronous but secular revelation. This revealed a continuous progression and an ultimate historical fulfilment, equally to be glorified, thanks to a continuing development of human reason (which was consequently elevated in a revolutionary period to Goddess Reason). Not only was there the secularized but otherwise completely identically oriented objective concerning the final denouement of the historical world drama with an "all's well that ends well". But, moreover, how much simpler, clearer, "more enlightened" and "more rational" was this substitution. The impenetrable, arbitrary and therefore apparently capricious action and intervention of divine Providence made history, by definition, entirely incalculable and unpredictable. Moreover, it had gradually come to be realized that there was not the slightest *certainty* any longer even about the time of the promised Redemption descending at a given historical moment, including the new heaven and earth and the lion lying down with the lamb. There was not even any certainty as to whether such a conception of the end of time and the last things could' still rightfully be maintained. Its place was now taken by a history of the future malleable and governable by human action, not only a Progress that could be sensed, but also and above all one that was reasonably predictable and even capable of exact calculation, continuously and systematically unrolled towards a final destination established by one's own future-directed determination of one's destiny.

On the analogy of Jesus' suffering as a substitute for the suffering of all mankind, the firmly convinced belief in this rational Progress, as a task now taken over by man himself of deliberately and purposively making his own history, itself became a *substitute religion* for mankind. The indestructible Sehnsucht for inner *certainty* was again fully satisfied. The now shaky certainty of man believing in Revelation was now exchanged en masse for the new proud and definite certainty of man gifted with Reason, at least as regards history, which from then on was to be governed by rational man himself. This was made possible partly by the fact that Christian theology felt obliged to stand further aloof from secular historical events, no longer identifying itself positively and actively with social structures developed therein. Too much crime and injustice had been committed, or at least had been concealed, in the name of the Christian Church. Further, according as the expectation of salvation concerning the return of Christ and the Kingdom of God on earth had had to be shifted ever further away from earthly time to a distant horizon of supermundane eternity and rather meaningless transcendency, the nearer was the coming and the more open the way for another, highly promising but, in appearance at least, more historically concrete doctrine of salvation.

The increasingly ebbing self-confidence of Christianity, the occurrence of more and more doubt, fear, uncertainty down to despair (Kierkegaard and his influence, extending far beyond the narrower Christian circles) had of course inevitably to penetrate historico-theological interpretation. All the more quickly and strongly was the growth of the authority of and confidence in a spiritual force working towards the Progress of mankind immanently and autonomously within history.

However, this idealism of progress, as it shot up, also drew nourishment from other and older spiritual roots. We must first glance briefly back at these. Otherwise we shall not be able fully to grasp how it was possible that gradually a practically silent revolution, but almost complete movement and replacement, was able to take place. This was a spectacular and fundamental shift, going from the original, *"jenseitig"*, supermundane and transcendental, invisible final destination of history, regarded as a natural law, to a *"diesseitig"*, mundane, tangible final destination of history ascertainable by reason but equally elevated. This practically unbelievable transformation proceeded almost imperceptibly. The initially unforeseen endproduct of this course of development, which in turn was regarded as a natural law, was, however, no less than revolutionary. *Christian* conversion with repentance and penance was replaced by *rational* conversion with inspiration and instruction.

Above all instruction! For it soon became a supplementary condition of the progress to be achieved, i.e. of the progressive perfection of mankind, that the course of *human reason* through history could be considerably accelerated and improved. It was also rational to develop Reason to its optimum. This was of course possible by education. In this development phase the idealism of Progress is coupled with Romanticism, especially in Germany, where this view was to culminate in idealistic philosophy, crowned by Hegel's World Reason (beginning of the 19th century).

However, this was by no means self-evident. In France, for instance, Jean-Jacques Rousseau, child of Enlightenment and father of Romanticism, proclaimed almost exactly the opposite. In his "Discours sur les Sciences et les Arts" of 1750 — the same year in which Turgot published his speeches on progress — he regards modern sciences and art as decadence. Admittedly, he proves to be an enemy of Revelation, but not of divine Providence as such, a Providence which, however, according to Rousseau, stands entirely *outside* historical time[7] and does not justify itself until the Hereafter. In historical time he sees the opposite of progress. He is an avowed enemy of reason and of all rational volitional activity. In his conviction as a sombre culture-pessimist all the misery in the world is attributable precisely to the use (abuse) of human freedom of will.

And yet the same Rousseau ("Emile") is regarded as one of the classic founders of education and modern pedagogy. But that is precisely opposite and contrary to the German view given above.

As the reader will be aware, Rousseau does in fact advocate a transition from enlightened rulers to enlightened people, notably by education. However, this is an in principle reactionary education (only for rich boys, the girls belong at home). The paternalistic, autocratic educator must restrict all liberty, cut short all free expression of will by the pupil and, above all, foreseeing everything, must take the vacant daily place of Providence (from the cradle to the wedding night and even thereafter). No pupil educated according to this thought model and coercive system could ever have developed into a Rousseau.

Rousseau's call for "back to nature" was definitely also of value and influence from the point of view of the philosophy of history. One might say as an inverted "model of the future", directed towards the past. More stress was laid on the historical intrinsic value of old, also primitive peoples (Rousseau's "bon sauvage"), as well as that of the dark Middle Ages, and needless to say also of the Renaissance, which after all was to a considerable extent precisely a revival of Antiquity and its values.

However, the nostalgic tendency towards the distant past clearly perceptible in Rousseau (who thus in more than one respect was spiritually akin to Nietzsche) was chocked, above all by the development of German Romanticism, which *did* ally itself with the optimistic rationalism of Progress, i.e. was in fact specifically and deliberately keyed to the *future*. It was in particular G. E. Lessing (not to be confused with the later, pessimistically minded philosopher of history Th. Lessing, murdered in 1933 by the Nazis) and Herder who contributed towards this reversal in the 1780's.

Lessing breaks through the dogmatic theology of history. Continuing to build on Joachim, he sees history as an advancing revelation and realization of the "eternal gospel", which thus finds its completion in a third, Joachimite age. In essence the established Christian revelation is consequently eroded and replaced by a human, increasing rationalism, though still founded on a broad religious basis. This progress of mankind is due to rational education in accordance with this eternal gospel and, according to Lessing, finally leads to the moral perfection of man. This reasoning was also entertained in France, especially via the Saint-Simonians. In Germany this line continued to Schelling and Nietzsche.

This break-through and also continued effect (despite the partial rejection by Kant) became even stronger thanks to the works of Herder. In his philosophy the dominion of reason in history explicitly occupies the foreground.

90

Another premise is the aim of history marching onward with the aid of this reason, viz. the development, taken to its end, of what he calls "humanity". This once again clearly *humanistically* directed orientation means a final break with the theological view of history. According to Herder, nature forms a kind of matrix, from which higher organisms repeatedly evolve up to the appearance of man (a biological-philosophical theory of evolution). Then man gifted with reason serves in his turn as an independent link in this evolution for the repeated attainment of spiritually more elevated phases. Every phase is predestined, in accordance with a teleological plan, to prepare a following, improved phase and so on, until the ultimate completion in the foreseeable future. In that ideal final state the laws that have already been existing eternally will have completely revealed themselves in earth's history. In his optimistic-idealistic view true humanity unfolds in this way (with a parallel reduction of destructive demonism), namely "nach inneren *Naturgesetzen* einer sich aufklärenden Vernunft und Staatskunst".

This is a pronouncement worth underlining. As one of the great and also one of the truly free spirits, Herder therefore likewise submits to the thought model then prevalent of the strict conformity of historical events with natural law. This lends lustre and coercion to it as an unconditionally reliable *prediction of the future*. Thus here too the historical circle is drawn and completed again. Not because God wants this completion, but because this aspiration towards the highest level of human values is contained inside human history and is active towards that end entirely under its own power. And without any opposing forces whatsoever being able to hamper this upward surge of development temporarily, let alone permanently. Once again a thought model, however elevating, nevertheless reveals itself as a *coercive model of the future*.

It would be most interesting to place such thought and future models in the schematic-graphical form that their devisers themselves evidently did not see as coercive, let alone distorted. Before I try to show in graphical imagery how images of the future ossify into obligatory models of the future and assume the shape of linear strait-jackets for the human mind, I should, however, like to outline a few other and last model variants. It is almost self-evident that, just as happened against the benevolent and all-wise *Providence* governing our destiny, at a given moment rebellion and resistance had to occur against the substitute idea of Progress. This was especially so when this was on the one hand overdrawn in an excessive and ultra-rationalistic manner into the irresistible, uninterrupted, automatically advancing Progress, which calmly ignored even all irrational opposition, and even obvious relapses, with closed eyes, or at least with blinkers on. While, on the other hand, the naivety and the irrealism of this idealistic but head-in-the-sand depiction — as had formerly been the case with the theological interpretation of history — were at least as obviously exposed. For undeniably the scandal and the rock of offence were publicly revealed precisely by the concrete reality of this horrible onward march of history, devoid of any true progress. For quite apart from the fact that the lion did not lie down with the lamb, the swords were not beaten into ploughshares, the blind could not see and the lame could not walk, weaping and lamentations never ceased to be heard, just as of old. Torture, crime, murder and misery, injustice, inhumanity and evil, wickedness, blood and terror, cruelty, revenge and salacious sadism remained characteristic of this earthly vale of tears and thus of the human evidently unchangeable condition and situation. That the exaggerated optimism and rationalism of progress could not but consequently swing to the *other extreme* of culture-pessimism, irrationalism and anti-rationalism (Schopenhauer, Nietzsche, Ludwig Klages, L. Frobenius, Oswald Spengler, Th. Lessing, Eduard von Hartmann), further continuing from there up to modern existentialist philosophy (with its great influence on the philosophy of history) was a reversal in thought to be expected of "necessity". Swinging as an extreme, by definition, likewise one-sidedly, to the other side. And of course again and pre-eminently *dogmatic* at and for that other side.

In the above we have witnessed the dramatic struggle between *divine* and *human* power, with now one and then the other gaining the upper hand temporarily. When human power at long last seems to be winning, it quickly grows into a self-satisfied mood of human superiority. However, this new fundamental attitude of the "bourgeois satisfait" already contains the germ of an immense new reversal and setback. If Progress forms an *automatism*, active in accordance with an immanent, historical force dictated by natural law, the application of human power is in essence completely *superfluous*. But when it is irrefutably evident that progress is neither automatically active nor even a real thing, human power gets the blame — which is in itself not incomprehensible — and the time is ripe for a predominant mood of human *impotence*.

From the point of view of the theology of history and the philosophy of history a number of the lines separately given above converge and merge in the world of ideas of Heidegger and Sartre. First of all, from Proudhon runs the line of human forethought and foresight, which Heidegger incorporates as central concepts in his "besorgen" of the world, of "Fürsorge" towards one's fellow-man. Another line leads mainly from Kierkegaard, that of elementary fear, spiritual sickness, existentialist despair, indissolubly bound up with a lonely, temporary existence, face to face with inevitable future death. And finally from Nietzsche comes the power-seeking ego, cast into and struggling in the existing world, which, as in Ecclesiastics, is subject to an endless, uniform repetition of history.

Heidegger's conclusion, resulting in the only possible recipe of life for adventurous, risky and dangerous human existence, is again — comparable with that of Nietzsche and also of Jaspers — that of the amor fati of the Stoa. In the existentialist philosophy of Heidegger the questions about the sense of human existence are interwoven as a Sein zum Tode with those about the sense of history and of Being in general. He once again postulates the essence of time (and also of future time) to answer these questions.

In the view of Sartre and his disciples, again characterized as atheistic, these trend lines are taken to their logical extreme and also to their furthest, seemingly ultra-pessimistic consequence. The absolute unchangeable and incorrigible history of mankind, in his view, contains only boredom and disgust, meanness and horror, without any hope of relief. This is a struggle always and eternally doomed to failure right from the start. There is *no divine Providence* caring for mankind and ultimately leading man along the right path. But equally there is no prospect, as rational, moral work of man, of any Progress to be realized at any time. There is *never* any *favorable prospect* achievable for and by man. Human existence is without hope, without any other prospect in the historical course of time than Death, which at the same time is for everyone the eternal return to the identical, to the bottomless abyss of absolute Nothingness. This futureless image of the future, applicable to man as such in his passage through history, is equally a coercive *model of the future.*

Historical models of the future translated into coercively prescribed graphical models

1. Curvilinear and rectilinear certainty

I think that the time has now come to attempt to survey the battlefield of history and of its conceptualization. Upon closer examination it proves that it is not so much history itself that is explained and elucidated as human thought around it. True, there seems to be an ineradicable human urge, satisfied by an endless series of philosophers of history and of the future, to overcome the course of history and, in order to conform the *certainty* thus conquered, to force the former into a strait-jacket, so to speak. In order to grasp the ceaseless Becoming or essential Being of history, these successive thinkers have employed all kinds of specially devised fixations, conceptions and interpretations. These various purposive auxiliaries of historical thought may be reproduced by or expressed in certain *causal relations* and *constants,* in fixed *laws of development* and *structures,* in clearly marked *phases, stages* or *periods* and, if possible, even in all-embracing overall systems.

If one were to try to reproduce these thought and future models with the greatest possible degree of simplification (i.e. not without abstract generalization) — an attempt which so far I have not encountered as a self-critical examination in any work on the philosophy of history — this schematic-graphical reproduction would appear more or less as follows:

(1) the cyclical representation of history, derived from cosmic metaphysics, prevailing among others in the Greeks, fully rehabilitated as the "eternal return of the identical" by Nietzsche, and — or so it seems to me — also present for instance in principle in Heidegger's methaphysical struggle with time.

(a) This cyclical representation implies the possibility of *prediction* which, depending on the given temporary position or appraisal of the historical situation, can be interpreted either pessimistically or optimistically, i.e.

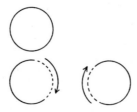

(b) A variant of this cyclical representation was encountered above in for instance Vico. As Vico leaves open the possibility of renewal in the eternal, in itself invariable circular course, he therefore at the same time excludes the possibility of absolutely exact prediction. One could depict this partly spiral interpretation of history more or less as in the left-hand sketch:

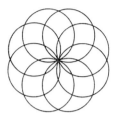 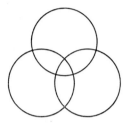

(c) In addition, the celebrated representation of the three interlocking rings in Lessing's "Nathan der Weise" (1779) has an admittedly important historico-philosophical and notably anti-dogmatic and anti-authoritarian background, which as such also contains a non-coercive, chiefly utopian future model of tolerance and free-thinking. And yet the form of expression chosen seems in this case to be symbolic and artistic in nature rather than to be intended as a scientific-philosophical scheme. On the other hand Lessing was definitely strongly inspired by the Joachimite upward endeavor of the third or eternal gospel. And to that extent there is all the same a clear connection with the historical view of the world given below under 2 which, however, in that case appears somewhat different in graphical form, e.g. circular or spiral as follows:

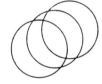 or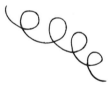

(2) As the second main depiction of the development of historical motion, which repeatedly appears in varying historical forms, we are confronted again and again with a certain three-phase conception. Set out graphically, it assumes on average the following form:

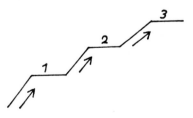

95

This upward trend, taking place in accordance with a three-stroke motorial movement of history, as stated, has been borrowed from Joachim of Floris. The latter also had his much older predecessors as well as his historical successors (as for instance in the culture-dynamics of an unfolding stone, bronze and iron age or of a successive nomadic, agrarian and industrial civilization). From him and through him this threefold and triune idea is transplanted to Lessing, and from the latter, together with Turgot, to Saint-Simon and his followers, and finally via this group to Comte's elaborated law of dynamic development (theological, metaphysical, positivistic).

(3) As a separate main variant of this three-phase theory the historic dynamics of the dialectical view of history may be detached. This is because the historical dynamics of these three phases, ultimately leading to progress, also incorporates decline. The presentation in graphical form — also as an image of the figure cast before — would look more or less like this:

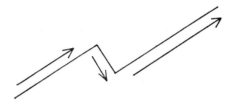

As is known, the scheme is that of thesis-antithesis-synthesis. In its rectilinearity it is more angular and more pointed, but above all simpler, than the threefold upward spiral already depicted above, which after all is not so very different in essence or resultant, except that of course there is also a threefold retrogression:

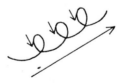

Under this scheme fall two views which, while externally practically uniform, are internally practically opposite:

(a) In origin this tripartite depiction is Biblical-theological, from both the Old Testament and the New Testament.[1] Led to the Promised Land, the Jewish people were to be driven out of it again (diaspora) though their own fault and decline but, by virtue of the Covenant concluded with Yahweh, confirmed by the prophets, would return some day gloriously restored. According to the gospel of Jesus (continuing the line of the Jewish prophets), in connection with the revelation of John (likewise linking up with a long series of older apoca-

96

lyptical representations), the old earthly time, after a satanic time of distur-
bances, would be recreated and completed, after the coming or return of the
Messiah, in a new heavenly time.[2] The revelation upon the mount in the desert
of Sinai (Exodus 19:11) reaches its climax on the third day. Jonah spent three
days in the belly of the whale. As regards the New Testament I need only
recall the symbolism of the resurrection on the third day (cf. also Luke 13:32),
the three wise men (the Three Kings) and the divine Trinity.[3]

In Christian theology neither the original tripartition nor a further refined
quadripartition ultimately held their ground. First they were narrowed down
to an essential bipartition, for instance by Augustine (the present earthly state
as against the Kingdom of God further spreading there, as the ultimate fulfilment of history). Finally, history gradually developed into one independent,
separate whole, the Kingdom of God then being elevated (one might almost
say "kicked upstairs") to form a matter beyond time, forming part of unearthly eternity.

(b) As we have seen, on the boundary between a Christian and a secular
view stands Hegel, whose rational World Spirit likewise operates in accordance
with a tripartite dialectical scheme used by the prophets of old. Unmistakably
on this side of the dividing line between sacral and profane, of "jenseitige"
and "diesseitige" historiography stands Marx. However, his tripartite law of
development, the product of natural necessity, has retained the pseudo-theological and apocalyptical-eschatological character of a doctrine of salvation.
But this promised salvation will again and above all be realized in conformity
with natural law in historical events on earth, by virtue of the materialistic
trinity of the successive systems of production, with a coercively prescribed hop,
skip and jump.

(4) New thought models, with corresponding images of the future, come into
being in the ages of Rationalism and Romanticism, of Enlightenment and
Progress. A distinction could be made between three variants:

(a) The at first still moderate proponents of the doctrine of progress, such as
Voltaire, had sufficient sense of history to remain thoroughly aware, for all
their idealism and optimism, of the movements and countermovements occurring in reality. In short, of the ups and downs in history which, if not purely
coincidental, were at any rate constant, wayward and inevitable. Hence the
following graphical depiction:

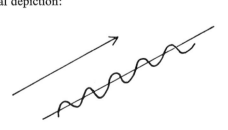

that is to say a line which, though fluctuating short-term, nevertheless in the long run moves steadily onwards and upwards though history. In the anti-clerical Voltaire there is in that respect little difference from the volitionally active pilgrimage of mankind moving ultimately towards the Christian faith, as depicted for instance by Bunyan. As explained above, this modern historical representation was at the time strongly influenced by the classical sciences and in the 19th century in particular by Darwin's theory of biological evolution as well. Viewed philosophically it is, on account of its automatism leading to good, cognate with old tenets of Epicureanism and eudaemonism and ulti-mately even with a deflection towards existentially optimistic and volitionally passivistic quietism (see the offshoot under c).

(b) We have seen a specifically evolutionistic variant in Herder (who was not alone in this). A simplified drawing would yield more or less the following picture:

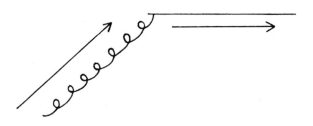

which may be described as a spiral moving upwards in conformity with natural law, continued until the highest plane of ultimate spiritual completion of the history of mankind has been permanently reached.

(c) The third variant of the belief in progress, which has gradually become the most ordinary one, finally destroying itself by an arrogance as excessive as it was naive, has the following appearance:

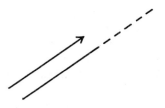

the picture of practically rectilinear progression as automatically active and meaningful Progress thanks to a strange, beneficial force of social dynamics. A visionary representation, which every professional historian (afterwards, but hardly if at all at the time) refutes as a-historical or unhistorical. It is incidental-ly an almost faithful copy and equally serenely secularized parallel, the pure counterpart, of the originally religious depiction of a benevolent Providence omnipotently active in history. The Providence of God who, though in His supreme wisdom and omnipresence often inscrutable, undeniably leads man on earth via His own mysterious ways from darkness to bright light, perhaps extremely slowly but absolutely surely, despite or perhaps precisely thanks to purifying struggle and suffering, leads him to the ultimate finale of His glorious Kingdom.[4]

(d) An opposed pseudo-religious world view never fully developed, although for some time it exerted a not inconsiderable scientific-philosophical influence. It was the model image of a variant going in exactly the opposite rectilinear or fluctuating direction from the preceding one:

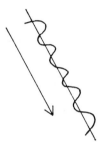

In this depiction too some influence is perceptible of modern science. However, while this culminated in Turgot, Herder, Comte, Marx and many others in optimistic views, even in the deepest essence and to a certain extent in Nietzsche himself, it leads here to the deepest pessimism. This could be attached to the second law of thermodynamics. The endlessly continued emission of heat during conversion into energy and the endeavor to compensate for this ought to lead to an ultimately maximum situation of the absolute, motionless zero, i.e. to an entropy death. Extinction of the fires of the sun would at last condemn all life on earth to death. It may still be argued whether in this way mankind would meet its end by an irreversible death by heat or by an inevitable death by cold. On the one hand this possible physical terminal lies so tremendously far away, while on the other hand nuclear physics has brought atomic destruction in pregnant fashion so close to hand that the line descending straightforwardly drawn here has so far been unable to play a part of lasting importance in the philosophy of history.

However, a philosophy of culture, starting from the historical peaks of the history of human civilization, does derive some support from this view of modern cultural degeneration. But the main impulses come from pessimistic romanticism and metaphysics, notably from the paradoxical, anti-Hegelian and negative nihilistic philosophy of Schopenhauer, making itself further felt in Klages, Th. Lessing and Eduard von Hartmann, among others. According to Schopenhauer this world is the worst of all possible worlds and will therefore have to deny, forsake and eliminate itself. There is also some connection with those views of an existentialist philosophy in which Death functions not only as the repeated, irrevocable, individual end, but also finally as the ultimate victory over all life and history.

(5) A much more direct influence on the philosophy of history was exerted by biology in particular and the idea of causal conformity with natural law in general. In the evolutionistic and anthropocentric progress models, whether moderately optimistic about historical development, or unworldly but unshakably optimistic about salvation, or optimistic about the world (as in the dogmatic, anti-humanitarian social Darwinism of Spencer) this influence, as is known, finds pronounced expression.

However, this biologism of Spencer, like any other strained extreme that finds expression in a returning pendulum movement, could, as we saw, with equal ease be deflected towards another finishing-point. As in the case of Spengler who, long fashionable, firmly held the attention of the Western world for his historico-philosophical and also physical and mathematical thought and future model. As an impressionistic sketch of the repeated historical development it looks broadly like this:

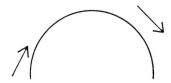

The curve reproduces every cultural-historical drama enacted again and again. It consists of the parts inevitably returning at all times, succeeding each other uniformly, which in essence must develop the exactly identical life-cycle of every organism. On each occasion the beginning is birth, then follows growth, and after that adult maturity, succeeded once again by the inevitable aging and senile decadence with a gradual loss of powers. Until, under nature's inexorable law, merciful or merciless death finally cuts the thread of life or releases the dying organism from its suffering.

In Spengler not only is this historical cycle between the beginning and the end of each culture fixed in advance, but in his view the same applies to the distances in time between the various phases, which therefore always occupy a fixed position on a curve that is almost a pure parabola. One could therefore determine exactly at what moment of the total course of time allotted, i.e. at what stage of rise, matured development or decline, every historical culture developing synchronously happens to be. Moreover, in accordance with the principle of this natural uniformity (and also, when making comparable historical cross sections, simultaneity), the *future* course, including the ending, i.e. the degeneration and the predestined doom, could be calculated with almost mathematical precision and predicted in causal conformity with natural law. This is again a characteristic example of a thought model that spins itself into the cocoon of a compulsory future model but does not further emerge from this.

The strange thing is that if a large part of modern existentialist philosophy were to be converted into this imagery, essentially the same line would have to be drawn. In this case one does not start from culture but from the identical and uniform life of every individual separately who after all, taken together, form the history of mankind.

This view is practically identical with the mythological picture used by Camus. Man, for ever wrestling in vain, is like Sisyphus given the lifelong task of rolling a stone (a part of the globe) uphill. Once this has almost reached the top it rolls back again in endless repetition, so that it returns eternally from the end in view to the same starting-point.[5] Historical man, released from his temporary existence not by suicide but only by death, can find his happiness only in this bitter despair. For Jasper too all existence — as in Heidegger — is a "Sein zum Tode", which cannot be transcended. According to him the meaning of life, and also of history, is "Scheitern", failure. As a result philosophizing is learning to die; every rising-time-curve is closed off at its final lower point by ultimate death, the border-post of life. In Sartre the ever-hopeless death.

Although in its form it has an outward resemblance, the picture emerging from the rainbow, symbolic for the Jewish people, is entirely different. The rainbow, which linked earth and heaven, which served as jacob's ladder for the angels, is the inspiring symbol for the believer in his dialogical relation to his own God, accompanying him through history, leading him irrevocably to the end of earth's time.

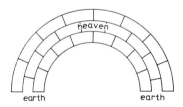

This picture contains the idea, as eschatological as it is utopian, of a historical gateway to a different and better future. However, it transcends each time the finite life of the individual Jew to that of the Jewish people as a collectivity. With a continuous, indestructible and unchangeably perspective outlook on that other world dawning some day.

2. Modern sacral future-models

However, the above illustrations do not entirely complete my brief historical review of the images of historical thought and future models.

The philosophy of existence (whether the religious or the secular version) has not yet pronounced the last word for our time.

It was almost self-evident that purely secular philosophy of history would develop further. However, in a much more surprising fashion the theological view of history, which had already been considered dead after the zenith of Bossuet and the nadir of Nietzsche, with his "Gott ist tot", revived.

Two leading figures acted as representatives of this new trend, separated by a wide gulf (and not only on account of their Protestant and Catholic theology or philosophy respectively), relatively soon after one another. The first, Toynbee, long lionized (and also sharply criticized) especially on account of his imposing work "A Study of History", as one of the last great architects of a historical system. The second was Teilhard de Chardin, around whom a quickly growing cult of enthusiastic, albeit sometimes uncritical, veneration has developed only since his death.[6]

I have already written at some length elsewhere about Toynbee's thought system.[7] I shall therefore confine myself to a few notes here.

In Toynbee, as in Spengler, we find a culture-pessimistic theory which at the same time presents itself as ultra-scientific, that is to say incorporating and interpreting history as an inevitably natural and mechanistic development. What is given with the right hand as the possibility of intervening human freedom of will, viz. contained in the now proverbial pair of concepts "challenge" and "response", is taken away with the left hand because evidently the imperfect human faculties of readiness and ability always fall short. In fact must fall short, because at the same time they are subject to the supreme law of constant change, already known from ancient Chinese wisdom as the uninterrupted movement between the poles of yin and yang.

Of course ten large volumes, with their brilliant composition, testifying to an impressive erudition and a splendid wealth of imagery, cannot possibly be reproduced in simple schemata without doing them an injustice, although D. C. Somervell attempted this in a particularly meritorious manner in his two-volume "Abridgement". Nevertheless, at least the broad trend evoked by Toynbee of repeated rise and fall of all the cultures analysed by him could be summarized in graphical form as follows:

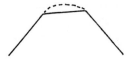

a picture which, further shortened, can be drawn somewhat sharper (or even contracted) to form:

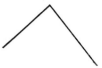

In essence this differs little from the cyclical, somewhat more rounded, truncated conical image or the parabolic projection of Spengler, which after all amounts practically to the same thing de facto. Vico's "corso" and "ricorso" can also be found in this pictorial reduction.

According to this view of Toynbee's given in abridged form, the climax temporarily crowning the rise of every cultural phase is inevitably followed by a breakdown. In turn this passes into a period of disintegration, which then again irrevocably heralds the end. This period of disintegration has been further stylized by Toynbee. It takes place, with irregular flare-ups, in a rhythm of "three-and-a-half beats". The end, for which the death-knell has sounded after an unmistakable collapse, could therefore be represented as follows:

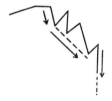

In our Western culture, according to Toynbee, the breakdown has already taken place, unstoppable disintegration is already active. Must we therefore abandon all hope? No, Toynbee stresses, transforming himself at that moment from modern historian to ancient theologian of history, and acting as a medieval theocratic Savonarola. Just as Leibnitz has chosen the divine miracle as an auxiliary construction in advance, Toynbee uses it after the event. People themselves can favor this miracle in well-nigh magical fashion by doing the only thing that still holds out hope of delivery and salvation, viz. by converting en masse to the true Christianity, praying fervently and uninterruptedly to God in order that history stops — like the sun for Joshua — and reverses at the last minute thanks to a divine interruption of necessary conformity with natural law. This reversal is therefore exclusively by virtue of the Dispensation of Providence, which in this sense may possibly be mollified and should be awaited in resignation.

Whilst, as we have seen, during the deism developing in the 17th century

God was still recognized as the original lawmaker, i.e. as the Creator of the laws of nature, He was at the same time deposed as the operator, acting in history, of a mechanism of these laws, which had meantime come to be regarded as further self-active. From then on God too was bound to these laws of nature.

In itself it is not so surprising — nor can one make any valid objection to it — that three centuries later a leading historian again discovers an absolute and unconditional conformity with natural law in history, even though preceding attempts to do so had always undeniably failed. However, it is all the more surprising, not to say paradoxical, in the light of the development of historical thought models, that Toynbee goes back to long gone-by, long dead and decomposed views from or even predating the Middle Ages. He does so in order to proclaim that God is able, and probably willing for once, to put these historical laws of nature, which according to Toynbee prevail with unconditional strictness, temporarily out of operation under certain conditions. Toynbee first goes to a great deal of trouble to demonstrate that the nature of these laws is in fact absolutely inexorable, and then concludes with the argument that for our case they are on the contrary pre-eminently "exorable" and, if God wishes, changeable this time — and this time alone.

This thought model is more coercive than any of its predecessors, and also the most strict and dogmatic. In so many words it is prescribed to God Himself. There seems to be no model of the future in the proper sense of the word: the forecast is, in accordance with the terminology of Antiquity, unchangeably "nefastus" (fatal, disastrous) and negative. For the future Toynbee fixes his gaze solely on Christ and the Cross, which of course he is fully entitled to do privately. Together with Lazarus, Toynbee rises from the grave of history. Closing the circle, he returns completely to the doctrinaire theology of history extending from Augustine to Bossuet. However, there is the characteristic difference that the divine completion of history is no longer an established fact a priori, but could be realized for our own time only by a New Testament miracle. Despite the demythologization of the present time Toynbee believes unconditionally in the historical reality of such miracles. But because he does not believe in the idealism of present-day man, he hardly believes in his heart that such a miracle can in fact still take place in reality.

However, Toynbee is also reconciled to that in advance and "sans rancune". For he is of the opinion that, as a historian, he has proved that every civilization is above all assigned a theological function. All perishing cultures, and therefore ours too, in that case serve only as "stepping stones to God". We too now have a "civilization on trial", with Toynbee and God together on the bench, so that a probable death sentence will not be open to appeal. Or is Toynbee the devil's advocate? Toynbee confronts God with a challenge with two possible kinds of response. Either people heed Toynbee's urgent and divinely inspired appeal, and then as far as he is concerned God may, with a clear conscience, cause a miracle to happen. Or they do not listen to Toynbee, but God does, and it is up to Him to choose a culture more in the spirit of Toynbee than the thoroughly degenerate Western civilization, which should then be ruthlessly abandoned to historical downfall. What will that new culture be like? God may decide that for Himself in due course, although Toynbee has a number of important suggestions for Him, which God will doubtless carefully consider. In any case, not a culture with Jewish taints!

In this sense Toynbee proclaims a new prescription, unequalled in its coercion and barely distinguishable from indoctrination and methodical brainwashing, also intended for God. If, as is extremely probable, people ignore Toynbee's admonishments and homilies and do not turn aside at the right time from the errors of their ways, a justly punishing God, rudely awakened by Toynbee from His good-natured snooze, may finally condemn their cultural barbarism, which deserves no better fate. This will have to make way for civilization more pleasing to God, a true (i.e. Christian) culture. As may be seen, the same interpretation — already given *in advance* — which Augustine felt that he had to give, *after the event*, rather more cautiously, in fact apologetically and decidedly less arrogantly, *after* the world-shaking, unforeseen and completely surprising downfall of the sacred but overnight barbarian Rome. Le roi est mort, vive le roi! Let Western culture, which is damnable because it is godless and ultimately abandoned by God at Toynbee's urging, sicken further and die its painful but deserved death. Another and better civilization — better in accordance with the theological criteria of Toynbee — may then arise like a phoenix from its ashes after combustion by the divine thunderbolts.

A theology of Progress which, however, no modern theologian inspired by a sense of social responsibility would dare to adopt today. A theology of Progress, at the same time as crude and repelling as that of classical liberalism. A theology of the optimum laissez faire, laissez aller, which concentrates Spencer's social Darwinism into a cultural Darwinism. This is based on the conviction that the strongest surviving civilization definitely will and must be (after all Toynbee, as evidenced by his gospel, has tried to make this clear to God as the leader of history) the more specifically Christian or, in somewhat broader perspective, the most sanctified culture, devoted to God and elected by His will. This is, however a rather paradoxical and unhistorical view, if only in view of atheistic world Communism spreading vigorously and the expansion of differentiated Oriental world religions coupled with the rapidly increasing growth of Asian and African populations. All the same, this view does in fact contain a specific *model of the future*. Or rather two models of the future for alternatively possible futures. The future thus revealed is on the one hand only possible, as far as our own culture is concerned, via a barely negotiable, very narrow mountain pass at tremendous altitude, through which only one man of God can lead mankind, provided that the latter is in possession of a valid passport stamped by him. On the other hand, even though *our* culture probably has no further chance, somewhere around the corner, still veiled from the eyes of common mortals, a new cultural prospect is already beckoning. For the time being God is still holding this back, and only Toynbee, as His sole true prophet, shows us it.

A greater contrast, in practically every respect, than with the view of Teilhard de Chardin is hardly conceivable. The latter was not a historian and theologian, but a paleontologist and biologist. Here there is none of the exact literary clarity of the decidedly fascinating imagery of Toynbee, but instead a style inclining towards the mystical and sometimes rather hazy in form. In Teilhard we find no deliberate historico-philosophical design in the proper sense of the term, but an approach which, though likewise strictly and narrowly scientific, gradually broadens and merges into a phenomenological treatment. The insight thus obtained, which Teilhard himself calls hyperphysics, is ultimately graspable only as an overall view borne by inner, cosmic experience and communicable by enthusiasm or at least affinity.[8] Now this view is specifically and even passionately directed towards the future. *Another* and *better future* to be realized through steady *human progress*.

Teilhard is in a class apart as an original thinker and an author going his own way. It is extremely difficult to classify and delineate him schematically. The two pillars of his view of history — for only the latter is relevant here — are dynamics and evolution. Here we are for the time being still in our own field. And here we therefore once again find some schematic representations of older date. For instance, with almost striking similarity, Herder's idea concerning an as it were spiral progress of history. Teilhard, as always, gives this uninterrupted process of development his own names: in this case as the product of ever-new aggregation, constantly leading to integration on a repeatedly higher plane. According to Teilhard, testifying to a modernized secular idealism of progress that is combined with renewed religious optimism, this biological evolutionism follows an unmistakably upward course, rising from a starting-point alpha to a climax omega — the completion.[9]

We also find again in his view the three-stage development which has proved to possess great viability since Joachim, Lessing, Saint Simon, Comte and Marx. In his language Teilhard describes this development as one going first from the Paleolithic period to the Neolithic one, and from there to our own time. In his opinion our time should be regarded, on the strength of a marked, complete caesura, as the beginning of an absolutely new time, which moreover is breaking new ground with a tremendous acceleration of the process of acceleration (Turgot). In this time a new, higher man[10] and a new, better culture will come into being. The higher and better is in no way, as in Toynbee, determined by Christian theology in the narrower sense. This higher and better will be reflected in the events of history in particular by an ultimate planetary unification of all men and of their separate subcultures. This movement goes from pole to pole. Just as the diversity of men and cultures in the phenomenon of the past, so the growing unity of mankind is the phenomenon par excellence of the future time and therefore for the first time of that *future* which is truly *humane* (Herder again!).

Up to here I might perhaps reproduce Teilhard's exposition in schematic form as follows:

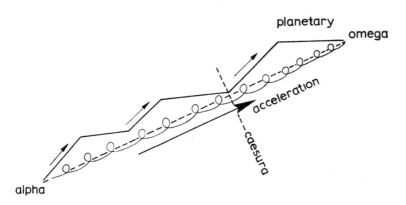

Now let me try at once to remove the impression that I may have created that "actually" Teilhard adds little or nothing new — except for the coining of a completely personal terminology — to ideas and images of the future existing before him. For this is by no means so, even though the new element is often the least obvious one. I shall mention only one addition, which is of particular importance in our context.

It was not without reason that Delfgaauw, an authority on Teilhard's work, selected the following sentence both as motto and for further elaboration: "Nous sommes parvenus à un point décisif de l'évolution humaine, où la seule issue en avant est dans la direction d'une passion commune". Now one might suppose that Teilhard, as a devout Catholic, meant by this one human, forward-moving force of a "passion commune" a Christian "foi commune", like Toynbee. But it was likewise not without reason that during his lifetime the Catholic Church imposed a publication ban on him, on account of his supposed deviations from orthodox doctrine. This, of course, only caused interest in his works to grow, sometimes beyond all proportion. It seems to me that Teilhard definitely did not have a dogmatic end in view with this passionate exhortation.

In a very important passage from his fundamental work "Le Phénomène Humain" Teilhard gives a clear commentary on Comte's motto: "savoir pour prévoir, prévoir pour pouvoir", namely as follows: "Pouvoir plus pour agir plus. Mais, finalement et surtout, agir plus afin d'être plus". In my opinion the most complete antithesis to Toynbee's theology of history occurs here.

Toynbee rejects every response that does not go completely back with him to the incarnation of God in Christ. In his opinion every other answer is absolutely ineligible and ineffective, either because it is archaic (pagan) or futuristic (un-Christian). Every human action directed towards the *future* that is not governed — and exclusively so — by the letter of the New Testament (according to his interpretation) is doomed in advance to inevitable failure, as a fatal departure from the only doctrine of salvation and from his Savior, the sole governor of history. This point of view, inexorably adhered to by Toynbee and, according to him, by God, holds good without any distinction. This negative condemnation befalls not only the martial "savior with the sword" but equally every other tried secular solution denounced by Toynbee as an irrational and irretrievable aberration. For instance solutions characterized by Toynbee in accordance with the platonic model of the "philosopher masked by a king" and also of "the creative genius as a savior".

The pair of concepts "challenge and response", in which the appropriate response is provided by a "creative minority", as depicted by Toynbee himself in particularly lucid fashion, nevertheless evidently relates only to pre-Christian cultures. With regard to the Christian culture he abhors every human, volitionally creative exercise of secular power for the purpose of determining one's own destiny, even if it is on a philosophical basis. Toynbee collides most sharply with what he typifies and ridicules as "the savior with the Time Machine". This approach is not only pernicious and completely hopeless, but moreover causes lasting, immense harm. The future is that of the Christian doctrine of salvation or, at least for us, is completely non-existent.

In the ancient conflict, running like a thread though the present considerations, between *divine supremacy* and a developing, future-oriented, consciously creative *human power*, with the supreme control of historical dynamics at stake, Toynbee comes down firmly on the side of the former, offering no other alternative. This view is thus at the same time an extremely illuminating and completely classical example in the purest form of the antithesis between *dogmatics* and *prognostics* discussed in this work and still existing today. That is also the reason why my opposition or protest has been somewhat sharper here than is usually the case.

Teilhard, on the other hand, building instead on the radicalism of Proudhon, attempts a viable synthesis between these two extremes of divine and human power, and also between material and spiritual progress. Furthermore, strangely enough, he tries for the first time in history, as far as I know, to establish a synthesis between sacral and profane historiography. As against the transfiguration and transcendence so strictly forbidden by Toynbee, effectuated thanks to the "futurism" practised by man and intended for man, for Teilhard human *liberty* and *volitional activism* are precisely indispensable instruments of at once historical and cosmic progress. It is these highest qualities of human dignity which, according to Teilhard, will lead par excellence to the ultimate transformation, desired and promised by God, of the completion of history to be pursued by *man himself* and to be achieved sometime in the future. Essential and fundamental both to human existence and to this future to be realized is man's purposive determination of his own destiny. In this way Teilhard opens up a very broad ecumenical path of evolution through human power to the future, which can also be trodden by unbelievers.

3. Modern profane non-future-models

Toynbee and Teilhard, however greatly opposed to each other in their theology of progress, nevertheless do agree in one respect. For modern historians they both represent as a rule a point of view that has already been overcome, an anachronism. Not so much on account of their theology, but above all because of their mechanism cloaked in scientific garb, which moreover is set in motion by the finalistic drive of a doctrine of salvation. In its deepest essence criticism is directed towards their methodology, however schematically it may be arranged, whether it is that of a semi-cyclical movement going continuously up and down or that of a steady forward motion, stamped in advance "Progress". Nor does it matter whether this concerns progress towards God, or towards true humanity, or towards a man perfected in the image of God, in whom God is reflected and in whom He recognizes or finds Himself, while man finds himself again in Him, finds the way back to Him.

Of course a set of motives can be pointed to for the new turn in thought. They are in close interaction with the development in, of and through history itself.

In the first place history, in particular that of the last fifty years, as already touched upon above, has not exactly supplied proof of the idea of an incessant, irresistible Progress. In fact actual historical progress has shattered the optimistic ideal picture of automatic progress.

In the second place past history, and even more so that which is now foreseeable, testifies to a steadily increasing dynamization, to an ever-greater acceleration, comparable only to the effect of an avalanche. Change has become the essence of the movement of history, the characteristic of human existence. The changeable now seems the only and eternal unchangeable. Change, increasingly designated as revolution in a steadily growing number of fields, with an ever-wider range of action, increased intensity and close-knit interdependence. In this process the grasp on the future is increasingly slackening. Historians are already over-occupied with incessant reconstruction of the equally changeable past. Social scientists are already unable to make much sense of their analysis and diagnosis of the present. There seems to be increasing confirmation of the prophetic words of the cynical statesman Walpole: "the wisest prophets make sure of the event first".

Meanwhile the progressing natural sciences have developed new thought models, which also serve as an example for the practice of science as such. Certainly for the science of history too, which has never been able to terminate the lengthy struggle for acknowledgment of its scientific status in a general recognition.

For the science of history this struggle has at any event resulted in the sacrifice of two things very dear to it. Both the objectives and the values have had to be cast out.

The modern natural sciences owe their phenomenal growth — since Bacon — to the empirical observation of facts. The historian too could therefore only pronounce on factual causes and effects, or factual connections between change and the movement of history, in a scientifically sound manner. So-called predestined or implanted objectives of the movement were not factually observable nor active in accordance with scientifically establishable and verifiable laws. The objective of progress had therefore to be rejected by a self-respecting science of history, both in the sense of a movement towards future salvation in accordance with sacral history and in the sense of a well-considered evolution by virtue of profane history.

Finally, how could one appraise change in any kind of scientifically acceptable and reliable way? The long dispute between the "anciens" and the "modernes" on progress was not, it was now found, essentially capable of settlement on the strength of any objective criterion, nor will that ever be possible. There is no exact measuring instrument which could already clearly divide today's change and movement into the retrogression and progress, decline or prosperity. Let alone — according to the continued present-day argumentation and interpretation — that future development could be appraised as such in advance with any kind of precision (instead of prophecy). Come to that, any appraisal is itself subject in its turn to historical change and fluctuation.

Philosophically speaking, the consequence of all this was that one was as it were impelled at the same time towards two extremes touching one another in accordance with a principle of polarity, both far *backwards* towards a certain type of philosophy of Antiquity and as far as possible *forwards* in an encounter with the modern philosophy of existentialism.

Backwards to Heraclitus, the spiritual father of the continuity of eternal Becoming, to struggle and conflict as the sources of moving progress, of endless progress, without a given significance, and certainly not provided with any definite purpose for the future.

Back, too, to the Old Testament and the pessimism of Ecclesiastes "there is no new thing under the sun". Back, willy-nilly, to the New Testament too and to the doctrine of original sin and the resultant ever-lasting (until redemption) imperfect, unchangeable human nature, which excludes a priori all change in the sense of progress during the still remaining time of history.

110

Forwards, returning to the same starting-point in a secularized sense, tying in with existentialism: hopeless Becoming, unchangeable despite all change, as nothing more and better than a "Sein zum Tode". Coupled with the eternal return and continuation of evil, meanness and injustice in this world. There too is no change for the good that could ever be regarded as fundamentally possible, no essential improvement or even stepwise progress.

Of all the historical schematic representations shown above, only two therefore remain on the whole after this slimming process:

(a) a fairly level, practically horizontal line of developing progress, around which only continual fluctuations of greater or smaller amplitude occur, which in the longer run can be smoothed out again, for instance more or less like this:

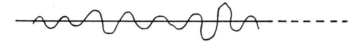

(b) a somewhat different picture is presented by the following representation. This again revives, though in highly abridged form, the idea of the pursuit of equilibrium taken from nature (seasons, tides, recovery after natural disasters, woman's periods, the succession of the generations, birth and death, etc.). In the legal system and the administration of justice, too, there is a constant search for equilibrium between opposed interests, parties and problems. It is thought that in the turmoil and the movement of history (revolution and consolidation, the conflict between progressive and conservative, war and peace, etc.) a repeated disturbance of equilibrium is likewise followed by a restoration of balance, as a result of which the scales may tip to the other side (may, but not must), i.e. as follows:

As will be clear, in this alternating interplay of movements the line drawn under (a), which on average remains level, would be continued and only the fluctuations around the "natural" equilibrium have been taken as somewhat larger (and longer-lasting) here, also with a greater range of the opposed action and reaction.

To that extent, then, one could attribute both schemata to a position of *realistic pessimism* or even *fatalism* with regard to Becoming in time towards the future. A faint spark of hope can still be cherished in that variant of the same view that possibly (certainly not necessarily) a somewhat higher ceiling could be reached in the restoration of balance (although it could also come to adopt a lower position immediately or some time afterwards).

In the latter eventuality the picture looks about like this:

111

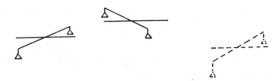

(c) But, apart from these unprecluded possibilities of reaching a higher (unfortunately also a lower) level, there is no predictability on this score. As a result we can hardly give this the label even of a highly tempered optimism; it would be more exact to say that it is a typical *present-day realism* with a *future-asceticism*.

I shall confine myself to a couple of examples to illustrate this final argument, which apparently rather peters out with regard to the future models in our contemporary thought.

In the first place that of the rightly famous Swiss historian Jacob Burckhardt, known above all for his studies of the Renaissance, a typical transitional figure towards our century. It is Burckhardt who consistently and resolutely rejects all theological, philosophical, Marxist or evolutionistic interpretations of history as "hineininterpretieren", as unsound and speculative. In his view history has no beginning, no development according to natural law, no progress or end. The essence and the only sense of history are continuous change. The real philosophy of history is therefore dead.

Insofar as this view lends itself to schematic reproduction, it could only be reproduced as a non-uniform, entirely fancifully undulating endlessly continuing line:

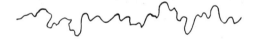

A basic tenet of Burckhardt's is that the future can never be derived from the historical past by rational inferences or via extrapolations. Moreover, in his opinion modern time is separated from Antiquity precisely in *that* respect by an unbridgeable gap. Not only because we no longer consult oracles or, being rational people, no longer turn to soothsayers and prognosticators to learn or to be able to foresee the future, but also and above all because — according to Burkhardt — we also no longer regard these practices as *desirable* or *wholesome*.

The future, Burckhardt argues, is and must be "blind". "Eine vorausgewusste Zukunft ist ein Widersinn". Here we have the characteristic change in attitudes of mind. Here we no longer find a coercive future model but, conversely, an equally coercive *non*-future model.

Burckhardt is convinced that the historian must leave the future entirely to the future. Prognosis is nonsense, i.e. from the historical point of view both impossible and undesirable and giving an effect opposite to the one desired.

112

On the other hand, precisely on the strength of his historical studies, Burkhardt testifies to a pronounced culture-pessimistic view with regard to the present and the future, a conviction founded on great knowledge of his subject, which has largely contributed towards his fame. This view of the future, for this is after all implied in it, can in my opinion only be reconciled with his pertinent abstinence with respect to the developing future as a return to the Stoic doctrine of resigned acceptance and "amor fati", which runs in a straight line from Nietzsche to the modern existentialist philosophy.

Over half a century later this view of history is still fundamentally unchanged in R. G. Collingwood. His argument is that history has neither sense nor purpose. His book, entitled "The Idea of History", is aimed straight at all historians like Löwith, whose work in its English edition was entitled "The Meaning of History", or Jaspers, who had still spoken of a "Ziel der Geschichte", and in actual fact against all philosophers of history. Only Vico is complimented by this authur. True, Vico's fundamental cyclical-historical scheme, like any other scheme based on a natural law, was untenable, but at least he adhered explicitly, on account of the renovations which he observed and regarded as probable in principle, to what Collingwood regards as an imperative basic principle, viz. that the true *historian never prophesies.*

Eschatological historiography (up to and including Toynbee) forms a particular black sheep for Collingwood. "Eschatology is always an intrusive element in history". Not on account of the doctrine of salvation itself, but because of the false introduction and incorrect injection into the science of history of a prognostic (in this case theological) substance. "The historian's business is to know the past, not to know the future; and whenever historians claim to be able to determine the future in advance of its happening, we may know with certainty that something has gone wrong with their fundamental conception of history.[11]

In other words, there is no inherent historical development as Progress. Even less so is there a possible prognosis of any kind of continuous historical process, but on the contrary an ever-procceding discontinuous and therefore unforeseeable change and renewal.[12] Is, then, no historical progress at all possible? Collingwood is in no way prepared to exclude this in advance, although his concluding section contains a detailed argumentation of the problems and practically insurmountable difficulties of recognizing it.

Strangely enough, the title of that section is "Progress as created by Historical Thinking". Not until the last sentences of the very last page[13] does the intention of this heading become clear to some extent. If we want to do away with something that is wrong, his argument runs, and replace it by something better, there is a considerable risk that, while we may destroy something, we may not be able to substitute something else, a better working system, for it. For instance: let us assume that it is desirable to abolish capitalism. Now how can we prevent a state of affairs in which, blinded by hatred, we act destruct-

113

ively and not constructively or, alternatively because we may love the system so much, only offer resistance to this process? In both cases only change would occur, but no progress. Collingwood offers the simple solution for this: only by good historical insight into and understanding of the growth of a system existing from the past up to the present day shall we be capable of creative progress (viz. of the capitalist system) ("a knowledge of the past conditioning our creation of the future").

To the fancifully undulating line of Burkhardt Collingwood therefore adds here a piece in the final instance in a rather arbitrary and sowewhat improbable fashion:

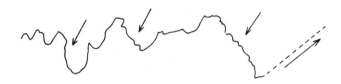

Here, therefore, the "évolution créatrice" is placed in the hand of the professional historian, and in his hands only. Moreover, these hands are tied, insofar as the historian might want to *think ahead* and *look ahead* on behalf of these conditions of progress which he is to create for the future. For this is strictly forbidden. Let us imagine how it will be: with his back turned permanently on the future, systematically compelling the spirits of the past to appear with regressively directed will-power, contemplating the navel of the present and of the established order with fixed, fearless gaze, this historian will proceed to supply us with a completely satisfying explanation of possible future progress. Thanks to his conservative and abstaining attitude towards the future, we may now apparently expect from him the decisive answer to the two main questions that have to be settled as priorities with regard to every progressive change: *where* will the movement now developing in history take us? What *can* we, *may* we and *must* we do in this respect? The naive optimism of progress has here been converted into a much naiver optimism tied to the reconstructed past. Without a purposive commitment in the future-dimension the model of the future evaporates in a one-sided historical fashion into a dogmatic *non-future model*. At best it narrows into a *model of the present* anchored to exploration of the past and extended from the latter:

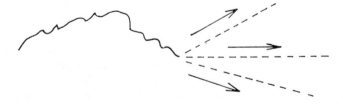

The last piece of the historical line may therefore equally well have the following appearance, i.e. remaining practically the same, or even dropping further; however, a deliberate radical reformation and improvement of the existing pattern of society could hardly be expected by this process.

If, conversely, we were to try again to trace the graphical models given here back to their orginal fundamental thought and future models, this could be done by means of a common formula: "The image is the message".[14] To remain in the modern idiom, I could add: the medium is the dogma. But definitely not as the mobile, supplying massage, but as the immovable and also unmoved mummy.

CHAPTER 7

Scientific models of the future

There is so much literature on the development of scientific thought models that I can more or less confine myself to reproducing a few main ideas as advocated by the great renovators in this field.

The advent of scientific thought models reflects in its historical development the incessant struggle against older, contemporary and even later coercive thought models of philosophical-religious belief and superstition. This is the case not only among the old, in part so-called primitive peoples, but equally so in Europe, until far after the Middle Ages. The irony of history again resides in the fact that precisely these new scientific thought models, liberating the mind from intellectual tyranny and terror in their turn and, at least at the beginning, in spite of themselves, were later to take over the role of the dethroned rulers of dogma, doctrine and orthodoxy. At first spreading a "more" scientific civilization, they were in the long run to elevate "less" scientific ideas to idols.

Human life in inimical nature was long governed by "totem and taboo". Disease, crop failures and natural disasters were ascribed to angry gods, malignant demons or accursed magical powers. Animal and human sacrifices, priestly rites and sacred mystery services could perhaps propitiate these powers, ruling with extreme arbitrariness and as a rule uncontrollable, in the only effective manner. They were thought to be able to ensure fertility of the soil and victory over the enemy, by an extremely meticulous observance of the regulations applicable in that respect and of "techniques" regarded as the sole effective ones. The catastrophes *predicted* in particular by comets and eclipses could possibly still be averted at the eleventh hour by a completely correct attitude of mind and by conscious good behavior towards higher powers.

As opposed to this, *scientific* thought develops in *four* main lines which at first were separate ones. The first and at the same time one of the oldest developments (1), that of the Babylonians, began precisely with the study of these eclipses and comets and the movement of the planets. The Chaldean priest-astrologers tried to explain these, and even to *predict* them, by calculating their change, course and appearance as accurately as possible. The three other main lines run respectively from the highly developed pure mathematical thought of the Greeks (2), from the specifically Hellenic mathematical-philosophical minds, which developed in Alexandria in particular (3), and last but not least, from another equally Greek and scientific, non-mathematical but mainly methaphysical intellect (4). It was the last one in particular that was to combine with Christian theology and to dominate thought rather one-sidedly for nearly twenty successive centuries. That is to say, until the three lines previously drawn were again to be extended into the forcefield of the spirit, viz. until the revolutionary mutation in the mental attitude of the then modern sciences (see below under 5 et seq.).

(1) It is generally known that the Babylonians are regarded as the inventors of astrology, thus standing by the cradle of Western science. Their predictions, although not always completely correct, were understandably famed on account of their astonishing accuracy. Tides, eclipses, floods, influences of the moon, the course of the seasons, the movement of the planets and other successions or changes in or of time — recorded in the "calender" of the "good" and "bad" dates or periods to be expected — could be calculated in advance and predicted as the *future*.

However, it was not the budding science, but in particular the *world view behind it*, linked with unscientific belief and superstition, that first enjoyed the privilege of being elevated to a very lengthy, almost ineradicable, reactionary and tyrannical, in brief pre-eminently *dogmatic* tradition. As a result people in centuries to come continued to regard comets and eclipses in particular as manifest signs of God's wrath and vengeance. They were the unmistakable harbingers of plague, epidemic, war, revolution, hurricane, famine or other divine scourge. For centuries the outcast and hidden Jews — who most conveniently could almost always be discovered somewhere — were given the blame for these scourges and thus made the scapegoats for them, at one and the same time by way of revenge and expiatory sacrifice. As was rightly required by the Lord Jesus, His name be praised, and the beloved Mother of God, ave Maria. The fact that the Jews usually did not offer the slighest resistance to their oppression and persecution was incidentally clear proof of their criminal intentions, still manifest in full force after their killing of Christ. This cried out for God's just punishment, with an ice-cold, unsparing cruelty which the God of the Old Testament had in any case Himself declared obligatory against those guilty of sacrilege.

Although the New Testament gave absolute primacy to evangelical love and Christian charity, it was precisely this strict Old Testament thought model, so long applied to others and dissenters, that for centuries found the greatest approval and offered the greatest attraction as the imitation of Christ. Should it happen that now Jews were not available for execution, other heretics, witches, magicians and alchemists, as almost equal stand-ins, had to take over the role of the Jews, and the pogroms were directed against them. The inevitability of this was always based on an intolerant, dogmatic thought model. If necessary, after the occurrence of natural disasters and fatal calamities one could always invoke thoughtful recollection by way of explanation, by pointing out that these disasters tallied exactly with warnings — unfortunately not taken seriously enough — of remarkable symptoms and indications augured in the firmament. There is no more malleable and suitable a subject for indoctrination or interpretation than a well-guided or misled human memory. With an appeal to heaven all the actions of authorities and vicars on earth, by the grace of God, could be rationalized beforehand or after the event, and thus manipulated as required.

The heavenly and universal macrocosm was a fore-reflection of the earthly and human microcosm. In the physician and natural philosopher Paracelsus (16th century), at the same time one of the great transitional figures towards modern empirical science and astronomy, a religic-cosmic interlacing of ancient astrology and undogmatic theology comes to the fore in the most elevated but now pre-eminently *humanistic* manner. For Paracelsus this comprehensive knowledge of the universe and of the heavens served to heal men and to restore the divine harmony on earth.

John Knox, pupil of Calvin, reformer of Scotland, however, still adopted in that same sixteenth century the classical view as evidence: he and his followers regarded such phenomena of the heavens as eclipses and comets this time as "a warning to the King to extirpate the Papists".

Similar feelings also prevailed among Cromwell's fanatical Puritans in the 17th century. His poetic servant Milton said of an eclipse of the sun that it:

> In dim eclipse, disastrous twilight sheds
> On half the nations, and with fear of change
> Perplexes monarchs.

While therefore Milton in *democratic* fashion treated peoples and princes more or less alike with regard to future astronomical disasters, Shakespeare had in his day made a rather sarcastically relativizing, *aristocratic* distinction:

> When beggars die, there are no comets seen;
> The heavens themselves blaze forth the death of princes.

Shakespeare must have been a contemporary of Francis Bacon and Galileo, and Milton lived to see the advent of Newton. These were thus times of great contrast in outlooks on and views of the world.

A considerably longer life was even granted to the original Babylonian astrology, even after the rise and branching-off of scientific astronomy. In Kepler the two branches were still almost inseparably combined.

Admittedly, opposition arose in the Church: Astrological prediction of the future granted destiny-determining power to the planets and to the signs of the zodiac dependent on these, a power which, however, rightly belonged exclusively to God. Augustine thus adduced even all the profane arguments of sceptics and pagan thinkers from Antiquity against it.

118

However, freethinkers, who no longer recognized the inviolability of the authority of the theocratic church and did not yet recognize the unassailability of that of modern science opted for Ptolemaic astrology. And, after and in spite of Augustine, so did a number of Popes, striving for personal or political reasons for well-founded prescience of the near future. But, of course, they also sided with ancient astrology for other reasons, since Copernican science and modern astronomy evidently collided in their pronouncements with Biblical and ecclesiastical teachings and doctrinal authority.

(2) A second main trend originates from the oldest Greek philosophical and scientific reflection. Once again the theory of numbers developed by Pythagoras of Samos and his advanced geometric research is general knowledge. It is not entirely certain to what extent there were links between the Babylonians and the Pythagoreans, especially as regards the numerical, arithmetical refinement of the theory of numbers. What is certain, however, is that Greek mathematics developed independently towards the side of geometry in particular.

For instance, a Greek adage, ʿο θεός ʾαει γεομετρει, may be literally interpreted as "God acts always as a geometrician". This is the Greeks' aesthetic view of God and the world, no less, but also no more. A view — we have already encountered it — of cosmos and harmony, of music and beauty, of geometrical dimension, order, completeness and artistic-mathematical configuration (circle and centre). Plato conceived of the composite movement of all heavenly bodies as the resultant of uniform circular movements, which it ought to be possible to describe and reproduce mathematically and geometrically.

De Solla Price rightly again stresses this difference between the mathematics of the Babylonians and that of the Greeks, which is in various respects a really fundamental one. The Greek world of ideas was one thought out with strict logic and projected in concrete images, i.e. not so much as with the Babylonians an abstract calculation which was later primarily to lend itself to fusion with a symbolic, algebraic outlook. Using my own terminology, one may also say that the Greek possessed not only a pre-eminently realistic *thought* model which could be depicted with geometric logic, but also a qualitative, ideal and partly imaginary model of the *future* as overall conception.

In itself it is interesting to investigate with Price how, throughout the ages, this contract between analytical calculators and geometric model-builders — incidentally already discovered and elucidated by Poincaré — has continued to exist among scientists and probably will always do so. It is also present for instance between the microphysical model-builders like Rutherford and those nuclear physicists who work mainly with symbolical relations only, with Bohr as the characteristic transitional and key figure between and in the two attitudes of mind.

However, in our context it is more important to see how the above-mentioned type of mathematical (logical-geometric) thought model and at the same time qualitative-imaginary future model of Plato's in the 4th century B.C. developed into the purest synthesis. This future model is unrealistic and for that very reason essential, since after all it is of cosmic and universal validity. On the other hand the essence thus distilled from it has not been absolutized to such an extent that it hampers *free thought* and *critical discussion* in relation to it. For it is these two main representatives of *un*dogmatics which, on the contrary, occupy a central position at many places in the Platonic dialogues.

Nor was this speculative approach to stand in the way of the further development of pure mathematics, especially geometry, since this reached its culmination in the Greek philosopher Euclid in Alexandria in the 3rd century B.C.

(3) About a century after Euclid a further radical development took place — likewise in Alexandria — preceding by more than 15 centuries the reasoning of Francis Bacon. It was Hero who discovered all kinds of scientific applications, including that of various automata and a preliminary design for the steam engine. He was far in advance of his time. The same applied in the 15th century A.D., i.e. the first similar great milestone about 17 centuries after Hero, to his in that respect kindred successor, but at the same time the greatest genius of all times, Leonardo da Vinci.

The most important new development — the third main trend — in the field of mathematics and physics, which had long preceded the one just discussed, began, yet again in Alexandria, during the 2nd century A.D., with Ptolemy. His work, the celebrated Almagest, is the master product of a grandiose synthesis between Babylonian, Greek and Hellenic scientific development. Usually all we remember about Ptolemy from our school days is that in his geocentric system the sun rotates around the earth. It is regrettable that for many years, except in expert circles, only this extremely defective picture of his work, which led to enormous astronomical and scientific progress, has come down to us. Despite the fact that Copernicus, in his revolutionary work "De Revolutionibus Orbium Caelestium", used Ptolemy first and foremost as the springboard for his new heliocentric view, Ptolemy was in no way a brake on but on the contrary the great and greatest pathfinder for classical science.

(4) This misunderstanding is due above all to the long-standing agreement between, or preparation of, this one wrongly postulated geocentric idea of Ptolemy's (not his eminent mathematical-astronomical method) and entirely different trends of thought. I mean its coincidence with a couple of other authoritative though non-mathematical-embracing metaphysics of Aristotle, the Stagirite, and on the other the logos, ethos and mythos of Christian theology.

Aristotle, the genius who was the pupil of another genius, Plato, opposes the Pythagorean and Platonic geometric-mathematical mode of thought. This ultimately places him fairly and squarely against the characteristically Hellenic, neo-Pythagorean and neo-Platonic spirit. Nearly six centuries before Ptolemy the geocentric view is evident in Aristotle. At that time it had for centuries been a self-evident and also completely understandable point of view, the product of general experience and apparently irrefutably confirmed by unanswerable observation. It is tragi-comic that the specifically unempirical thinker Aristotle had to be wrong on that very point on which he did *seem* empirical.

It is not difficult to collect all kinds of nonsensical pronouncements from the works of Aristotle. For instance, his thesis that women have fewer teeth than men, which is yet another proof of his anti-empirical attitude of mind, a fortiori since he was married twice. He is also said to have posited that children are healthier if conceived in a north wind. "One gathers", says Russell with his usual biting sarcasm, "that the two Mrs. Aristotle both had to run out and look at the weathercock every evening before going to bed". But it is equally easy to derive from a study of the works left by Aristotle very great wisdom and even to place him in a number of respects above Plato and Socrates. But we are not concerned here with the transient or lasting value of Aristotle. What interests us in the main is his method of thought with regard to science, and more particularly the way in which this was later rightly or wrongly used, through no fault of his, and, above all, made *compulsory* for all scientific thought.

One of Aristotle's convictions was that the heavenly bodies are moved by the gods by virtue of postulated objectives. This view, and that which was later to be called the Ptolemaic, i.e. geocentric world view, fitted beautifully into the Biblical world view. And so Aristotle — in a manner which he would presumably not have wished — was elevated in the Summae of the medieval, theocratic scholasticism on to an unassailable pedestal of absolute authority. This authority was completely confirmed by a divine authority, which was itself confirmed just as irrefutably through an ingenious twist by the theological interpretation and re-creation of the philosophical thought of Aristotle intended for that purpose, and also refined.

In brief, in all those centuries, this invulnerable bulwark of scientific thought — though of course there were exceptions even then[1] — rested on three immovable pillars: 1. the authority of philosophical pious thought as against observation, 2. the authority and the autonomy of God's will with respect to all events and movement in nature or in the universe with the earth as its centre, 3. the final entelechy imparted by God to His Creation, a purposiveness forming part of creation, and thus expressing itself accordingly in every natural event (on earth and in heaven) and developing in accordance with His postulated Plan or in accordance with His repeated Dispensation, with a progressive movement towards the Completion predetermined and revealed by Him.

121

(5) It is against all these three views that modern science was to rise up in opposition, at first in many cases unconsciously, unknowingly and, as regards the consequences, usually unintentionally.

The new era is generally considered to begin with Copernicus, although of course he too had his important predecessors in thought. Just as much from a symbolic point of view his work in the "heavenly revolutions" is in any case decidedly pregnant for the spiritual revolution of human thought. Copernicus' work was dedicated to the Pope, whilst according to a letter printed in it it was recommended by a cardinal and was provided with a foreword by a well-reputed Nuremberg theologian. Whilst the first part still contained the then usual mystic-cosmological observations, according to this same foreword the pure mathematical-astronomical elaborations that followed in the later part were also in complete accordance with the doctrine of Thomas Aquinas.

And yet Copernicus would definitely not have escaped the physical consequences of theological criticism if the work had not appeared shortly after his death in 1543. In 1616 it was placed on the Index.

One should not forget the time in which he lived. The scientization of medical research, for instance, was still considered to be related to witchcraft. Disease and above all lunacy, or what was considered to be such, could be healed only by a cruel treatment for the purpose of driving out the evil spirits from these persons possessed by Satan. Vesalius, the physician from the South Netherlands, was the first to dissect corpses, to the horror of the church. Only through the personal protection of Charles V, the Holy Roman Emperor, whose personal physician he was, did he escape persecution for some considerable time. After the Emperor's death (in 1558) he was however, accused of witchcraft and condemned.

It is therefore not surprising that Giordano Bruno, who not only took over the Copernican system in all its explicit clarity but also, attaching to it the Christian God and the Bible, as against Aristotle, adopted a particularly free-thinking attitude for those days, had to pay for such a doctrine by death at the stake (1600).

Nor is it surprising that Kepler was refused (Lutheran) communion and that Galileo had to renounce his scientific pronouncements on the orders of the Inquisition, in order to escape Bruno's fate after conviction and re-imprisonment (1632). Although historical legend has, by way of consolation, left us his famous last words with regard to the motion of the earth, "eppur si muove" as an aphorism.

(6) For Copernicus, who again largely turned back from Aristotle to the Platonic thought model, the essence of the world, which in him again emanated the visionary, imaginary Hellenic intellectual strength and aesthetics, consisted in a mathematically determinable harmony.

Kepler, inspired by this Copernican turnabout, also based himself largely on the extensive, excellent observations of the Danish astronomer Tycho Brahe, who himself, still largely bound to the Aristotelian way of thought and the Ptolemaic system, did not dare to draw from these observations the radical conclusions arrived at by Kepler.

For Kepler human reason was cognate with divine reason. Mathematical thought was the highest, godlike power granted to man as a rational being by God. All true knowledge is mathematical in nature, which Kepler now interprets as meaning that all that is known consists exclusively in quantitative relations. The geometric mathematics revealed to us by Euclid is the sign and the guarantee that "the human spirit is the circle in which the plane of this worlds intersects the sphere that is God".

In the thought of Galileo, the founder of mechanics and physical dynamics, the mathematical method likewise occupies a central position. As he argued, "the Book of Nature was written in mathematical language and signs". He rejected authority as a source of knowledge and as an argument. Like Baco, he advocated the systematic use of experimentation as a source of experience. However, as a symptom of a typically dogmatic attitude of mind, people refused to look through his telescope to verify his findings.

It is well known how Galileo formulated the task of natural science: "To measure everything that is measurable and to render everything measurable that is not yet so". Only such science was first-class science, dealing with primary properties of nature and of events — all the rest was automatically secondary. A new *coercive thought model* had budded, to liberate science from the theological-methaphysical thought models that had previously shackled and Christianized it for centuries.

Only one further philosopher still tried, by a completely split dualism, to escape the already clearly apparent, threatening and practically inevitable consequences of the new science developing into an autonomy for the Christian doctrine of salvation. Descartes argued that a "mathesis universalis" did in fact apply to movement and all relations of matter; they were completely subject to mathematical relations. However, all matters of the spirit were excluded from this. For this ultra-sceptical philosopher, who subjected everything conceivable to his independent and self-assured rational doubt, the divine, which is revealed to all as established forever, was therefore also excluded.

For Newton this exception made for the divine, detached from critical thought, did not hold good at all. New Copernican thought, which had shot up via Kepler to Galileo, and had been further elaborated by Descartes, Gassendi and Huygens, among others, was combined by Newton into one mathematical-physical dynamics. The mechanistic system, in which all processes were governed by one and the same mechanical law, seemed to have been perfected by him for good. Only, in this dynamics a mathematically calculable force at-a-distance operated, that of gravitation. The question could not but arise as to who or what moved this force, a question which mathematics itself no longer

123

seemed capable of answering. As stated, for Newton this formed no problem, but on the contrary, insofar as still necessary, precisely an irrefutable proof. His new theory, the integrated system of law of nature and force of nature, confirmed for him theologically-philosophically with the greatest possible emphasis the existence of God, the ruler over these laws and forces.

(7) However, Newton could not prevent his adherents and imitators from thinking differently about this. This went in stages, with at first God still being recognized as original creative architect and cosmic lawmaker, but no longer as daily engineer and clerk of the works, and finally with complete autonomy being granted to the whole world of physics and astronomy. The law of nature, which grants knowledge to man's own power, gradually displaced prayer, in which God's will and sole power was recognized. For the result of the law of nature gave man absolute and exactly calculable *certainty*, whereas prayer always remained completely uncertain in its result, being entirely incalculable as dependent on divine whim or at least impenetrable power.

Needless to say, this development did not go smoothly. Between Descartes and Newton there stands for instance Hobbes, proponent of an enlightened despotism. He it was who said that thinking is reckoning in words. It was in his day, three centuries ago, that Charles II founded in 1662 the Royal Society, which was to make modern science fashionable.

However, at that time the English Parliament was by no means as modern as its king. The House of Commons set up a committee to examine the causes of the Plague and of the Great Fire, dating from 1665 and 1666 respectively. True, both successive disasters were generally felt to be due to God's displeasure, but it was not certain what particular offence had led to them. Russell has the following comment on this: "The Committee decided that what most displeased the Lord was the work of Mr. Thomas Hobbes. It was decreed that no work should be published in England. This measure proved effective: there has never since been a Plague or a Great Fire in London. But Charles, who liked Hobbes because Hobbes had taught him mathematics, was annoyed. He, however, was not thought by Parliament to be on intimate terms with Providence".

(8) But the victory of the new over the old thought did not go all that quickly. The two predecessors of Charles II, James I and the Lord Protector Cromwell, had both still been fanatical persecutors of witchcraft. Even Bacon, as a Member of Parliament, had personally worked on an intensified anti-witch legislation. His contemporary Shakespeare had likewise given a large part to witches in "Macbeth". The last laws concerning witches were not officially repealed until 1736, and even so for instance John Wesley, the theological leader of the Methodists, still fulminated for many years afterwards against witches. Meanwhile, in France the Encyclopédie had already started

publications in 1751 as a "dictionnaire raisonnée des sciences", in which New-tonism was preached as an atheistic gospel, which in its turn would drive Rationalism and Enlightenment along.

(9) In 1772 the last volume was published. By then the mathematician-astronomer Laplace had been for a few years a professor, though one of the youngest, at the Ecole Militaire, which in 1787 was combined with the Ecole Normale Supérieure, France's highest institute of scientific education. Laplace was the founder of the mathematical theory of probability, and later a friend of Napoleon I. Tradition tells us of his answer to the Emperor's question about his "Traité de Mécanique Céleste", in which the Creator Spiritus was not mentioned: "Sire, je n'avais pas besoin de cette hypothèse-là".

However, perhaps of much weightier influence was Laplace's equally cele-brated world formula, as he called it, according to which one could, thanks to the knowledge of laws of nature acquired and still to be gained, completely fathom and survey the cosmos, including even the *future*, which would then become entirely predictable.

Thus Laplace, incidentally building on Leibnitz, created a new *future model*. In his own words, which still deserve the greatest attention today, after 150 years, this picture is sketched as follows:

"Une intelligence qui, pour un instant donné, connaîtrait toutes les forces dont la nature est animée, et la situation respective des êtres qui la composent, si d'ailleurs elle était assez vaste pour soumettre ces données à l'analyse, em-brasserait dans la même formule les mouvements des plus grands corps de l'univers et ceux du plus léger atome: *rien ne serait incertain pour elle, et l'avenir comme le passé serait présent à ses yeux*" (my italics).

Here we have, from the beginning of the 19th century, the ideal definition of the *nomothetic-physical* (or in German terminology physikalisch) *thought and future model*. It was nomothetic-normative in two respects: it laid down the law to nature; by applying this law, man could completely govern nature. However, just as much at least it also laid down the law to science itself: only strict application of the method connected with this ideal of knowledge could lead to true, future-predicting and empirically verifiable science. Only through that was well-founded practice of science susceptible to reliable and exactly calculable technical application.

(10) This thought model was based on an initially original but gradually in-creasingly absolutized axiomatic fundamental principle. A postulate which was not critically examined, i.e. which was traditionally authoritarian, in short dogmatic, to which finally eternal value was once again accorded. If in that case God (despite violent opposition to this by among others the 17th century physicist and opponent of alchemy, Robert Boyle) no longer was the daily ruler and intervening governor, indeed even had to be driven ever further back

125

into a first beginning lying infinitely far behind as Creator and designer-law-maker, then this must ultimately have consequences for current thought. For if it was in fact true that after His Creation God, modestly content with the "rühmen des Ewigen Ehre", evidently by Nature itself (cf. Newton), had withdrawn in solitary isolation from the hurly-burly of the world as Emeritus with an otium cum dignitate, the *ancient* Greek conception gained largely in authority again. The newly formed scientific tradition of thought thus led in that respect not *forwards* but, at least in part, *backwards* again. For in that case a self-active cosmos had been unmistakably discovered, a cosmos of well-ordered law and regularity, of unequalled and metrically artistic beauty. The observable, scientifically established, exceptionless uniformity and strict natural necessity then represented an indubitably objective reality of universal validity, fulfilling itself in complete autonomy.

Conversely, since this scientific, indubitably true disclosure — or, one may say, new revelation — unquestioning obedience both of the strict laws of nature and of the equally strict scientific method formed a secular twofold commandment for the exploration of the present and the future. An extremely strict commandment to abstain from offences just as unprecedented, indeed almost inconceivable and therefore severely punishable, as those stated in the First and Second Commandments of the Bible.

(11) For nearly a century this orthodox dogmatism, later developing into what is sometimes called scientism, was to prevail practically undisputed over the whole field of the "globus scientarium". Its future-monopolizing character in particular formed a typical characteristic. It might even be said by way of a paradox that, like Christian theology itself (Kierkegaard) it was to be confirmed all the more strongly in its unshakable certainty precisely by some doubt and uncertainty.

This doubt began to crystallize around 1875. It is often wrongly believed that it was decisively strenghtened by a speech given by the famous French-Swiss-German physiologist Du Bois-Reymond on "Die Grenzen des Naturerkennens". The opposite was rather the truth. This speech related to our possible, limited knowledge of the first and last things, and also a verdict which he attached to this as to whether knowledge of the future was possible in principle or not. Now strangely enough only his concluding words with regard to certain last future-questions of finity or infinity, viz. the "ignoramus, ignorabimus" (we do not know and we shall never know) have stuck in people's minds as a constantly repeated adage. However, in the same speech in 1872 he proclaimed with no less self-assurance, indeed even more boldly and exuberantly than Laplace, that an astronomer could not only exactly predict the day on which a fallen comet will again shoot up from the depths of space (an old Babylonian idea), but also that from his scientific equations the exact moment could be derived on which Britain (geological-energetic) would burn its last

126

coal and moreover that moment at which (theological-historical) the Greek Cross would again adorn the Aya Sophia. Never before had the characteristic future-fixation found such pertinent expression in this scientific ideal. The scientific thought model was elevated with the most absolute self-assurance to a practically all-embracing *future model.*

Some ten years later the celebrated physiologist and physicist H. von Helmholtz also stressed the strictly deterministic, *future-determining* character of science as an objectively existing, inescapable "foreign power". "Wenn wir uns vergewissen können, dass die Bedingungen eingetreten sind, unter denen das Gesetz zu wirken hat, so müssen wir auch den Erfolg eintreten sehen ohne Willkür, ohne Wahl, ohne unser Zutun, mit einer die Dinge der Aussenwelt ebensogut wie unser Wahrnehmen zwingenden Notwendigkeit".

Such sounds could be heard in the second half and even in the last quarter of the previous century from the mouths of thinkers of very different plumage, but all of equal prominence, also in France, for instance the physiologist Claude Bernard, the historian-philosopher Taine and the chemist Berthelot, with his well-known pronouncement dating from the turn of the century: "le monde n'a plus de secrets".

Opinions could differ as to whether the very last and the deepest riddles of nature would remain mysteries in the future, would continue to be insoluble for the time being or forever. Was it true to say that, the more the problems of nature were unraveled, the more new mysteries loomed on the endlessly receding horizon of a possible "creatio continua", an endlessly continuing, even expanding creation? This too was, by the way, a sentiment that had been current in Antiquity. It is exactly this which is expressed in the line from Virgil which many regard as obscure but which to me is completely clear: Numero Deus impare gaudet — the odd numbers are pleasing to God. Pleasing, because the incomprehensibility of at least the odd numbers would compel highhanded man to return to and retire into God's inscrutable supremacy.

Virgil, however, had miscalculated! Leopold Kronecker, who helped to build the modern mathematical theory of numbers (including the negative, complex, irrational and imaginary numbers much more difficult to understand than odd ones) again gave God in this respect too a much reduced territory. As he put it in his famous saying at the end of the 19th century: "Die ganzen Zahlen hat der liebe Gott gemacht, alles Andere ist Menschenwerk".

Just as Euclid was overtaken by the later non-Euclidean geometricians, so his pupil Archimedes (2nd century A.D.) was left in the rear as a theoretician of numbers (among other things he invented the number $\pi = $ pi) by the more modern mathematics and physics, with its greatly expanded, modern theory of numbers. His eureka upon discovering the law of hydrostatics surrounded by a legendary aureole in Antiquity, likewise formed merely a first introduction to the discovery of all later, universally valid, so-called classical laws of nature.

Needless to say, the general theory of science and methodology gradually

127

linked to the prevailing natural sciences and identified with them, culminating in the extremely deterministic and mechanistic scientism, could not but provoke a reaction, just like any other ism. And this was soon to come as the 20th century dawned. In the German-speaking area it was ushered in by the works of Kirchhoff and Mach, in the French one by those of Boutroux, Duhem and Poincaré, among others, and in the Anglo-Saxon one in particular by the repeatedly reprinted book by Pearson (("The Grammar of Science"), already preceded almost a quarter of a century before by that of the economist and logician Stanley Jevons ("The Principles of Science", 1874). Together they formed the undogmatic reaction to another and new doctrine, which was itself ultimately to degenerate again into another dogmatic ism, namely that of the initially liberating neo-positivism (of Wittgenstein and Neurath), in turn merging with the symbolic, formalistic mathematical logic (with which the names of Carnap, Hilbert, Russell, Whitehead and Reichenbach, among others, are connected), ending in logicism.

Via this mathematical detour as a special branch a highly important facet of the original, more widely comprehensive idea of the natural law, whose absolute necessity had at least gradually come to be doubted, was strangely enough indirectly strengthened, and indeed with still more force than before. In that respect even scientism was exceeded and ultimately overdrawn again. This was with regard to the aspect of a strictly normative scientific doctrine, with prescriptions that had to be followed quite unconditionally, likewise connected with this causal conformity with natural law. For the universal validity of the natural law entailed that one could count on it completely and absolutely, that, to put it another way, scientific *explanation* had to be entirely identical with scientific *prediction*. Through the strictly mathematical development of formal, deductive logic this evident agreement between an eternally repeated past and a future that could be derived from this with certainty was again ensured. The aprioric identity of coercive *thought* and *future* model was perfect.

By way of example I may mention the American physicist with the French name, Lecomte du Noüy, who, according to the Introduction to this his "Human Destiny", which became a best-seller, proceeded from everybody's responsibility for the future of our Christian civilization, but now based on, and made to tally with, modern science. He continued to define the task of science in general in this as follows: "The aim of science is to foresee, and not, as often has said, to understand. Science describes facts, objects and phenomena minutely, and tries to join them by what we call laws, so as to be able to predict events in the future". Here the scientific model has again been generalized, on the strength of one given scientific attitude of mind. A random quotation, which could be effortlessly supplemented by many other along the same lines, even dating from today, as will be discussed in detail below.

In brief, the practice of science is, in this view, *prediction* on the basis of

128

established conformity with natural law. Accordingly, all that can be recognized as the practice of science is the possession, thanks to an established conformity with natural law, of a capacity predicting with such *certainty* that, precisely as a result of this, after empirical observation and experimental verification, it proves to possess a universal, objective validity. Physics and mathematical physics were themselves developed into a model of learning and knowledge prescribed by way of general norm, a model that could serve for every science as an example of this highest, inherent, *predictive* qualification.

Such a coercive model was bound to have far-reaching consequences. Pierre Duhem, an erudite cosmologist and historian of science, who was himself, to judge by various many-sided works, a declared opponent of exaggeration in a coercive sense of the inevitable outcome of the operation of natural law, had already stressed one of these consequences. Before his later mathematical colleague, Oswald Spengler, Duhem already drew attention to the fact that again and again so much striking *affinity* was perceptible between on the one hand the prevailing scientific image of the world and on the other hand for instance the contemporary systems of government, architectural styles, forms of art and literature, philosophical thought models, etc. In his opinion the only explanation can be that above all this image of the world gave substance to a certain vitality bound to time and space, and evidently as a result found multilateral expression.

This is a theme of particular interest in itself, but one which must be confined here to a single but extremely important main variant: the tremendous influence of this scientific world view on *general scientific thought* as such.

In this concection the phenomenon which A. N. Whitehead vainly typified as "the dogmatic fallacy" emerged with particular clarity. With a lack of historical knowledge and sense, people repeatedly prove — precisely in this objective practice of science — to fall into a *dogmatic* trap which closes and crushes the subject of study, or at least temporarily hampers progress. Now what *dogmatism* does is to freeze all possible and conceivable meanings into one sole admissible meaning, immune to criticism. It is forgotten again and again that the heresy of yesterday is to become the dogma of tomorrow, that the established scientific code of today will be regarded as incorrect, premature or even ridiculous by posterity. Again and again people fail to expose the ever-present methaphysical foundations of modern science; they are opposed to the never-absent implicit postulates of the practice of science being made explicit.

Only thus was it possible that practically everyone, if not for ever then for a very long time, was led astray in almost every field of science by the awe-inspiring expansion of natural science. Unfortunately, so far nobody has attempted to draw up a general *theory of relativity* for the *practice of science* itself. Scientists are — and act like — the people who *know*. In general the history of science, including the countless, oft-repeated scientific aberrations, as the lasting warning of an intellectual "memento mori", is not over-popular with them. They do not even find sufficient consolation in the discovery that not infrequently the latest scientific error formed the first impetus for new scientific truth. They have reluctantly to admit that in the *past* a constant change in scientific truths and values, in theses, norms, codes and doctrines has occurred, in view of the historical facts and repeated changes of view. However, as regards today and the *future*, this possibility and desirability of an uninterrupted, indeed relentlessly progressing change and conversion is usually not anticipated. They are too easily inclined to cling to the existing (or at least assumed) scientific *certainty* (preferably derived from classical science).

Many scientists are completely unaware that this prevailing, conservative attitude of mind is mainly determined by the past and that they are constantly guilty of an unscientific prejudice. Even less do they possess the requisite capacity of scientific imagination enabling them to realize that posterity will probably take their in part still primitive views no more seriously than we often do in many a respect with regard to our ancestors. In brief, they fall short, as a result of obstinate adherence to what is assumed to be a fixed datum here and now. Despite or perhaps because of the status and authority granted them, they are inadequately equipped with the ability to see things relatively, from a distance, with the humility and self-criticism that are qualities required for the true practice of science. It is the celebrated irony of history that, upon closer examination, the good desired at any price and pursued with all conceivable means, the scientific *certainty* regarded with such envy and leading to such irrational attitudes of mind, is the very first to collapse.

It might seem superfluous and even rather arrogant to lecture some scientist or the other and to hold out to him the mirror of history, including the history of the future, were it not that in a special branch of science an extremely great and not infrequently unfavorable influence can be and also is exerted far beyond the narrower professional circle by a dogmatic attitude of mind. For that is very much the case with the social sciences and their relation to, or impact on, the development of social reality. The future models discussed so far have all had a farreaching effect in their interrelationship on the social sciences. In their turn the future models of the social sciences thus formed have been of an importance to the development of social dynamics that can hardly be underestimated — they still are, too, even emimently so. In the following chapter we are therefore confronted again with the intense emanations of other and above all of scientific future models in this field. The relation there between dogmatics and prognostics is of the very greatest importance to our time and to the future.

We are not concerned here with a kind of original sin committed by science,

130

but a sin committed by the neglect or maltreatment of a legacy of the future entrusted to science in good faith.

This legacy of the future is by definition the arch-enemy of every "ancien régime".

Scientific technology is entirely uninterested in the past; it is exclusively oriented towards the future.

Are socio-scientific thought models capable of absorbing and integrating the new dimension, the mutation of this future?

It is of crucial importance whether, and to what extent, social sciences are really able to anticipate the permanent revolution.

CHAPTER 8

Socio-scientific future models

1. The law of the copying machine

If one considers in broad outline the history of economic and social doctrines, and also that of socio-scientific methodology, one becomes aware almost at a glace how the lines of development and turns of thought there run more or less parallel to those of the natural sciences. One is struck by a surprisingly similar use of corresponding terms and analogous ways of explanation and, mutatis mutandis, of practically identical thought and future models. In the first instance, therefore, it will practically suffice briefly to review these successful and now highly fashionable transplantations in the socio-economic field.

Here too we find again after centuries of stagnation the same turning-away from medieval thought, which as faithful handmaiden of Christian theology had been directed towards understanding the purpose of the world's creation and the metaphysical significance of man's existence contained therein. Once again we see at a given moment a break in this development, which then concentrates on understanding and governing actual events in cosmic nature, including human nature, individually and collectively reflected in the socio-economic pattern of the satisfaction of wants and the organization of society. Here too God's transcendent rationality is put on a par at first with an in essence equally rational, now immanently active human nature, which in turn, as God's image, is again envisaged as eternally unchanging and therefore capable of being grasped and reproduced in essential, universal and uniform, in brief natural and evident, basic principles.

Next there is again a gradual turning-away and liberation from such a given, established natural order, or one based on natural rights, towards a whole regulated in conformity with natural law and, on the strength of that, systematically controlled.

Sometimes the difference or the transition is subtle and almost imperceptible, through a mingling of old ideas about natural right (often originating from Scholasticism) with more modern scientific ideas. But gradually *both* elements of the latter mode of thought begin to stand out more clearly in the socio-scientific field: on the one hand an ever-greater autonomy accorded to this system governed by natural law, and on the other hand a much greater stress on the *empirically* observable fixed regularity in the whole of socio-economic events from which this prevailing *conformity with natural law* may and must be constituted.

Then, and following on the former, a turning-away from God's incalculable will and from events which are inconstant, or at least unforeseeable, because they are subject to the change in His almighty dispensation which is unknowable in advance, towards events which are in causal conformity with natural law, constant and, for this very reason, determinable in advance.

Following in turn on this the idea unfolds that, though the divine-rational prescription has now been replaced by an independent natural course of events, the prescriptions connected with the latter are certainly no less imperative. For one thing the conformity with natural law placed in the economic and social order is of an unmistakably normative nature. These are absolute norms to which man is tied hand and foot, to which indeed God Himself is subjected for good. These norms are consequently also automatically conservative; through the sanctions imposed by their operation they confirm and protect the existing order.

If the norms are followed, this leads to happiness, progress and cosmic harmony. Transgression is punished by misfortune, misery and chaos.

Meanwhile, these prescriptions have also become *normative* for the scientist. Faithful and strict compliance with the nomothetic-physical ideal of knowledge reproduced above also elevates every non-natural science to the peak of Parnassus. Infringement of or departure from the corresponding thought and future models declared binding is heresy and leads irrevocably to expulsion from the consecrated scientific temple of Solomon.

At the end of this development, which occurred during the 17th and 18th centuries, the claimed revelation in the 19th century of kinematic and dynamic laws of development confronted socio-economic events. This largely repeated the preceding development from Copernicus to Newton, which is as systematically extended as that running from Condorcet to Laplace. Physical mechanics not only led, as was to be expected, to social mechanics. It likewise favored a mechanistic copying process of the stereotyped scientific model by every self-respecting social science, down to every phase, component and process. By means of an exact and minutely copied process of development of modern science, that of the social sciences could in fact have been exactly and accurately predicted. It could also have been foretold that none of the socio-economic laws "discovered" to satisfy the thought model accordingly prescribed would prove tenable in time. The perhaps sole development law of the social sciences themselves — at least the only one that it has been possible to prove so far — is that of the literal imitation of the admired natural sciences, though without its having led to anything like a comparable result.

The development laws also drafted for socio-economic events by this slavish imitation on the part of the social sciences, if they were in fact to be of the same value as the classical laws of nature, had to testify to a similarly strict necessity and an absoluteness brooking of no exception. Consequently their strictly deterministic nature was unconditionally necessary. Only on that basis could the possibility of *predictability*, which truly crowns the work, be inherent in this conformity with natural law. For it would be this reliable predictability that essentially perfected a theory into a strictly scientific, objective explanation, instead of a series of unrelated facts, accumulated figures, arbitrary hypotheses and subjective opinions. Only the stenographic formula, if a, then b, forms the secret of this in causal conformity with natural law which strings together events in time and finally projects them with indisputable certainty on to the future.

2. Physiocracy, social mechanics and social physics

Now the development process briefly outlined above, in which all the successive links in the mechanical copying process are interconnected with logical and consistent necessity, can be clearly seen, with all its historical stages and transitional nuances, in the actual trend of the developing social sciences.

It acquires a clearly defined form notably in the birth of physiocracy in the first half of the 18th century. This was later to merge into the development of a social physics, which in its turn reached its climax in the first half of the 19th century. It is, of course, anything but a coincidence that the two names reflect the world picture of modern physics as it developed. Even if this terminological association is gradually eliminated (during the course of his publications Comte replaced the term social physics by sociology) this definitely does not mean a loosening of the ties between the natural and the social sciences. For Comte the sociology in accordance with his model meant nothing less than the crown on all preceding exact sciences. Comte's development laws, just like those of Marx, bear the stamp of 100 percent Newtonian Laws of nature. They are equipped with an unescapable natural necessity and, for reality, a determinateness just as strict as that once accorded to divine predestination.

It is almost frightening to see that, though the religious and metaphysical starting-points or objectives are subject to historical change, also as spiritual bases of the practice of social science, despite all change one thing in fact hardly alters, if at all: the dominating influence exerted by the natural sciences and the coercive nature derived from this. It is particularly remarkable — and even now it has still hardly penetrated — that, for all the change and difference in mentality in the triple process, spread over some two centuries, of switching from physiocracy to social physics and, finally, to a socio-mechanical system of development laws, in essence nothing has really changed.

It is, of course, by no means my intention to give here once again the history of economic and social doctrines. I merely wish to detach from it, as an all-prevailing methodological fact, the transplantation of the coercive scientific thought model and to outline this broadly.

134

(a) Physiocracy

Founded by the physician Quesnay, at the beginning one of the writers of the Encyclopédie, whose influence he underwent, the initially physical picture of this doctrine is still chiefly that of physiology. The famous "Tableau Economique" is an exact scientific model showing "circulation" (as of blood in the human body) in economic life.

His pupils Dupont de Nemours and Mercier de la Rivière further scientized the socio-economic picture. The socio-economic order is an "ordre providentiel", i.e. a divine and supernatural order. For divine-human reason this order is evident, essential and invariable. A universal order, the same for all people of all times, since it is in accordance with, proceeds from, the essence of human nature. As an expression of God's will the laws of this order are irrevocable and universally valid.

This order is therefore normative. Everything should proceed in accordance with the basic principles of this ideal order if the economy is to remain "normal" and "healthy". Economic life should behave in accordance with the partly natural, partly scientific laws. This occurs automatically in an established order of protected property. A regime of enlightened despotism (Quesnay regarded himself as the Western Confucius), protecting property and freedom, ought to lead to the healthiest economy. Hence the maxims of "laissez aller, laissez passer", and "le monde va de lui-même" resulting from the "recipes" of this doctrine, and at the same time providing the existing order with a scientific basis. In this way Quesnay, at first a member of the "philosophes", founded a new school of "les économistes". For this new sect, which is how it was originally regarded, this economics founded on conformity with the natural order was a "science exacte". However, for the adherents these tenets formed a dogmatic catechism. Despite the sarcasm of Voltaire and the criticism of other contemporaries this Messianistic gospel aroused great enthusiasm in France, not only in Mirabeau but also in Turgot, who made the doctrine the basis of the economic policy to be followed. What rendered the new science particularly popular at the time was its unshakable, rosy *optimism*: God was not only an omnipotent but also an omnipresent, all-wise and pre-eminently benevolent God. Just as the moon had been created to light the sky at night, so human nature had been given the gift of achieving natural harmony and the summum of human happiness in an extremely simple manner, via the reason granted it and the natural order of things derived by physiocracy with the aid of this reason.

What was later to make this doctrine precisely so unpopular, indeed ridiculous and pre-eminently *fatalistic*, was the coercive fixed nature of this eternally invariable order. For the physiocrats strict obedience to the laws thus discovered could not but lead to recovery of paradise lost and to re-opening of the Garden of Eden. But, precisely because of this natural-scientific dogma of immutability, thanks to a fully guaranteed natural freedom and fixed order,

135

and therefore, as people gradually came to realize, unchangeable injustice, inequality, lack of freedom and exploitation, this dogma could not but ultimately become a thing of hatred, the abhorred exponent of conservatism, passivism and oppressive *pessimism*.

For the first time we see here too that the normative character of conformity with natural law in the natural sciences acquires exactly the *opposite* meaning when borrowed uncritically by the social sciences. For, according to Bacon's motto, the acquisition of knowledge regarding the events of nature and obedience to the natural laws thus discovered mean a tremendous increase in the possibilities of human control of nature: *"knowledge is power"*. On the other hand, normative interpretation of the laws in socio-economic events means at most a ratification of the power of the established order, and in a more general sense in no way an increase in man's power but, conversely, a scientific confirmation of *human impotence*.

The real laws of the natural sciences can never be infringed by man, but he can use them for his own benefit, notably via applied science and technology. This is *not* the case with the normative legal prescriptions of the social sciences. It is true that the same strict determinism applies here, but in essence it is a negative determinism. These prescriptions *can* be infringed by man, but never with impunity. And in fact at all times they have been and still are being infringed by people acting unwisely, irrationally. But the disastrous consequences of violating these dogmas have never failed to make themselves felt, irrespective of whether they took the form of a punishing, avenging divine justice or the scientifically predictable reaction of a violated secular order. According to this doctrine, such an economy or human civilization in conflict with the naturally prescribed, only true order or organization would automatically be doomed to disease, misery, economic depression, disharmony, if not to all kinds of possible and potential catastrophical developments. On the other hand, however, it began to dawn on critical, progressive minds that unconditional obedience to these so-called laws in complete subjection would chain mankind forever to the existing order, which in reality could be regarded less and less as ideal for people as a whole.

(b) Social mechanics

The interpretation of society as a system of social mechanics also originated from natural rights, on gradually a scientific stamp was likewise impressed. The stress is somewhat different, but the principle differs little. British empirical philosophy in particular elaborated this parallel. To cite an example, Hobbes already regarded people as being as it were identical with atoms and therefore, by virtue of their nature, just as subject to fixed laws as all existing nature. These strict Newtonian "laws of nature" had to be rigorously obeyed by man as "rational commands". They are, once again, strictly normative legal prescriptions derived from the essence of human reason.

136

To the enlightened philosopher Locke, too, human society was still a part of a fixed, immutable plan existing for the whole world. The "laws of nature" governing human society were prescribed by God.

Almost a century after Hobbes one still finds Berkeley depicting man as a social atom. Society is the resultant in the social force field of these atoms attracting and repelling each other in accordance with natural law. Even the sceptical Hume, who on the one hand violently disputed natural rights could not in this respect escape science's causal conformity with natural law. On the strength of uniform, invariable human nature, in his view too, the same consequences would repeatedly follow from the same causes of social action and events in accordance with certain fixed principles and constants. The social sciences ought therefore to discover and apply these general rules.

Right down to our century repeated efforts were made — in vain — to found a social mechanics of this kind, in which society is made to function like a machine operating systematically and in conformity with natural law. However, this trend has become particularly important through a branch leading from it to a more specific "social physics", which ultimately produced in its turn sociology.

(c) Social physics

It is said that the term social physics was likewise originated by Hobbes. And indeed this term was current in Britain among various authors like Berkeley, Ferguson, Mandeville and Shaftesbury, who, however, also occasionally speak of a "natural history of society". It will be recalled that Vico, as the predecessor of such a view, had already concluded in his "Scienza Nuova", on the strength of an extensive collection of factual material, that historical and social events were governed by fixed laws that had to be ascribed to God as lawmaker and governor and which were supposed to be proof of the supreme command of His Providence.

However, it was neither the philosophical physics in the British style (which incidentally is difficult to separate entirely from social mechanics), nor the historical "new science" along Italian lines that was to give social physics its own scientific doctrinal authority. In my opinion social physics really first acquired a fixed universally accepted basis thanks to a separately developing science or, at first, auxiliary science, viz. statistics.

The celebrated "Political Arithmetic" of Sir William Petty, published in 1960, sought a kind of socio-mathematical conformity with natural law (by which even in those days anything could be proved). Two German theologians, Neumann and Süssmilch, from the first half of the 18th century, both considered the statistically observable, immutable conformity with natural law in society a decisive proof of the workings of divine, merciful Providence in the running of the world. People were subject willy-nilly, inescapably and invariably, to these laws established in accordance with God's will.

However, the greatest impression was made by the Belgian astronomer Quételet in his "Essai de Physique Sociale" of nearly a full century later (1835). It proved the strictly determined conformity of social action with nature, not only through the fixed tables of birth and mortality, but above all through criminological activity, which proves unchangeable in every field. Each number of crimes was constantly determined beforehand. Destiny (or fate) predetermined one as a criminal. Consequently, the most that could depend on human liberty was "whether one stole on foot or on horseback".

Later, in his two-volume "Physique Sociale", Quételet expanded this inevitable criminal conformity with natural law systematically to cover the *whole* of man's life and social behavior, including his moral and intellectual activity. The long-sought proof of the exclusion of human free will seemed to have been given in definitive form. For in this view all human actions belong to the same field as the phenomena of physics subject to natural laws. This scientific legal concept, sparing nobody and nothing in its strictness, was to exert great influence on later economics and sociology through the response it met with among the public. And also of course a destructive influence on human, individual and social responsibility and on the power of man to determine his own free personal and collective destiny.

3. Economics and sociology: from "dismal science" to asocial science

In matter-of-fact Britain the romantic-idealistic doctrine of physiocracy had never made much of an impression, although there too philosophical reasoning was initially strongly influenced by natural right, and also by the related system of social physics.

However, Adam Smith, himself a moral philosopher and a friend of Hume, succeeded with his "Wealth of Nations" (1776) in converting the natural order of the physiocrats into a new system conforming to natural law. Although it was just as naively optimistic, it managed to conquer the world from Britain — together with the first industrial revolution that had begun there, i.e. thanks to a combination of theoretical natural science and practical technology.

The organism of Quesnay et al., governed by finalistic entelechies, was transformed by Smith mainly into a mechanism (influence of the earlier social mechanics) that chiefly displayed a causal connection with natural law. Of the weighty "ordre providentiel" only a slight and rather vague suggestion remained metaphysically and religiously. This was the "hidden hand", which automatically merged the free self-interest arising from human nature with the public interest, thus ensuring the economic optimum of its own accord, completely in conformity with nature. This system was equally normative: true, it no longer said what had to happen, but it explained what had in fact occurred. But man was not permitted to tamper with this: negative determinism

138

again. If one followed this rule, abstained from artificial intervention, the mechanism worked automatically and well. In that case God was literally only a "deus ex machina".

In France it was Smith's follower, J. B. Say, who drew the inevitable consequences. Once again economics, as with Quesnay, became an exact science of strict natural laws. Repeated reference was made to Newton and the laws of gravity to clarify the nature of these economic laws. Their universal validity was sharply put: they applied also to lawmakers and rules, "et jamais on ne les viole impunément". It was Say who reforged these economic laws of nature based on a "homo economicus" (in this sense little had changed since Quesnay) into a normative legal prescription for the economist. The latter had to behave as a "spectateur impassible", on pain of accusations of scientific misconduct. In this way Say became the pioneer, but equally the first rock of offence, of that neutral economics without values that was later to be branded "the dismal science" by Carlyle.

Say represented with Adam Smith a branch of *optimistic* quietism. The best that can be done is do nothing more than what one is usually automatically and naturally inclined, and therefore also obliged, to do — what's good for me is good — indeed is optimum — for everybody. Later this "optimum optimism" established a link with for the rest entirely opposed views of conservative, or revolutionary, progress-optimism. On the one hand that of classical liberalism, on the other hand that of classical Marxism, both views equally appealing to a course of development completely in conformity with natural law, both equally guaranteeing a *predictable* socio-economic optimum as mechanical automatism.

However, another ramification came into being, this time one of *pessimistic* quietism, which in no sense held out hopes of the Promised Land. On the contrary, in the socio-economic field it was just as dogmatic and stressed human impotence vis-à-vis the course of events determined by the course of nature.

As the reader will be aware, this development began in Britain, after Adam Smith, with Malthus (a contemporary of Say), who constructed a socio-mathematical model that collided head-on with earlier notions of for instance a Condorcet and, in Britain, a Godwin. This model contrasted the geometric series of human reproduction with the arithmetic series of the food available. Apparently Malthus left his "homo biologicus" a free choice, viz. moral restraint. In actual fact this is again a form of negative determinism: if you transgress the law of sexual abstinence imposed upon you, you will either starve or suffer moral ruin through the use of other forms of contraception. There is only one commandment as against two prohibitions.

Ricardo built up a complete scientific system, with immutable natural laws regarding the distribution of income. Wages ought to display a steadily decreasing tendency. Later Lassalle derived his "iron law of wages" from this. Even Von Böhm Bawerk arrived in his famous essay "Macht oder ökonomisches Gesetz" at the conclusion that human power always had to give way to economic law.

It was inevitable — I might almost say in conformity with natural law — that opposition would grow to this basic tenet of human *impotence*. Strangely enough, at first people were entirely unaware that the thesis had acquired its strongest fundamental confirmation through the diligent emulation and uncritical worship of the goddess of natural science. For through the same knowledge in conformity with natural law it was being endeavored in the social field too to acquire the same human power as acquired over nature so as to be able to control society. People had no idea of the paradoxical effect that, according as scientific methods were applied more zealously and strictly, the remaining human power itself had, on the rebound, to be reduced to all the smaller proportions. This led to tensions and logical contradictions of which, remarkably, even the greatest and most philosophically trained thinkers seemed hardly aware on occasion. It seems difficult for human minds to grasp why scientific laws constantly increase human *power* (over natural events), while on the contrary socio-economic laws of nature fetter human power (with regard to social events) in unbreakable chains.

This attempt to sit on two stools at the same time might be described as the adoption of intermediate position which are barely possible in themselves. Barely possible, because one wants to combine the strictest conceivable action determined in conformity with natural law with a certain degree of indeterminism, i.e. of human freedom of will and of choice. To put it another way, because one thinks that a fixed maximum of human impotence can be combined with an indispensable minimum of human power.

When a thinker like Goethe takes this liberty, and so speaks on the one hand of the "ewigen, ehernen grossen Gesetzen" and on the other hand of the "wer immer strebend sich bemüht, den können wir erlösen" applicable to man, nobody will quibble at this possible contradiction.

But when thinkers like Marx (in emulation of Hegel) and Comte insist on and persist in this iron necessity of natural law and the inescapable conformity with natural law of their thought models, one begins to wonder how they themselves, when they above all fervently plead the exercise of human power, can ever free themselves from the self-forged iron clamps of this dogmatics.

Machiavelli could have taught them something about seeking an intermediate position. De Valk rightly places him in the forefront as one of the pioneers in the early 16th century of scientific thought (avant la lettre) in social sciences and as one of the spiritual fathers of sociology. According to Machiavelli, social phenomena should be regarded as natural phenomena. For instance, the cycle of forms of government is based on an iron law of nature. One can only try one's best to extend the good phases of these somewhat and to shorten the bad ones to some extent. Just as one can prepare in advance for an inevitable flood to some extent, or afterwards can try to limit the damage done by it where possible. Since human nature does not change, these laws have a coercive character according to Machiavelli. Man can do something in social life, but only within fairly close limits, on secondary points, and only with any chance of success insofar as this is in accordance with the fundamental, immutable laws of society. Thus, according to this view, which is consistent in itself, one can never hold back the cycle, let alone change it at will.

As is known, Marx bothered little with the epistemological incompatibility of his development laws, which he furnished with an inescapable necessity, and of his requirement of philosophers that it was their task to change the world by their own efforts. Class struggle and revolution were, in his reasoning, required in any case as the fuse to explode the powder-barrel of his natural development process and to actuate the then following scientific explosion and dynamics. One can continue to rack one's brains on the subject of whether in Marx' view this development ought to have happened in any case at a later date without these weapons, or whether the use of these weapons was also already determined by nature, and thus included in the development mechanism itself. His brief comment that a midwife should assist in the confinement and that the inevitable birth pangs must be shortened and can be alleviated to some extent has a rather vague and cryptic ring to it.

Not until Comte did the scientific thought model take complete possession of sociology. He too uses concepts like inevitable necessity, complete social determinateness, constant and invariable laws of nature. And yet in Comte, as in Marx, the fiery will to reform society had long burnt, although towards the end of his life he became just as strongly dogmatic and conservative. "Nature is stronger than theory" says De Valk, rather laconically, and endeavors to show that Comte incorporates the dualism referred to above in his theory. However, the result is a rather poor one. For in essence Comte does not get much further than Machiavelli did nearly four centuries before. He too must admit that the phenomena determined by nature can only be influenced to a limited extent, at most smoothed a little. Both the inner ambivalence and the philosophical and methodological conflict between strict law and human power remain unsolved in their deepest essence.

That is why, when after Newton a Darwin arose and natural science was enriched by biology, so pre-eminently active in conformity with natural law in its theory of evolution (in Comte only sociology takes pride of place to biology), the balance could not but swing again to the most extreme position of human impotence. According to a view that then appeared on the scene again with renewed vigor, the same inexorable, merciless conformity with natural law prevails in social life that is found in physical *and* biological events. The social Darwinism of Spencer et al. is the extreme logical consequence of this negative determinism radically transplanted to the field of social science. On pain of defeat in the struggle for life, which leads only to continued evolution, any kind of interference with the automatism of social mechanics is strictly forbidden. No social legislation, no philanthropy. Only by the natural selection of the socially stronger and the total abandonment of all the socially weaker to the natural process of development could human society flourish as a totality. The "homo homini lupus" (the one man is like a wolf to the other) of Hobbes is here elevated to an omnipotent, all-wise and all-good law. The evil, pain and suffering of the theodicy, as a justified divine necessity, have returned here as the natural law of the social jungle. An evil to be accepted and loved as an unavoidable necessity, an evil which only in that way can lead to the "summum bonum", the highest good of human society, as the first aim.

4. Socio-scientific thought model: fully scientific

What Marx and Comte had really wanted could be achieved by later sociology only by opposing the scientific coercive thought model, or rather by drawing attention to society itself and its needs through, before and still more after Spencer. A period came about of socio-critical and explicitly reformatory practice of sociology. But what could it do without the force and the supporting foundation, the encouraging methods of the dominating scientific ideal of knowledge? For the time being, nothing!

It is therefore not surprising that once again there had to be a reaction to this reaction. But now it had deeper roots. For some time previously an epistemological theory of science had been devised, which of course itself also bore clear traces of the scientific revolution. For that we must first look back, though not in anger.

As already outlined, social science too had turned away, at first halfheartedly, then resolutely, from a cosmic, natural order for the social phenomena, a fixed order supposed to be founded on God's will and wisdom, proving His omnipotence and benevolence at one and the same time, an established natural order which, if there were unconditional submission to its existence, would contribute to the greater glory of God and the greater happiness of man.

True, social science had ultimately relieved God honorably of His lofty post in social life and, with due respect, furnished a walled-off corner of heaven for Him as a safe and sacred home for the aged. Nevertheless, after this sinful rebellion demanding autonomy, it adhered just as firmly to an identical, pitilessly dominating strictness. An iron necessity, an exceptionless conformity with natural law, had to apply to social phenomena, as if they were physical phenomena. God disappeared, but Nature, with a capital N, remained as before. This Nature assumed the place and the task of God as lawmaker almost unamended: its lawmaker now became Natural Science.

Leading thinkers immediately swore allegiance to this new but equally rigorous and absolute despot, viz. the new scientific pattern of thought, compulsorily imposed upon all. This implied that the laws to be discovered for social life had unconditionally and fully to comply with the requirement of the inexact predictive capacity proceeding with inexorable logic from this new intellectual approach. But moreover, on the strength of this assumption of power, strict obedience had likewise to be paid henceforth to a second explicit requirement, viz. that of a verification in due course.

In other words, socio-economic laws could only be and remain of value if they predicted a certain movement with sufficient precision, and if they did so with undeniable correctness in comparison with the development that then followed. Thus every possible future social development had been and was assiduously predicted: revolution, progress, retrogression, downfall, three-stage development, circular course, etc., etc.

Unfortunately, these predictions afterwards proved in part to have been of the type of self-fulfilling prophecy (e.g. class struggle and revolution) deliberately set into motion and disturbing precisely the natural course of events, and to a larger extent of the type of prognoses that proved entirely untrue. Malthus and Marx who, for quite different reasons, had formulated a prognosis of misery and pauperization, were first of all proved wrong by the actual development. In the opinion of many, long-term events could prove Malthus right, while the collapse of capitalism, admittedly in another way than dialectically foreseen by Marx, might yet take place some time as the result of a lengthy continuous or also discontinuous process, chiefly by gradual erosion from the inside. The iron law wages of Lassalle, drawn in the tracks of Ricardo and confirmed by Von Böhm Bawerk, met its end against the economic power wielded by the unions, public opinion and parliaments.

Not a single law of social or economic movement or development previously postulated has so far withstood the ravages of time. Unless it is the tripartite development prescribed by Comte for the practice of science itself: from a theological to a metaphysical and finally to an equally coercive positivistic stage.

For in fact, of the normative and coercively prognostic legal prescriptions for social events, only one remained: the sacrosanct dogma, cultivated by the theory of social science on its own behalf, for the small esoteric sect of select, consecrated practitioners of science. While on the one hand society increasingly liberated itself — as it had to — from the cruel iron chains of inescapable conformity with natural law, nevertheless — in accordance with the historical irony of fate — on the other hand a number of the most gifted social thinkers, with a masochism as incomprehensible as it was merciless, were voluntarily to cast themselves into chains strangulating their own flesh and to confine themselves in this dungeon with its unbreachable walls of most stringent legal lawlike prescriptions.

It is quite understandable that a number of leading thinkers, also in the epistemological field, in a line running from for instance Locke to Kant, were strongly inspired by and therefore particularly oriented towards the scientific revolution starting with Copernicus, and provisionally completed by Newton. Kant, the truly wise philosopher, was very well aware of the fact that in his time, the 18th century, no social science had as yet found the philosophers' stone. Conversely, he was optimistic enough to expect that social science had still to find its own Kepler and Newton, and thus would definitely do so.

Since then a not inconsiderable number have considered themselves called upon to become the Newton of social science. On the other hand, *not a single* conformity with natural law in social life has been discovered yet that is comparable to the Newtonian system of physics and thus demonstrably functioning. As stated, not one social or economic law of the same strict validity has so far proved tenable as such. The freer and stronger the individual movement of social dynamics is, the less chance there of course is of grasping it in a natural system.

This has often placed social scientists before a dilemma, and sometimes caused perplex consternation, but nevertheless it has not in general caused them to stray from the prescribed path of doctrinaire and dogmatic orthodoxy.

To concretize this argument further, let us return — rather arbitrarily — to that point where over a century ago the already established sciences of economics and logic clearly merged for the first time, supporting and scientifically elevating each other. That is without a doubt the case with the polymath John Stuart Mill. With his "System of Logic" (1843) he exerted a far-reaching influence long after his day, indeed far into our present time, likewise in sociology.

Relatively soon afterwards, in 1858, the American sociologist Carey attempted to build up a sociology along the lines of exact natural science, in which people were moved like molecules in accordance with a sociological law of gravity. He acquired mechanistic, energetic, biologistic, organicistic, climatological and once again psychologistic imitators in America and in Europe. With the possible exception of the unproven psychic-social "laws" of Tarde, later already rather watered down in the partial structure laws of Durkheim, their systems are practically forgotten. But certainly not the method that they pursued as an ideal, even though another notable English economist and logician, Stanley Jevons, had already protested against this in 1874 and prophesied an unavoidably lasting disillusion.

And yet, as recently as 1951, to mention only one example, the German-American methodologist Hans Reichenbach argued just as dauntlessly that the difficult search for sociological laws must be continued untiringly. In his opinion there is not the slightest reason to doubt the ultimate success of such socio-scientific endeavor by emulating and matching the triumph already achieved by the scientific procedure, which in essence is no different. "If the possibility of prediction is regarded as the criterion of scientific method" says

Reichenbach, again explicitly postulating this *predictive* capacity, "the social sciences can be made as scientific as the physical sciences, without requiring any logical principle other than those which have brought to the physical sciences overwhelming success".

American scientific sociologists, such as Lundberg, Dodd and Lazarsfeld, and also a number of congenial sociometricians, have tried — completely in vain — to write this success story. None of them will enter history as the sociological Kepler or Newton.

At present we certainly cannot sign the death certificate of the dogmatically coercive thought model of the classical natural sciences in its claim to apply to the social sciences. Even though the newer natural sciences already seem to have abjured for good this antiquated thought model for *their own* use in the last twenty-five years. For all that, the old idol is holding its ground, also as a socio-natural future model. A future model giving power over the human behavior to be predicted, and for this very reason condemning this behavior to lasting impotence, and at the same time confirming the established order — deliberately or willy-nilly — for the future predicted, extended and therefore, in that respect, unchangeable in accordance with natural law. In this way the *future*, as a different and better future, is once again *deadlocked*.

5. Socio-scientific thought model: semi-scientific

After the evidently completely unsuccessful series of attempts at a slavish imitation of the natural sciences for the social events propelled onward by the human spirit — attempts which, despite severe admonition, were apparently predestined to endless failure — a vacuum occurred at a given moment. Some, supporters of the historical school, turned their backs on these natural sciences that evidently led in the wrong direction and sought refuge chiefly in a study of the past. Others, though they stressed the essential difference between natural sciences and the humanities, did not wish the present brainchild to be thrown out with the historical bathwater. Under the influence of a German group of philosophical, partly neo-Kantian thinkers, such as Dilthey, Windelband and, above all, Rickert, they did their best on the one hand to make the limits of the scientific thought model visible and on the other to work out an at least partially independent methodology for the social, cultural or human sciences.

One of the greatest renovators of sociological thought, the many-sided genius Max Weber, went to considerable effort, in the footsteps of Rickert, to extend these attempts at mediating and bridging into an integral, systematic synthesis. In this system the former strict laws of nature were replaced by purely rationally constructed but fictitious ideal types. In addition he conceived of a steadily progressing "homo sociorationalis", through whose medium the development of social reality would gradually conform to these postulated, in part still unreal schemata and structural tendencies. They would do so with a consequently increasing probability (designated by him as "Chance") of conformity and identity. Ultimately they would in this way acquire the nature of abstract "vérités de raison" (to use Leibnitz' expression). The strict causal-logical conformity with natural law thus lies as it were first in purely rational thought and only later — it is hoped — in the concrete social reality con-forming to this thought.

But now the socio-scientific investigator following this method had to be prepared to make a large but unavoidable sacrifice. The classical scientific thought model originating from Newton himself had relentlessly to be stripped of all old finalistic elements of a divine or natural order. And not only Newton's personal theistic or deistic notions about a universal system that was God's will and that was moved or guided as a pacemaker for certain ends. No, all conceivable objectives, norms and values, whether religious or humanistic, transcendental or immanent, eschatological or utopian, ethical-idealistic or socio-reformatory. The absolute standard to be set for every socio-scientific investigator, i.e. a seeker of causal connections, was that of a complete and unconditionally anti-normative attitude. The mental disposition of freedom from values, of a strict limitation to the actual "Sein", free from any kind of "Sollen", of a pure "Wissen" entirely liberated from whatsoever "Werten". All that matters is the reality constructed in an empirical basis, as it is in actual fact or at least could be rationally thought out, and not how it ought to be ideally. For that was exactly how the modern research scientist set about things.

This sociology, which attained great but completely lonely heights with Max Weber, slumped in the hand of his epigones. One of the cleverest and most original followers, Karl Mannheim, attempted another coordination, in which he no longer sought universal laws applicable always and everywhere, but "principia media". A new kind of limited laws, applicable to certain historical situations and periods of limited duration, to social structures of a type prevailing in time and space but subject to fluctuation. In this way the absolutism of natural law was somewhat relativized and historicized.

But, just as not a single natural law has ever been discovered for social life, or rather confirmed after the event by future-history, so the work with ideal types after Weber and that with principia media after Mannheim did not bring much joy or prove very fruitful. Except perhaps for the interested but dying-out historian of science or unproductive methodologist.

The result of this was at first considerable confusion, irresolute discourage-ment and, worst of all, tottering uncertainty. Thereafter — I am passing over a few links — the ranks reformed to the best of their ability. A rather para-doxical situation had arisen: strict conformity with natural law (including its rather attenuated replacements) had practically ceased to exist for social

146

science, since in the course of time it had of its own accord fallen into decay as fallacious.

What was left? Gone was the fixed providential or natural order, gone were the cycles, the constants, the schemata, the systems, the models. Gone was the uniformity, the immutability, the universality. Gone was the basis, the mainstay, the closely fitting doctrinal structure, in short certainty.

Conversely, the reality of social dynamics stood in sharp contrast to the once beloved geometric figures and constructions, now either of a regular circular motion or of a stepwise, linear or parabolic evolution. Not only did change now prove as such an essential feature of all social events, but moreover a still more strongly accelerating change of a completely irregular and discontinuous nature.

Instead of the familiar future-image of a restabilized harmony, a kaleidoscopic picture forms of unstable, sometimes chaotic, not infrequently disharmonious configurations and radical transformations.

As if to give the last, toppling push to the once cherished picture of the world and of society, in this almost endless chain of pronounced and accelerated change, another phenomenon, largely responsible for this but highly inconvenient, developed throughout history. For this history had been forcibly penetrated by human power, now of age but acting as a permanent mischief-maker. As Schiller had already written, "Die Welt is vollkommen überall wo der Mensch nicht hinkommt mit seiner Qual".

Since the Reformation and the Renaissance, Rationalism, Enlightenment and Progress, and above all thanks to applied scientific thought as well, human power has developed increasingly further, more strongly and more rapidly. It is the irony of fate that the natural sciences worshipped by the social sciences made the most direct contribution to that development, and that as a result it had indirectly to be these very natural sciences which had to knock out of the hands of their faithful socio-scientific worshippers and foot-soldiers practically all the weapons for similar or to some extent comparable scientific achievements.

What was a modern sociology, and what could it ultimately be, confronted with this overwhelming flood of social events tempestuously stirred and swept along by human power? Had not Parmenides now in fact finally been defeated by Heraclitus? Was it in fact still possible at all to find one's socio-scientific bearings in this tangle or maze of an eternally intrinsically changeable Becoming which, moreover, to make matters even worse, is also subject to arbitrary and deliberate outside change (revolution, battle, conflict, reform, planning)?

The opposition of the historical school to the dominating scientific thought model, and its complete surrender to the past, which was at least still intuitively and psychologically graspable, had meanwhile been resolutely rejected. This empathic and understanding method was considered to be denuded of objective

147

criteria offering real certainty. Finally, its scientific result was rejected fairly universally as unscientific, since it was unreliable, uncertain and therefore invalid. Thus all that remained was the way back to Parmenides, a renewed refuge in natural science, even though it was only halfway or half-heartedly, as the sole "ruhende Pol in der Erscheinungen Flucht". One could choose a certain half of natural science: either its logical system or its empirical validation.

Accordingly, social scientists wanted to try one of two things: either a purely abstract, timeless theory, still rooted in classical natural science, as a purely formal statics of rational deduction, derived from a number of axiomatic basic theses (or hypotheses);

or an equally undynamic, but now purely empirical theory, based as in natural science on inductive, usually statistical observation, limited to the present reality of the here and now, and trying to find a rational explanation for this, as a rule still subdivided into small segments or microanalyses.

Both types of theory had of course evident and not inconsiderable attractions for their users. The first is, at least provisionally, in its rational-discursive set-up, immune from disturbance by confused and confusing reality. After all, this theory stands completely aloof from time and space. For the time being the changeable material events hardly affect its system of formalized relations, if indeed they do so at all. The pure abstraction protects it, safely ensconced in an ivory tower, against the impure hurly-burly of the world and the fluctuating violence of the flow of reality.

The second kind of theory is at least fairly well protected by its firm, empirical, descriptive foundation against a possible charge of lack of resemblance to the reality which it describes and reproduces as accurately as possible. Anyone who wants to may check and verify its result. In broad outline this must tally, if the data were sufficient and the processing of them statistically sound. Crouching in the trench of the excavated part of the concrete environment, a sense of reality protects it against the unworldliness and meaningless vagueness of all invalidated or unverifiable, i.e. verbal, theorizing.

However, both types of theory (and one can continue to seek sensible combinations like Diogenes with a lantern) equally have their less evident but much more regrettable disadvantages. Unlike Buridan's ass, both do in fact choose between two bundles of hay, but they "make no hay". They are both ultimately gored by the horns of the dilemma for which they are themselves responsible, and which is in essense insoluble. They have manoeuvred themselves into the impossible position of detachment either from variable social reality or from future-oriented social dynamics.

6. Socio-scientific thought model: wedded to the wrong other half

The first type of sociological theory mentioned is a retreat to the rather faint-hearted, fruitless position of Archimedes, who despairingly implored the advancing enemy forces not to disturb his beautiful mathematical-cosmic circular models drawn in the sand ("noli turbare circulos meos"). But the enemy armies of disrupting human power and accelerated change advance relentlessly with overwhelming force. The timeless theory has no chance at all against the jerky movement and drastic intellectual changes of this present (and still more of the future) time. In this ultra-dynamic period of time any form of statics is pointless right from the start. Maintaining this aspect of classical natural science in modern social sciences is not only unreal but nothing short of asocial.

The second type of socio-scientific, purely empirical and microsociological research is exposed to dangers which, though quite different, may ultimately lead to an equally unacceptable result. In essence the same process of absolutization is applied; a piece of complete fictitious permanence is imprinted on a purely momentary event in an artificially demarcated part of a comprehensive whole. The fleeting moment is preserved, the part of matter dealt with is regarded as a representative "pars pro toto", as illuminating for the totality. But while the investigator is painstakingly examining his part of the whole, it runs away through his hands, so to speak. It does so because the relation between and interaction of all coherent parts of the whole are subject to lasting, intensified change. And because, moreover, the totality itself of contemporary society is uninterruptedly subject, within ever-decreasing periods of time, to a violently fluctuating, radicalizing and revolutionizing process of development. By the time that the partial study, undertaken with years of persevering industry and fully documented on an empirical basis, has been published or only shortly afterwards, it is already in danger of being wholly or partially outmoded. Insofar as it is still of value, this study will be ephemeral, will evaporate beyond recall.

Both types of modern socio-scientific theory suffer from one and the same fault. They have removed the time dimension. For the one, time does not exist at all, or only as a stationary eternity. For the other, time lies completely enclosed in a cross-section of a part of the fading today. Both of them have tried in their own way to master time, but both are being irrevocably subjugated by the very time.

Both have unanimously excised the future as an unclean and infected thing. As already stated, both types of theory are semi-scientific. The other half has been docked with the tail. For from the scientific point of view it was necessary, indeed the criterion of the scientific value of every theory, to be able correctly to predict the future.

However, so far, despite all historical attempts, social scientists have proved absolutely incapable of doing so. It is more than paradoxical, it is even more than significant, indeed it is no less than tragic, that the social sciences chose the *wrong* half of the natural sciences as *their* half.

But they have proceeded to oppose the *other* half, that of study and forecast of the future, with intensified dogmatism, indeed almost rabidly. Attracted as they had been to the future, they had repeatedly been rejected with their various methods and laws, causal and constant relations, fixed schemes, etc. The psychological reaction to this series of failures and frustrations was an extremely dissenting attitude towards *any* contact with the future. Now, conversely, future-research became strictly forbidden territory for the social scientist. Any attempt to anticipate the dynamic movement of social events was now regarded as evil or as proceeding directly from the Evil One. Any approach to the future prospects or the future forms of society was suspect and, from the outset, unfounded. Every forecast of the future of society could testify only to a scientific aberration. A future-vision was by definition woolly, wild, muddle-headed and arrogant.

In emulation of the British physicist and novelist Sir C. P. Snow, the term "the two cultures" is often used today, by which is mainly meant the gulf that has grown between the natural sciences on the one hand and the cultural sciences (the social, mental or behavioral sciences) on the other. In fact this is not just a simple antithesis, as is often assumed, also by Snow himself; the actual relationship is much more complicated.

The present social sciences are not in a state of complete antithesis to the natural sciences; instead they draw a marked caesura which now runs right across the scientific model of the classical natural sciences. Their present methodology is still almost feverishly based on a part of this model, clinging to it without rhyme or reason. As such they behave "plus scientifiques que les sciences exactes".

The empirical-factual or formal-logical research aspect of the natural sciences was placed in the limelight, but its predictive character with regard to probable futures was, conversely, completely blacked out, pushed out of sight. On the contrary, the future is now as it were phenomenologically "placed outside brackets" (Husserl). But had the social sciences chosen the right half of the natural sciences as the sole monogamous other half for an indissoluble marriage?

The new, normative code of social science now ran more or less as follows: *First* commandment: wedded for ever to classical natural science, thou shalt not commit adultery nor even behold another woman, in whatsoever scientific garb she may be clad. *Second* commandment: honor thy father and thy mother, i.e. thine own past-present reality. *Third* commandment: thou shalt not worship strange changes or dynamic phenomena as other gods. *Fourth* commandment: thou shalt not covet or enter thy neighbour's scientific field. *Fifth* commandment: thou shalt not kill time once it has been born. *Sixth* to *tenth* commandment: thou shalt not make graven images of the Future nor presume to create or re-create these in thy image, as if thou wert thyself a natural science.

Only now can we fully see that the gradual widening of the gap between "the two cultures" goes much deeper as a controversy, differs from and means more than was apparently intended. The simultaneous return to and renunciation of the natural scientific thought model by social science contains a contrast between the two main categories of natural science or of science as such which is as diametrical as it is paradoxical, and which goes to the heart of the matter.

For natural science, precisely owing to its scientifically gathered and applied knowledge, gives and creates *human power.*

Social science, on the other hand, conforms with an explicit testimonium pauperitatis its own powerlessness and bears the clear stamp of *human impotence.*[1]

Natural science remains constantly predictive, or at least prognostic. The whole of technological development, the ever-progressive unfolding of scientific theory and techniques, or practical application, are based above all on that predictive power, are oriented towards that permanent and completely reliable, or at least highly probable prospect.

Social science examines and confirms existing reality, whether it wants to or not. Its tendency, its essence and operation, are mainly conservative by nature. It freezes the explanation of what, in its view, to the best of its knowledge and ability, has been previously introduced into present reality. In an almost automatic fashion this alienates it from and even places it on inimical terms with any change that may rudely upset this explanatory interpretation, and a fortiori against a deliberate changeability and reform aimed at programmatically or politically, and highly manipulable. For, if not, remaining uniform and up to date even to some extent is a practically endless task. The "spectateur impassible" once treated with scorn in economics gains new understanding, even luster, in sociology.

Starting from this attitude, social science cannot but adopt a sceptical and ascetic attitude towards the boiling motion and change that nowadays do their undermining work in social events. Social *dynamics,* which really ought to be its key subject, lies abandoned almost motionless. Who dare reasonably interfere with it? Whatever Marx may say about philosophers, it is certainly not the task and the responsibility of sociologists or of any kind of practitioners of the social sciences — so they argue — to change the world. On the contrary, they only bother to explain it and make it understandable. But, while the ground is constantly sinking away under their feet and social events have entered a state of turbulence, can they still grasp something lasting? Apparently they can only try to detain time, as it hurries by, in framework so far regarded as effective by clamping it in outmoded thought models. Thought models that truncate and mutilate social dynamics, in particular by systematically snipping away the movement of the future. Thought models whose parallel we saw in the philosophy of history, which are ultimately non-future-models.

The matured and gradually ossified conviction about the infallibility of the inseparable mating or crossing of the socio-scientific thought model with the *wrong* half of *physics* not intended for that purpose has of course again found or produced its own inspirer, apologete and prophet: the *prophet of non-prophetism*, Karl R. Popper.[2] His methodological work, while invoking modern physics contains a systematic and fiercely critical attack on any predictive capacity of social science. Coupled to this is a consistent, fiery plea for "piecemeal social engineering", as an improvising control of society as it is today, cautiously progressing step by step. In his opinion all socio-cultural prediction has, from of old up to the present day, been an expression of the most fatal dogmatism. So great is the influence of this ultra-liberal contemporary thinker that, absurdly enough, even a modern socio-progressive future-thinker like Dennis Gabor cannot begin his work[3] without expressing his gratitude towards the anti-future-seer Popper.

A social science as proclaimed by Popper is auto-destructive and counter-selective. Its passive attitude towards and abstention from the future ends in a nihilistic desertion of the future rushing towards us. This compulsorily prescribed mating of half a physical horse and a whole sociological ass must lead to the biological variant of an extremely stubborn but nevertheless inevitable sterile mule. Literally and figuratively futureless.

In my turn I regard the prejudiced today-thinkers, such as the neo-positivistic Popperites, as the true dogmatic arch-enemies of our free, future possible and most desirable civilization. For our enormous social future-problems can no longer be solved by an improvising muddling-through from the one moment of the present to the immediately following one, but solely by means of a socio-scientifically founded future-prospect and endeavor. Oriented, with periodical revision, towards the long term of several decades, perhaps even with the attempted anticipation of half a century or even longer.

7. Socio-scientific thought model: a primitive attempt at psycho-analysis

The above might possibly be misunderstood — through a mistake of the author — to mean that all kinds of decidedly evil intentions and wicked plans were imputed to the social scientist. The actual situation is perhaps much worse, namely that all this is done with the very best intentions. And so definitely not just out of pure stupidity, ridiculous self-conceit or wanton conservatism. An invocation of Schiller's "mit der Dummheit kämpfen Götter selbst vergebens" would be completely off target. True, the unbroken thread of a religio-dogmatic foundation, with unassailable taboos based on it,

152

is also present here in optima forma, though usually in a sometimes unconsciously secularized version. However, very important and thorough thought has preceded the attitude of mind adopted. It can also be motivated entirely rationally. In doing so one reverts — though often as an implicit presumption — to the dualism of Descartes, himself a great proponent of thinking that was "clare et distincte", between body and spirit, in this case between matter as the subject of the natural sciences and spiritual consciousness as the determinant force of the behavioral sciences.

There is then a well-stocked arsenal of arguments for deepening and adequately explaining such an inherent contrast between the natural and cultural sciences as regards the code of social science connected with this and criticized above. Without in any way endeavoring to be exhaustive, but on the contrary with a preference for reduction to a few primitive but primary motives, one could classify these arguments according to their nature in two main types. The first argues "we *cannot*" — the second emphasizes "we *may not*". This irresistibly poses the psychological question whether (and, if so, to what extent), when digging deeper down to the heart of the matter, the most weighty but also most disputable reason ought not to be briefly rendered by "*we don't want to*". However, if the answer should be in the affirmative, this would again compel us to pose a last question, penetrating and illuminating still further, regarding the "why not", and also concerning the possible implications.

153

PART TWO

Counter-dogmatics and continuous dogmatics

CHAPTER 9

Deviations from dogmatic thought and future-models

It is apparently in the nature of the human mind that in the majority of cases it not only chooses bondage (the "escape from freedom") but at the same time again and again chooses freedom and thus, at regular intervals, revolts against dogma and authority which at these moments have obviously outlived themselves. However, it also seems to be a natural process that, in due course, the initially sharply anti-dogmatic and nonconformist mental attitude, in its turn, displays at regular intervals an apparently almost irresistible inclination to harden into dogma itself. As a result of the "horror vacui" (the abhorrence of a vacuum) the empty place is quickly filled and new vassals, courtiers and worshippers or followers-of-the-latest-fashion gather around the new despot who then sits on the throne. Till a new swing, revolt and coup d'état take place, another anathema is pronounced, the despotically reigning science-monarch is violently dethroned and the monopolistic science model, after having received the finishing stroke, suitably reformed, etc., etc. This is an unending historical chain of science, always with the same linkage of conformism-deviation-rebellion-renovation-intolerance-conformism.

We can clearly see this double contrast effect and cycle of scientific reformation and counter-reformation in three main areas. We see it historically, and almost as a matter of course, in the theological-religious field, and also in the metaphysical-philosophical field. This is especially so because precisely these two fields lend themselves pre-eminently to domination by a dogmatic mental attitude (albeit that this affects theology more easily and for a longer period than the essentially free philosophy) and, as a result, to repeated swings in modes of thought. This reaction, however, can also be found, especially in the field of natural scientific thinking. Precisely this natural scientific thinking has freed itself and, in interaction, also put its independent mark on modern religious and philosophical thought. In addition to the normal anti-dogmatic swing in every field of thought regarded separately, this mental change, which spreads from one field to the other, and the inter-connections of such mental revisions or reconstructions are equally important.

Precisely in view of these very important interactions and connections, it is not feasible to point to an exactly correct, chronologically and logically valid sequence or simultaneity. If we adhere to the respective order: religion, philosophy, natural science, it is not because we want to follow a well-known Comtean scheme of order. Above all, it is a didactic sequence meant to draw special attention to a specific point with relation to the future (or, respectively, with relation to the non-future!).

At a given moment, from the point of view of Weltanschauung, almost everything enters into motion and breaks loose. Old certainties are lost or rejected. While a completely modern, strongly deviating natural science gradually emerges from the cocoon of the classical natural sciences, which one can clearly recognize in kindred developments in modern religion and philosophy, the socio-scientific thought model, on the contrary, displays strikingly motion and a certain amount of stagnation. Where society itself is energized to an increasing degree, and where this accelerated motion is reflected in every field of thought and also has repercussions, as feedback, on everything that happens, socio-scientific thinking, strangely enough, continues predominantly to fall back on orthodoxy and invariance. From the viewpoint of the sociology of knowledge, it has hardly been investigated so far, let alone explained, how and why it is precisely and almost exclusively socio-scientific thought that has been willing and able to cling practically unhampered and completely uncritically to once dominant attitudes of mind, notably to a classical but now, in its turn, antique model of natural scientific knowledge which for natural science itself has long ceased to be anything but a historically indispensable transition phase. At the same time, religious and philosophical thought wrested itself free more or less simultaneously, or at least not too long afterwards, by mutations in leaps and bounds.

1. Transformation of natural science

It is not only the Christian religion and western philosophy that have been displaying major, mostly radical and fundamental renewals, especially since the turn of the century; this also applies to the whole of the natural sciences (mathematics and logic included). Indeed, the intervention or breakthrough here may even have been the most revolutionary, the transformation the very greatest, with a powerful feedback (though not further examined here) to almost all other fields of the human mind, certainly those of religion and philosophy. With perhaps the only exception, as noted before, being precisely the almost aloof, unmoved social sciences. Thus, one of the principal aims of the examination made in this volume is to contrast the dogmatics social science maintains with this totality.

The classical thought model of the classical natural sciences, let us say from the period of Copernicus-Kepler, Galileo-Newton and Descartes-Leibnitz, has been completely outstripped and partly pushed aside by the concepts and inventions of modern science. The laws of kinematic and

157

mechanical motion, the electromagnetic laws of Maxwell and Faraday, Boyle's gas laws, the nearly 2,000-year old theory that atoms are the smallest and last indivisible nuclei of matter, the biogenetic law of Haeckel, the ether contraction theories of Lorentz and Fitzgerald, etc., etc., were, as far as necessary, absorbed, corrected, complemented or substituted.

Nowhere did such a free-thinking, undogmatic, indeed definitely permanent revolutionary spirit develop as in the natural sciences. All certainties were subject to criticism, all axioms to rejection or amplification, all accepted theses could be unmasked as untenable hypotheses.

Of course, here I am moving far beyond the area of which I could claim to have a modest amount of personal knowledge. I have therefore to rely on impressions derived indirectly from others, and, I hope, understood correctly. This applies a fortiori, because the explanations still comprehensible for the layman are, in a kind of proportion to the steadily more complicated development, becoming scarcer just when this scientific progress is developing with steadily increasing power and application. This is understandable, and I think, we do not have to be too ashamed, within certain limits, of the chance of lagging further behind in this time of both scientific explosion and, in spite of the importance of information theory, often still extremely imperfect internal and external communication. Even less so, because not only the obscurity and incomprehensibility, indeed even the mysteriousness, to the outsider, but also, as it seems I may say, the theoretical complexity in the smaller circle of the practitioners of the natural sciences in certain fields, appear to be increasing. This means an extremely fast aging process, especially for the interested laymen coming from other fields and still remaining as outsiders at a distance.

On the other hand, it is precisely the demolition of outmoded, dogmatic thought models with which we are concerned here. We do not even need to know exactly what the newly developing thought models look like in detail at the moment, or which form they will probably be able to assume before long. Now to my way of thinking enough is broadly known about the break-through and transformation processes already performed to allow me to touch very quickly upon the character and direction of thinking of these phenomena as anti-dogmatic intellectual products. However insufficiently this task might be fulfilled, I still feel called upon to do it, proceeding completely on my own responsibility and steering on my own compass, the more so because I am sure that, as a rule, there is not enough insight here, especially in my own field.

Of course, I cannot give a responsible treatment of the whole field of the exact sciences in one single section, because this area is much too extensive. But that is not required at all. An illustrative and definitely not an exhaustive treatment is called for. Plenty of striking examples could be borrowed from almost every special field or specialistically subdivided field.

158

The revolutionary developments of chemistry and biochemistry already play an important role in everyday life. On the one hand, synthetic materials, man-made fibers, plastics and polymers; on the other hand, antibiotics, tranquilizers, cortisone, oral contraceptives, psychedelic drugs, and also a series of chemotherapeutic preparations and products, the application of which stretches from virology to psychiatry, from immunology to surgery.

Soon, perhaps, the new discoveries of biogenetics and molecular biology, connected with the continued deciphering and influencing of the genetic code, will cause even greater mutations, just as biomedical research, possibly coupled to electronics and computer cybernetics, might be able to set even further-reaching changes in motion than are known now. This applies to all fields and specializations of medical science: diagnosis, therapy, anesthesis, transplantations, replacement of sick or damaged tissues or organs by their artificial counterparts.

In addition to this, astrophysics and radio-astronomy are penetrating steadily deeper and further into the universe with the aid of perfected apparatus, including automated space laboratories. Cosmogonic and cosmological research into the mysteries of the beginning and the end (or infinity), into the mystery of life, are driving forward with increasing power. Theories about continuous creation, about primordial masses of gas or the chemical components of original matter, about the "big bang", about quasars fleeing from us with their still incomprehensible red shifts and light intensities, come and go. They may all still be highly speculative, but again and for the third time — after the Babylonians and Ptolemy, after the Copernican change — the motion of the universe has set our brains into equally strong motion. It happens almost every day that old thought models are traded in for daring new ones.

The uncertainty and changeableness of theory is, at present, greater than at any other time in the history of scientific thought before or after Newton. This uncertainty expresses itself in the absence, as yet, of any generally accepted, exact and logical mathematical description of fundamental anchorage of what is observed. Surprisingly enough, this uncertainty detracts in no way from the effective certainty with which, on the basis of this always shifting foundation, applied sciences and technology still keep shaping and renewing our industrialized society, rushing forward with equally big strides or even leaps and bounds, thanks to ever-new, never-ending wonders of ingenuity and inventiveness.

Often these results may be ascribed to close cooperation through team-work between a number of branches of science, which are beginning to have a steadily increasing number of more extensive overlapping aspects.[1]

However, I have to leave this highly interesting interdependence of the developments of natural science out of consideration too.

I want to limit myself predominantly to some selected developments in modern physics with an addition concerning the mathematics, or mathematical logic closely related to these. There are several reasons for this, all of which are important to the purpose set here. In the first place, it may be said that about 450 years ago, physics, considered in the broad sense (i.e. with the inclusion of the mathematical and scientific astronomy of that time), had a very special place in the development of classical natural science. So special that, as we have seen, a model of physical-nomothetical knowledge was gradually chosen as the pre-eminent model and, as such, was finally made compulsory for the practice of all science, especially, and certainly not least, for social science too.

It would, of course — as the second principal motive — likewise be of extreme value if it could be established that this same model, or an important part of it, continued to dominate, dogmatically, *outside* natural science for a long time — perhaps even up to now for a large part. While on the other hand, precisely *within* natural science, especially within physics, it was slowly but surely, or also with rather sudden, radical changes of habits of thought, discarded and fundamentally transformed. If we look at ultra-modern physics, this seems at first sight extremely probable, if not self-evident. I am thinking of the most recent, revolutionary developments of nuclear physics, astrometry and astrophysics, spectrum physics, plasma physics, the high-energy physics of cosmic and electromagnetic radiations, the physics of the fluorescence of solid matter and of semi-conductors, of crystallography, physical cosmology, biophysics, electro-chemistry, etc., etc. But it is not even necessary to be informed precisely and completely up to date about these ever-renewing, wonderful, sometimes dizzying very latest developments, to state that the conservative status quo for physics belongs to an absolutely finished and played-out past. Nor to make the suggestion that only the future "whither" is still relevant: the "status ad quem" which we are continuously attempting to unravel further, and which, for all its mystery, is still progressive.

For in such an analysis we are strongly supported by a fortunate, attendant and facilitating factor, and this, therefore, gives us the third decisive argument for the choice made here in favor of physics. This reason is that the basic, critically renewing research started here somewhat earlier than in most of the other fields.

The greatest pioneers in the field of invisible radiation and radioactivity (Röntgen, Marie Curie, the two Joliot-Curies, and De Becquerel) already made their contributions before the end of the last century. Max Planck is about at the transition from the 19th to the 20th century[2], a transition also to quantum physics. Einstein wrote his first pioneering article, a pre-announcement of his theory of relativity of 1916, in 1905. Rutherford and Bohr built their respective, although wrong, atom models before the First World War. The concepts which followed afterwards, testifying in their

160

successive nuclear physical observations to an ever-strengthened revolutionary and radical mental activity, of De Broglie, Schrödinger, Dirac, Heisenberg and Fermi, are from about the period of the 1930's. Since that time, almost all physical research has happened pre-eminently in the farthest and most advanced front lines. As a result of that research, all the borders of a previous "terra incognita" are crossed undauntedly. One is always prepared for the discovery of new wonders of the world. The pioneers who are renewing, changing, turning everything upside down and inside out, opening always wider dimensions, are possessed of a fundamentally, absolutely free and creative mind, essentially unlimited by any axiom or dogma.

All the fourteen above-mentioned renewers of classical physics are Nobel prizewinners.[3] They participated in this honor from 1901 to 1939, i.e. before the Second World War. At the end of that war and during the decades which have passed since then, the results of their theoretical renewals have become, in more than one respect, tangible, palpable and visible because of all kinds of applications. They, and others, have thought profoundly about these renewals and have published a great deal about their significance and consequences. I certainly do not mean to suggest that the further elaborations and inventions in the field of modern physics have been of less importance or of a less revolutionary character. For that is not the case at all. I do mean to say — and that is more than enough for my intention here — that, in the half century from 1890-1940 alone, the image of the world and the thought model of physics have undergone, in overwhelming measure, size, depth and range, a complete metamorphosis. In fact almost so unrecognizable that, except for some additions and retouching, every aspect of the practice of science ought to have experienced its enormous impact. Even more so if and insofar as it had been predominantly influenced by the earlier thought model.

If, however, this imposed change appears to have had no obvious, or strikingly little effect, I could try to give only *one* explanation of this paradox, namely that these renewals, outside the real professional fields of the natural sciences, had not become common property before the beginning of the Second World War. After the end of the war, the philosophical and methodological discussion on the fundamentals as the central problem within the circle of natural science initially halted or decreased: the latter was as familiar with the subject as if it were evident and had never before been otherwise. Besides, almost all attention, for the present, was concentrated on big points of controversy, such as with reference to A- and H-bombs, to the peaceful uses of nuclear energy and the institution of nuclear reactors, to the continuously expanding number of new nuclear particles, and, in connection with this, about the building of ever "bigger and better" particle-accelerators.[4] With reference to the renewal of physical fundamentals as such hardly any more reports penetrated to the outside world than about a strongly continued development of microphysics, which come to that was regarded as self-evident. For that matter, just at that time most practitioners of social science were too busy themselves, either with making up and eliminating, as quickly as possible, obvious arrears in their own professional field which had arisen during the war-years, or with the study of specific social, structural changes summoned up during and because of the war. It goes without saying that the Babylonian confusion of tongues between what I may call for the sake of convenience the practitioners of the exact and other sciences, which already dated from before the war, had in the meantime if anything increased, but definitely not decreased. The idea of the necessity of an interdisciplinary approach, which would have to comprise *both* categories of contrasting science, is still young and, certainly in Europe, still only an idea.

2. Elementary and fundamental change

For the non-scientifically minded reader, therefore, it might still be *useful* to gain some more insight into the far-reaching changes, especially of the scientific thoughts model. I will define as far-reaching all those changes which absolutely collide with the building blocks of centuries-old historical thought models which emerged as elementary. A point-by-point, compact summary follows:[5]

(1) For thousands of years, there had been a physical image of the world regarding which there was complete disagreement on a number of things, but the theory was rather generally adhered to that the atom was the last and smallest indivisible unit of matter, as it were a solid and hard little sphere.

In addition to this, there was major disagreement about the essence of matter. For centuries it had been believed that there was an absolute dualism between mind and matter. In the 19th century, monistic ideas gained many followers, either as materialistic monism (everything is matter) or as psychic monism (everything is mind, world spirit, Holy Ghost, etc.).

However that may be, one was fairly certain for a long time that substances or bodies, which were composed of these atoms, could display the phenomena of motion only through the action of certain forces (falling, throwing, friction, oscillation, gravity, work, energy, etc.). Also, that this motion changed under the influence of calculable dynamic acceleration after the insertion of a fourth non-spatial and therefore non-geometrical coordinate: time.

Several fixed, unchangeable laws which were based on this had been discovered: the law of inertia (no motion of solid bodies at rest without friction, etc.), the law of conservation of mass (by destruction or creation, the totality of matter always remains the same), the law of conservation of energy (the emission of energy is addition elsewhere, and vice versa). In addition to these, a second, somewhat mysterious law of thermodynamics (the emission of energy to generate energy is always coupled to loss of heat; loss of heat in the world inevitably and incessantly continues from an originally higher level down, finally, to zero = entropy).

These views and laws of the world (the depiction of which here should not of course be taken as purely scientific but as illustrative) have all been radically overthrown. This often means that, though they retain a relatively limited value for certain situations, they have no universal, absolute validity under all conditions.

(2) The first big shock was, I think, caused by Max Planck, in two respects. In the first place, he discovered that heat radiation is only transmitted or received in certain small portions of something that he called quanta. To put it differently, radiation behaves in contact or interaction with matter as if it consisted of such small portions. Moreover, this energy could be further defined or approached via Planck's constant (formula $h\nu$) valid for all mass and velocity.

In the depiction of these portions the concept of the atom as the last, solid main particle already suffered a major setback. Indeed, so did the concept particle as such. An almost endless discussion arose on whether one should consider these quanta as a collection of particles or as a phenomenon of waves.

(3) This discussion really got going when Einstein proved that Planck's discovery regarding heat radiation also applied to light radiation. There too there was emission and absorption of quanta, in this case called photons. Gradually there developed alongside — or if need be diametrically opposed to — the new quantum mechanics a mathematical wave mechanics.

(4) This development was also strongly influenced by the mathematical-physical formula (now known even to the layman) of Einstein, building in this on Planck and Lorentz, $E = mc^2$. This gave a strong impulse for the expansion of wave mechanics likewise as a system of mathematical equations (De Broglie, Schrödinger, Dirac).

(5) In the meantime, quantum mechanics itself had been extended and refined too, through the atomic models of Rutherford and his co-workers, but especially by the models of Niels Bohr, the revolutionary Danish physicist. On the strength of his fundamental research into the structure of atoms, the real nuclear physics as such was really constituted. The public

163

then learnt that the atom, basically, was like a small solar system. Certain numbers of electrons were rotating around the nucleus of the atom in separate, discernable shells, while they moved in comparable, fixed, circular orbits (later amended to elliptical orbits around that nucleus).

As a result, the atom or the atomic nucleus, though it had not been dethroned as the center of the universe, as had happened to earth, had definitely lost its place as the smallest, fixed particle of matter. Moreover, attention then moved mainly in four separate though connected directions. On the one hand, to the shell, the nature and behavior and also the composition of these electrons and likewise of particles of matter added later and also considered to be fundamental and elementary, such as protons and neutrons, or of their component or opposed elements. On the other hand, to the further analysis of the heart and the structure of the atomic nucleus itself. In the third place, to a completely new direction, in which even the genius of Einstein came up against a brick wall for the time being, namely the fascinating question, intensified by the unstoppable discovery of ever-more particles and counterparticles, of whether all these seemingly inconnected, almost innumerable, spontaneously and stably behaving particles could be linked together in a certain way on the strength of a common foundation. It was conceivable that there was ultimately *one*, Atlas-like physical substratum, explicable and predictable in *one* law for the whole universe. In the fourth place, a drastic revolution begins to break new ground with respect to the connections and contrasts in the still valid basic considerations of physics. This especially concerned the laws of the inertia of matter and of motion both within microcosmic matter and outside of macrocosmic matter, such as this now seems to be divided over and to form the supposed filling of the universe.

But the research by Bohr already caused a highly important deviation from the classical thought model. Fixed orbits of motion and rotation seemed to be prescribed for the electrons according to the shells in which they were. However, there appeared to be impulses through which electrons could move on their own from one orbit into another. The dogma of the continuity of motion was breached as a result: motion and change by leaps and bounds were compatible only with a principle of *discontinuity*.

(6) In the meantime, uncertainty developed about more and more factors. What was really known about the phenomena and elements of nuclear physics? The different atomic models only formed an auxiliary for approximating a reality which gradually became unimaginable. The more this merged and evaporated into systems of mathematical equations, the more concrete reality as an objectively determinable reality vanished out of sight. While particles were still something tangible, this could hardly be said of mathematical waves. What, scientists wondered, are we really concerned

with? Are we really doing anything more than deriving formulas from formulas? What exactly do these mathematical symbols represent?

After much discussion, scientists finally arrived — if I might put it this way — at two compromises. In the first place, one would no longer speak onesidedly of particles, nor of waves, but of phenomena which occurred or could be imagined now as particles and then as waves. In the second place, it was now possible to satisfy everyone by speaking henceforth of wave particles. Both parties were therefore equally right and wrong.

However, a price had to be paid for this compromise. In the mathematical calculation and prediction of the behavior of these wave particles the basic idea of a strictly causal-mechanical conformity with natural law, as known from classical physics, had to be abandoned. The idea already introduced earlier by Boltzmann of statistical *probability* had to be adopted for the whole of nuclear physics. The behavior of *one* or of several particles could not possibly be predicted exactly, but this could, with a very good possibility of a foreseeable result, be done with very large numbers of particles. Individual and irrational behavior, contingency, accident and chance entered the microcosmic, gradually over-populated world of the atom.

(7) However, an additional but extremely hard blow was struck at the old thought model by Heisenberg in 1927. The causal determinateness in strict conformity with natural law had already changed fundamentally into a system of *indeterminism* which was protected from chaotically falling apart by the application of the law of large numbers, the regularity of probability theory which set everything aright again. A further considerable correction and reduction had now to be made to this, however. For Heisenberg proved irrefutably that the spatial position and the velocity of certain particles could not be calculated simultaneously — not even for larger numbers of particles. His famous principle of *indefiniteness* or *uncertainty* taught that one could calculate their spatial position in advance, in accordance with criteria of probability as distance covered, but in that case definitely not their velocity or impulse, and exactly the same the other way around. It is possible to calculate the speed, i.e. the time of change, but then not the final destination attainable on the strength of this development of energy.

(8) A point-by-point, condensed account naturally disturbs both the chronological and the logical connections. For, throughout all this, Einstein's titanic renovating work was active. His formula mentioned above did indeed create new order and certainty. On the other hand, it disturbed the last remains of the classical thought model and thus caused an enormous new uncertainty too.

According to the classical thought model, there were at any event two constants, as solid as rocks in the surf: the conservation of mass and the

165

conservation of energy. In the new image of the world presented by Einstein, however, mass (or matter) could be transformed into energy and, conversely, energy into mass. It was as if, suddenly, because of this transformation, matter could not only definitely be destroyed or decreased, but even provided with a purposeful mental energy. Moreover, the old, unreal dream of the mystical alchemists about the possible transmutation of elements — which were, for a long time, also considered as the last unchangeable building blocks of matter — still seemed capable of being realized concretely. For, with all kinds of experimental operations, large numbers of discovered small and ever-smaller particles of matter and anti-particles could, without difficulty, be transformed into each other or into something else. Thus, matter was not only just inert matter; even at *rest* its components contained a potential, indeed even an unprecedentedly powerful, all-surpassing energy of a virtual working-power, motion and *change*.

(9) But this too was only part of the brillant vision of Einstein. Now, changing from the *micro*cosmos, which had had to abandon its old certainties and laws because they did not apply to it, there followed the even more daring jump to the *macro*cosmos. Special and general theory of relativity. The laws of Euclidean geometry too were no longer universally valid, nor applicable, under all circumstances, to physics and astronomy. Einstein created a fourth dimension, a time-space continuum, which was not flat but curved and could, therefore, be reproduced mathematically only with the aid of non-Euclidean geometry.

However, from this *relativity* the most remarkable consequences resulted which inexorably sentenced several other *absolute*, and therefore fixed and invariable, magnitudes of thought to death. In the situations described and covered by Einstein, the magnitudes of measurement, mass and time could no longer be regarded as given, invariant units.

(10) Perhaps the most interesting aspect of this is the wild storm that burst in particular about the *non-existence*, or rather the no longer *established reality* of our earthly clock *time* measured by the second. This was an attack on the exactly divided time-calendar which had been adhered to almost unchanged since Babylonian astrology. Dilation and contraction of time were now possible. Simultaneity of non-simultaneous happenings was theoretically feasible. The time of a certain kind of space traveller might, according to his speed and the distance he travelled, pass considerably slower than here on earth sot hat, on his return, only a little older biologically, he would perhaps find a completely renewed world quite different from the one that he had left only a relatively short time before.

All philosophical-scientific thought was in great commotion and confusion.

166

This much was certain anyway: a strict separation between the observing *subject* and the observed *object*, as firmly assumed in the past, could no longer be made. This had already been implied in the Heisenberg uncertainty principle. For, precisely by the use of strong or weak impulses of light radiation, the observer faced the dilemma of whether he wanted to determine time or place beforehand. This influence was now generalized. For the observer, the results of his research were relative to his location, his system of notion, his own speed, and also the kind of instrumentation he used. Consequently, the Heisenberg uncertainty acquired much more sweeping consequences than was originally suspected. For, with extremely strengthened high-energy impulses and therefore enormously accelerated forces of motion, one could create all kinds of new particles of matter, but also make them disappear because of their mostly particularly short duration, measurable in tiny fractions of seconds, of a movement traced as "life". This extremely fast creation and destruction, apparently without trace, of these particles conjured up by high-energy physics, however, came into conflict with the law of the conservation of energy for solid matter physics.

(11) In one respect, new courage could at least be drawn from this. So far, the law of entropy had always been explained as a harmonic endeavor in the whole of nature towards a restoration of equilibrium as a result of the loss of heat at an ever lower level, until finally the absolute equilibrium or the zero point had been reached of a cessation of changeableness, but equivalent to a death by cold which would one day inexorably dawn. Who knows, one could now reason, perhaps this future-law too has only a relatively limited validity? In other words, perhaps the addition of heat, resulting from certain compensating situations, to the on the other hand assumed, inescapable and continuous reduction in heat could take place in the universe, on the strength of conversion of the forms of energy known to us? After all, it is far from inconceivable that as yet unknown sources of energy could become available in the still mysterious and uncomprehended universe through explosion, radiation or other means.

(12) Such unorthodox ways of thinking also received support from quite a different quarter.

Until then, classical physics had concerned itself only with matter which could assume one of three forms: solid, liquid or gas. True, efforts had been made to find a fourth basic state which, however, escaped every firm grasp like, in chemistry, the substance which for a certain time was called "phlogiston", a volatile stuff which could not be held in the fingers or trapped in a test-tube, or like a virus assumed by bacteriologists which managed to elude every attempt to classify it.

Maxwell and even Lorentz — just before Einstein's refutation — had still worked with the hypothesis of a substance, existing in space, which had been designated as ether for a long time, and which was believed to be subject to certain changes.

In the 1920's a new view was advanced, namely that the universe largely consisted of a fourth, quite different and peculiar material, which has been given the name of plasma (Langmuir). This fourth state of matter can be obtained by heating gases to thousands or even tens of millions of degrees with certain techniques. This plasma is said to constitute the basic material of stars and to fill up space between heavenly bodies, in various concentrations, but of less density than man on earth would be able to accomplish in an artificially created vacuum. In short, a new picture of the universe started to be formed with respect to the primordial matter, in which continuous, unimaginably large and awe-inspiringly powerful nuclear reactions of still incalculable consequence were happening with all-surpassing temperatures and overwhelming speeds.

A swirling and blazing mass of particles, supplied with a still indescribable amount of charge, was said to occur. These particles were, it was claimed, observable by their radiations, waves, resonances, etc. As far as one has been able to establish up to now these plasma particles roam the cosmos in a manner still completely obscure, unimaginably disorderly, individualistically independent, blindly groping, to our way of thinking. However, we do know for sure that if these particles were combined with other matter, for instance hydrogen, an amount of controllable energy would be released billions of times greater than that of all coal and oil taken together, which would last for tens of billions of years. Radio-astronomy and the techniques of magnetohydrodynamics are intensively studying this at present.

(13) It thus seems as if both the macrocosmos and the microcosmos can be broken down into particles, waves and wave particles. The question "What is matter?" can hardly be answered any more. An all-embracing physical theory, such as Einstein tried to find throughout his life, is no longer or not yet existent.

However, the number of particles found in an atom by nuclear physics is still steadily growing in the meantime: there are, I believe, already more than three hundred nowadays. We may probably expect that rather identical findings might result from the further growth of plasma physics when its research is passing through the same stages of development.

(14) But we shall have to be firmly and consciously prepared in principle, if necessary, to move on to a new, fundamental, even more radical unorthodoxy of scientific future-thinking. For, however extremely speculative (for obvious reasons) one might consider this to be at the present time, it may

very well be that, for instance, we shall also have to put behind us the laws of the Einsteinian universe and pass them by with purposive thinking for extragalactic worlds yet to be discovered. Imagine that in the cosmos the extreme limit of the speed of light, set by Einstein at 186,300 miles per second, should be reached or even surpassed by certain objects moving away from earth with a phenomenal expulsive power, whether or not controlled by an intelligence unknown to us. That would again overthrow all the existing laws of time and might give to temporal events a completely different, as yet almost inconceivable, even reverse direction. To mention only one example, then, for instance, the heavenly bodies in the cosmos furthest away from us and still withdrawing further would not be the oldest ones (on account of the distance of the number of billions of light years — imaginable only in mathematical terms — possibly being larger in itself than that radiated since the calculated origin of earth) but perhaps precisely the youngest.

At present, attempts are everywhere being made with very great and concentrated effort to receive and interpret the luminous and accoustical signals from this tremendously distant extra-galactic cosmos. These speculative interpretations of the "singing of the stars" are, of course, widely divergent. The discovery that certain signals are stronger and weaker with regular alternations has given rise to the hypothesis that such "messages" are being broadcast by extra-terrestrial, intelligent civilisations in the cosmos. Such a comparably regularly intermittent, half-yearly change in the intensity of strength and weakness of radiation, as from a lighthouse, has also been established with regard to the quasars (quasi-stellar radio sources). In this respect we are faced by different and even greater mysteries. These cosmic, radiomagnetically radiating objects, which are not stars but, on the other hand, could not be bigger than a star, nevertheless produce an explosive energy greater than that of a "thousand suns", greater than a whole galaxy of a hundred billion stars together. Thus, something incomprehensible, indeed even unimaginable, is happening with mass and energy, and also with matter and speed of motion, in that part of the cosmos, which is possibly in a state of continuous creation or procreation and evolution. Do these quasars, if they exist, bring us closer to understanding creation and, therefore, to the origin and structure of matter, and to the limits of awe-inspiring infinity? What new physical-mathematical laws, what comprehensive but different theories could be applied to this cosmic creative field? As yet, we know nothing for certain.

As soon as we have learnt more about this, and also with more than a purely hypothetical probability, within the next decades or centuries, mainly thanks to radiotelescopic observations and new, still to be invented, methods of research, we shall probably have to rethink all the existing thought structures drastically and, again, have to submit all the contemporary views of

169

the past and future to a reorientation as fantastic as it is revolutionary. Moreover, why could there not be other cosmic heavenly phenomena and extragalactic objects, hidden even further away behind the horizon of these now discernable "quasars", whose probable existence is still invisible to us, and to whose messages our most modern instrumentation is still blind and deaf? It does not really matter whether the contemporary, extremely bold, science fiction type of fantasies about cosmic objects traveling back into the past or, conversely, acting as forerunners of a not-yet-existing, extragalactic civilization of the future, prove to contain truth in any respect. Nor whether the gigantic nuclear explosions contain the true secret, as it were in laboratory form, of the origin and decay of cosmic matter. The heart of the matter is really the special caution we must observe and the distance we have to maintain, even with regard to the Einsteinian transformation of classical physics. This ultra-modern metamorphosis is probably not the *last*, permanent one of the ultima ratio, but, on the contrary, possibly the *first*, completely non-dogmatic step on entirely new paths again leading us much further.

(15) Summa summarum: we have to try to rid ourselves of the primitive and unhistorical arrogance which is repeatedly manifest in a number of scientists, however irritating or ridiculous this might be for our descendants. Our present knowledge, and we can already be sure of this, is no longer the be-all and end-all. In the year 2000 or, if one prefers a greater distance, in 2000 or 2500, a non-Einsteinian physics will probably be named after physicist X, which, in due course, will have to make way in turn for other physics, ad infinitum. We are not at the end, but only at the very beginning. The physics of the 30th century will perhaps be comparatively further away from the 20th century than the physics of the 20th century is from that of the 10th century. Much would be gained if we could accustom ourselves more to the continuous replacement of existing, prevailing thought models and the irresistible, undogmatic break-through to ever-new future-models. These cannot be permanently excluded from the social sciences either.

3. The way of thinking about the change in thinking

(1) It does not really matter whether my above interpretation of the basic transformation from classical into modern physics is completely accurate. At a non-professional level, imperfections and misconceptions can creep in easily. This treatment aims less at the letter and more at the spirit. Indeed, in this case and for this set-up, most specifically at the spirit. It is my conviction that in the first place it may definitely be said that the classical, Newtonian thought model which, de facto, has reigned supreme in all

170

areas of science with sovereign majesty, has been dethroned from that position, though not entirely destroyed. In a relatively limited field of partly changed validity, it has been incorporated in an immensely wider and also much more elastic, pluriform system of thought. In my personal language of thought, this means two things. On the one hand, unquestionable witness has indeed been borne to human error and to complete or at least partial untruth in all fields of human knowledge, without exception, in the course of time. These are errors and untruths which were repeatedly mingled with conscious or unconscious fallacy and with wishful thinking and which, after that, hardened into ideological, dogmatic, and almost compulsively neurotic, universally valid concepts, indeed obligatorily prescribed ways of thought. On the other hand, it seems to me, it can be stated that the natural sciences in general and physics in particular, finally proved to be the first branch of knowledge that was both repeatedly willing (and later the most willing) to introduce undogmatic emancipation and unprejudiced liberation, and clearly able to do so case for case.

In the second place, however, it definitely does not only matter *that* the old thought model has been repeatedly replaced and reviewed as often as necessary, and expanded into new, unprecedented dimensions of width, depth and distance. Within our context, it is of almost greater importance to understand *how* this occurred.

With this, too, we can separate and distinguish two highly important factors.

(2) To mention the first greatly differing magnitude, the time factor came into physics in completely new images quite altered from those during the time of Galileo and Newton. The speed of light, 186,300 miles per second, has not been surpassed so far. But the smallest imaginable units of time have been tremendously decreased and the largest equally increased.

Ever-larger and more powerful particle accelerators are being built. Scientists work with micro-seconds, nano-seconds (1 billionth of a second) and pico-seconds (1,000 billionth of a second). Some resonant wave particles do not seem to live longer than one hundred-quintillionth of a second and many no longer than one ten-billionth of a second.

The most recently discovered quasar, which is said to move away from earth into the cosmos at a speed of about 150,000 miles per second, is, now, as far as we know, probably the most remote heavenly body from us.[6]

Time has been decreased, increased, bent, made uncertain and relative. In spite of this, the capacity of modern natural science to predict the future has not been basically decreased or even increased. The modern applications of computers, transistors, super-conductors, super-magnets, lasers, generators and linear accelerators, etc., are based on mathematical probability theory of modern quantum and wave physics. The same is true of space travel for satellites and rockets, as well as of the huge arsenal, mostly still secret, of

171

offensive and/or defensive weapons, such as hundred-megaton atomic warheads, radiation sensors, high-energy shields and interceptors, or airborne multispectral reconnaissance instruments (which work both on earth and under water).

Even without the coercive, dogmatic, nomothetic thought model of classical physics, thanks in part to the very construction of deviating and also mutually differing thought models it was possible to keep one's finger on the pulse of the future. A not inconsiderable measure of theoretical uncertainty, contradiction and restlessly swirling motion or feverish research into the most varied, most remote directions are setting their mark on modern physics. At present, physics no longer has an inclusive general theory, compulsorily prescribed on every point, in a number of fields. Yet this physics still sets the trend, despite its changed, partly still shaky bases. Some recently discovered particles exhibit odd, strange, jumpy, almost clownish behavior, and are still incomprehensible and incalculable. In addition to that, for instance, the ordered connection between uncharged neutrinos is not entirely explicable. But there is more than enough insight in the whole field to continue building on this foundation. The concept of *time* of this physics may have been narrowed, extended, changed, refined and ramified; the concept of the future has not suffered at all. On the contrary, this modern physics, more so and also more purposefully than ever before, is definitely, emphatically oriented towards the future, both in its fundamentals and in its applications.

(3) In addition to this, I attribute exceptional importance to the way of thinking that has led to this phenomenal, truly gigantic shift from old to new thought models.

Probably this renovating way of thought is not only most visible to the outsider once again in Einstein, but in addition it was the latter above all who critically and reflectively considered it. He always took a great deal of trouble to penetrate into the essence of creativity, both in general, and in his own personal case in particular, with characteristic modesty and wisdom. His concepts, which were absolutely revolutionary for science, and which had begun already during his menial employment at a patent office were, of course, (this is almost a truism), the result of a creativity that contained the unique combination of speculative powers of thought, visionary and artistic imagination, intuition and inventiveness. But, most of all, they were the fruit of an undogmatic mentality and also of the energetic courage of his convictions to dare to run counter to accepted ideas and were combined in fortunate fashion with a specifically talented capacity for explaining his new ideas in the language of mathematics. He never set foot in a laboratory to create the structure of his theory of relativity, nor did he himself ever do any experimental research. But others, for some decades, indeed for

172

almost half a century, have verified and confirmed his theories with an endless number of patient, laborious experiments and, on the basis of them, built further.

(4) It is above all this same purely speculative power of thought, this creative fantasy, this imaginative vision — which can think beyond existing axioms, fixed legal prescriptions and absolutized bonds — which is today attempting to find a way out of the obscure mysteries that arose just after and because of the fact that the new physics had come closer to solving a large number of existing major problems regarding the heart of matter and the essence of the cosmos.

As regards the atomic nucleus, the counterparts of for instance fission and fusion are no longer of primary importance, nor are the chain reactions which must be controlled for them. The speculative spirit now singles out the very nature of the counterparts. Nuclear physics had already clearly proved that positively and negatively charged particles exist in certain symmetrical proportions and connections, in short that for all the particles discovered there are complementary anti-particles (or wave particles). An investigation of cosmic radiation, however, has proved that there too electrons have their own anti-particles and that, if they meet, they destroy each other, emitting energy.

Does this mean that a universal law of counterparts, functioning at the same time as an endless source of energy, has been discovered? Is it still pure science fiction or already modern physics to speak, for instance, of anti-gravity, or of an anti-matter, even of an anti-world, an anti-galaxy and even an anti-cosmos of spontaneous collision, destruction and explosion, of an energy pouring forth, associated with a still impenetrable restoration of harmony and equilibrium, in short, of modernized, Heraclitic eternal Becoming and creating?

To ask the question is not to answer it, at least, not with respect to its content. As regards the form, however, a pertinent answer is definitely possible and desirable, namely that, as we can foresee, from such a speculative, *unorthodox* and *undogmatic*, creative mental attitude, a continued, radical renewal of physical thought will, in time, definitely emerge. This is, at all times, the indispensable *condition*, the sine qua non, of scientific *progress*. Hence the repeated *resistance* of the established order, also and precisely in official, doctrinaire science.

(5) In my conviction, it is definitely not an exaggeration to state that modern physics and other natural sciences active in its fringe areas have undoubtedly arrived at a transitional phase to a third, more comprehensive revolution, compared with which the two previous ones which reached a climax with Newton and Einstein respectively will seem only forerunners. This can be concluded in particular from what I believe is the already per-

ceptible shift into another, more and more centralized area of problems in about the last ten years. I shall like to devote a few words to this here because precisely this fundamental shift is in its essence closely related — also philosophically — to the same *problems of the future* which are our primary concern in this work.

Three separate, although of course in a deeper sense interrelated points are involved here. In the first place, people have begun to wonder — quite rightly — whether modern physics, especially the new principles of nuclear physics and corresponding chemistry, are valid or applicable with regard to either mental phenomena or organic forms of life: both of these, of course, are typical of human society and social events. Is it necessary to call a halt to the applicability of modern physics and chemistry? Are they powerless in that respect, or will they have to be radically revised?

In the second place, attention has begun to concentrate more deeply on the phenomenon of the steadily increasing number of particles of matter. This attention is mainly focussed on three questions. First question: can certain particles be considered as fundamental, that is, as elements of all matter? For instance, some time ago the hunt started for the elementary particle known as a quark which, though postulated, has never been indicated or recorded by any instrument. This particle is said to be of an even more essential character than nuclei, electrons, protons and neutrons, let alone muons, pions, neutrinos, or chemically grouped ions, or light-radiating photons. This hypothetical quark (incidentally a name derived from an invention by James Joyce in "Finnegans Wake") is claimed to be able through certain combinations to form all the subatomic particles known so far. In addition to this, of course, the question touched upon of the possible infrastructure or substratum which also, in itself, would be fundamental for all fundamental particles, is being asked now with even greater insistence. The third, final and most decisive question: which particles, in comparison with all the others, may correctly be considered as fundamental? This could, it is supposed, only be concluded from natural low-energy processes. For, it is adduced, the artificial high-energy processes achieved by researchers themselves create all kinds of other short-lived particles thanks to splitting (by means of heating, acceleration, bombardment, pulverizing, etc.); these new particles, however, cannot be considered as pre-existent, but only as part of complex, elementary components of matter.

(6) This already comes very close to the social problems of the future. For here too we are concerned with an independent creation or personal manipulation, correction and direction of the existing, autonomous development into another and differently oriented movement, possibly even transformation, of social dynamics. Another, equally central shift in the problem of modern physics further reinforces this naturally broad analogy. An ex-

174

tremely complex, partially philosophical reflection on fundamentals is concerned here. In popular language, a cardinal controversial area of modern physics could perhaps be reproduced more or less as follows. Is it true that only one, single combination is conceivable between the earthly and cosmic laws now found? Is there only one, exclusive means of existence for the evidently present divisions and observable processes of motion of the matter found everywhere? In that case, extending one of Leibnitz' concepts, we should have to come to the logically unavoidable conclusion that this *one* universe that is known to us in the sole imaginable possibility.

In the other case, it might very well be possible to imagine a number of different, logical, consistent "universes" differing fundamentally from the universe which we are accustomed to explore, including an anti-universe. It is obvious that this problem — mutatis mutandis — runs parallel to the view, which the present author defends, of the existence of various possible futures about whose creation and destruction or re-creation, earthly mankind would be able definitively to decide by using human power, intervening in accordance with man's own personal destiny. This could be achieved — after imaginative exploration and the most exact scanning possible — by choosing between the possible, alternative futures, attainable within certain limits, in a purposeful and well-considered manner, acting in the matter in a future-oriented manner.

(7) The above illustration, woven around the figure of Einstein, may possibly gain in strength by confrontation with another of the great renewers of physics, the New Zealander Ernest Rutherford. Here we encounter a typical representative of experimental physics. In 1909, some experiments conducted by Geiger and an assistant in Rutherford's laboratory concerning alpha particles fired with high power at a thin metal foil did not conform at all with Rutherford's positive expectations. For, in absolute contrast with his expectations, these particles were reflected and deflected. In 1911, after repeated experiments of this kind, Rutherford published a new theory about the structure of the atom having a small, positively charged nucleus around which electrons spin continuously.

But again, something in this theory did not fit, and Rutherford was very well aware of it. For, according to classical physics, the electrons, in their spinning motion around the nucleus, in perpetual motion, so to speak, should definitely emit energy as light or other radiation, which was not the case. A few years later, Bohr dared to take the step, at variance with the classical thought model, of allowing the electrons to circle quietly without the release of energy and, according to his new theory, to let them radiate light only if certain portions (quanta) passed discontinuously from one orbit into another.

Rutherford could correctly predict, likewise on the basis of his continued experiments into the structure of the atom, that there must be a neutron particle as well. But here, too, remarkably enough, he continued to look backwards. As early as his own brilliant researches in 1911, but especially in the Twenties and Thirties, speculative and normative thinkers had suggested that it should be possible, especially with the help of these neutrons still to be discovered, to achieve nuclear chain reactions of both fission and fusion. However, as late as 1933 Rutherford spoke scornfully about these fantasies which, according to him, would never be realized. About the characteristics and function of neutrinos in particular he had quite different views. However, he was not only the pioneer, but gradually also the infallible pope of nuclear physics (thus the staff of his own laboratory called him "papa") and nobody could, at the risk of his further career, really permit himself to contradict Rutherford's authority. His pertinent and absolutely negative attitude with regard to a controlled or controllable splitting of the atom was also, until not long before his death in 1937, practically prohibitive with regard to both theoretical contemplation and practical research. Except in 1935 for the unbelievably opinionated Frédéric Juliot-Curie, as witness his speech of acceptance of the Nobel prize. By the end of the Thirties the latter, and also Hahn, Meitner, Fermi, Szilard, Teller and others, made further experiments which were to result in the famous letter by Einstein, again appealing to the imagination, in which these new forces were brought to the attention of President Roosevelt.

(8) Do not misunderstand me. I certainly do not intend to belittle Rutherford's renovating greatness, or to measure it again and compare it with that, for instance, of Bohr, Einstein or the Juliot-Curies. I only wish to offer a comparison of different types of thinkers and thought models.

It is consequently irrelevant that Bohr's atomic model, which corrected the earlier model of Rutherford, was not completely correct either. Now, about half a century later, we have, for the present time, come to the conclusion that the circular or elliptical orbits of electrons do not give a precise picture either, and that perhaps, in principle, an exact picture cannot even be given. One now speaks of a "cloud of probability" in which may be found, with a rather considerable degree of uncertainty, electrons whose number, place (in one of the shells of the atomic nucleus) and shape of the wave motion are also dependent on the chemical composition, the temperature and the level of energy present from case to case. The essentially important point is not, however, this depiction itself, but the imagination that underlies it.

It might be that this imagination, as with the theories of Einstein, is fundamentally confirmed by later experiments. But it might also be that this imagination, as with Rutherford's experiments, is strongly restrained or led astray. To be fair, we have of course to admit that persons such as Rutherford and Lorentz, remaining just within the existing frameworks, nevertheless, through their experiments and interpretations, lead to these frameworks being exploded by somebody like Bohr and Einstein. Nothing is more fruitful for scientific progress than the important mistakes of the giants operating in the front lines of the valid theories. Provided that such geniuses of reflection dare to take the decisive plunge and break through into the totally new and try to cross the frontiers of the Promised Land lying in a distant haze.

4. Mathematics and logic

(1) In order to complete the picture evoked of undogmatic revolution and shifts, we now must explore some by-ways, parallel paths and crossroads. For the transformation from classical to modern physics was not completely independent, but took place, as we know, in close interaction with a renewal of mathematics and logic. It is of course impossible — with regard to both space and competence — to give an extensive survey of these related developments here. For this reason, I shall restrict myself to this summary and moreover again to those salient points which seem to be important to this sketch of undogmatic deviation and renovation.

(2) It will therefore not come as a surprise to the reader that, for the conclusion of my arguments in this direction, I once again take as my starting-point the revolutionary renewals of the physical image of the world, especially as effectuated by the thinking of Bohr and Einstein.

It has already been pointed out that Bohr had to sacrifice the classical idea of the continuity of radiation particles in favor of a discontinuous process of leaping portions of radiation (packages of quanta collected or held together some way). However, there were also far-reaching, logical consequences connected with this. Quite simply, the principle of *identity* (still bound to solid particles bound in turn to place or time and space) had to give way to the principle of *complementarity*.

The logical principle of identity is based on a exclusive either-or: either something is true or it is untrue. The principle of complementarity supplements this with a both-and. In this case, with a concept of radiation which could alternately or successively have the characteristics of a particle as well as a wave, or which was to give a partly coinciding new concept of wave particles which was, however, difficult to imagine on account of its inner contrasts.

Einstein, building on this new science, then found himself obliged to revise the logical, theoretical ideas and images of space and time such as they had reigned in physics since Newton and Kant, no longer just for nuclear microphysics but equally for cosmic macrophysics. Once again, he used different, at the time usually less appreciated, but highly revolutionary

177

concepts evolved by the practitioners of fringe areas of science. This time geometry, viz. the Russian mathematician Lobatshevski and of the German mathematicians Riemann and Minkovski. Einstein projected as being the most appropriate a non-Euclidean, multi-dimensional geometry, and adapted it for the study of space and the theory of relativity based on it. Independently of what else this implied, it is immediately obvious that a relativization of the valid, logical systems of thought was inherent in it. Inde illae lacrimae: hence the many tears and the initially highly emotional, pre-eminently refractory resistance of the dogmatics.

In actual fact, older experiments, for instance by Michelson-Morley in 1887 and Fitzgerald and Lorentz several years later, had already shown, quite otherwise than might be normally expected or explained according to classical theory, that the speed of light was not impeded by its motion through space. The real meaning of this could not be fathomed until Einstein rejected the idea of the existence of a solid, motionless, ethereal space. On the contrary, as we know, he postulated that everything in this space moved at relatively different speeds. Except light, which had a constant speed, as such also independent of measurement, measuring instruments and measuring observer as well. In other words, one could not measure light by means of itself, i.e. by means of the constancy of light.

Considered logically and mathematically, this meant that one could not gauge any measure by means of the same measure. This has also been called the zero-effect which, for instance, is equally true for the law of uniform motion because the chronometer of every clock itself moves uniformly with what has been accordingly measured.

(3) It is immediately obvious that this places us fairly and squarely in the area of the notorious paradoxes which, from of old, have afflicted the search for purely logical solutions to logic, of purely mathematical solutions to mathematics or of a logical reasoning for mathematics or a mathematical reasoning for logic. Yet this has been attempted again and again along different lines of attack and from different starting-points, I might almost say in a most stubborn way. It is particularly fascinating to observe how dogmatic trains of thought and undogmatic ideas repeatedly come into conflict with each other, and to what incessant transformations this pursuit of remarks has led here as well, without as yet coming to rest in any perfectly satisfactory conclusion.

One would argue that classical, strict logic (either Eleatic or Aristotelian) has gradually been transformed into a much more flexible modern logic.

(4) From the mathematic side, this process began in Britain around the middle of the 19th century with the work of Boole, Morgan and Jevons and was continued in America by Pierce and his pupil, Mrs. Ladd-Franklin, with

an extension into our time by Reichenbach and Susanne Langer. It acquired its first and provisional conclusion in the fundamentally Anglo-Saxon work, the "Principia Mathematica" of Russell and Whitehead.

Cutting across this development, and also related to it, is the work of the scientifically oriented neo-positivism, primarily stimulated by the Wiener Kreis, of which Wittgenstein, Neurath, Schlick, Carnap and Frank can be counted as the most influential members. In addition to mathematical logic and logical mathematics, lines have been extended to analytical philosophy, significs, semantics and the mathematical linguistics of syntax and grammar which, in turn, are closely related to the development of logic itself.

All these directions and branchings, which have or have had the separate names of logicism, logistics, logical empiricism, symbolic logic or algebraic logic, encounter basically the same difficulties over and over again. The question always remains of how it will ever be possible to explain a system of logic by a system of logic and how it will be able to pull itself out of the quicksand of thought by its own pigtail, like Münchhausen. Hence, again, the effort to build a metalogic or matamathematics.

(5) As we know, these classical problems already began with sophisms and paradoxes[7]: the famous paradoxes of Zeno and especially the Cretan paradox: if a Cretan says: "all Cretans are liars", is this statement true or false? Logic always leads in the last resort to seemingly insoluble aporias, antinomies, anomalies, contradictions or whatever elegant word one wishes to use to indicate or eliminate these problems. It always seems as if the last proof is missing when one wishes, by reasoning in a circle, to prove a thing with itself (expressed in learned terms: circulus in probando or the petitio principii). Hence the indefatigable attempts to prove logic with mathematics and mathematics with logic in which, however, a non-mathematical foundation of logic and a non-logical foundation of mathematics always seems to hamper the construction of a sound system.

Remarkably enough, one also encountered a problem which was already known in Antiquity, that of the natural numbers, or in other words, that of the foundation of mathematics on the itself unfounded arithmetic. One of the most important reformers, insufficiently appreciated in his day, was Gottlob Frege who, at the same time, was one of the founders of formal logic with his "Begriffsschrift" of 1879. He contested Husserl's "Philosophie der Arithmetik" in which a search had been made for a psychological foundation of logic, and tried himself to find a basis for arithmetic in logic. Beside his fellow-German and contemporary Richard Dedekind, we should make separate mention from a somewhat later period of the Italian mathematician Peano who also tried to compose an axiomatic doctrine for natural numbers.

(6) Yet, precisely from the circles of logic and mathematics, continuous

179

criticism was uttered of this methodological reflection on fundamentals. One of the oldest is that of Bolzano, who was dismissed as a Roman Catholic theological professor in Prague in 1820 because of his liberal ideas. Among other things he described the paradoxes of continuity and infinity, which were also agitating mathematics. A century later (1931), K. Gödel proved that no arithmetical system of axioms which would provide proof for every arithmetical thesis could ever be conceivable. In other words, a complete deductive and consistent mathematical theory can never be constructed on the basis of the opinions of arithmetic because the proofs admitted to maintain the consistency of this theory would encounter fundamentally insoluble problems. Several years later, in 1936, A. Church proved, in connection with this, that there are arithmetical theories or suppositions, the correctness or incorrectness of which will have to remain problematic forever.

The Dutch mathematician-philosopher Brouwer then started from the unpresentable proof of the non-contradiction of the basic principles of mathematics because a never-provable non-contradiction of arithmetical assumptions would have to be taken into account. According to him, these contradictions could not be considered impossible, even in Russell's sign language. Thus, in contrast to logicism, he became the founder of the intuitionistic school. One could only accept certain basic theories as true through intuition or by means of evidence. Against that, of course, is the fact that axiomatic systems of non-Euclidean geometry or of a deviating algebra (for instance, where *ab* is not equal to *ba*) can definitely not be called self-evident.

According to Brouwer's system, we should already drop one very important principle of logic as being mathematically untenable, namely the principle of the excluded middle (tertium non datur): something is either *a* a *b*, but there is not a third possibility. Every indirect demonstration was based on this: once one had proved that something definitely could not be untrue, it was therefore automatically and by definition true. As we saw above, Bohr had abandoned this either-or principle (identity) for a both-and principle (complementarity) in quantum physics, logic and mathematics had to follow. As a result the narrow, exclusively bivalent, eleatic logic of Parmenides (with the exclusive choice between being and not-being) was surpassed by a logic which, for instance, could include becoming and being different.

Here lies the beginning of multivalent logic. But at the same time an *irrational* element inevitably enters. One can have a personal preference for a particular logic; this preference can depend on a certain situation, a supposed greater utility or appropriateness, or be based on acceptance of certain conditions and rules for certain applications.

(7) It is understandable, that from the side of logicism, attempts have been made to close this breach, to save what could be saved of the existing system and to maintain it as basically unassailable. However, in order to

escape from the repeatedly appearing paradoxes and contradictions, some strange contortions were required. I may mention some of the attempted escape routes from the dilemma:

(a) One could try to avoid the complications by incorporating, as it were, certain prohibitions in the logical system itself, by excluding certain matters (as had been tried before with the unsuccessful exclusion of the excluded middle).

In quantum physics itself, this direction had already been taken with the so-called Pauli exclusion principle. This meant before jumping to another orbit, an electron was in principle allowed, so to speak, to follow only one out of the different possible orbits. Because of this, every combination of quantum numbers can occur only once.

Russell and Whitehead started from the old robber paradox in a somewhat comparable way. If the robber in question spoke the truth, he would be beheaded on the scaffold; on the other hand, if he lied, he would be hanged on the gallows. The robber said: "I shall die on the gallows". Of course, if this is the truth, it excludes the possibility of his hanging; however, if it is a lie, he would have to be hanged, which, however, by that very fact would then be converted into the truth, etc. This paradox can be supplemented by or changed into the one of the village barber. He has to act only according to two related rules: every man has to be shaved by the only barber in the village, nobody may shave himself. The barber may therefore not shave himself, but, on the other hand, he himself has to be shaved by the only barber, too, i.e. by himself.

This paradox merely expresses in comprehensible language that no system of logic can pronounce on that system of logic, cannot apply to itself and therefore has to be impredicable. To avoid such pronouncements about what, by definition, is impredicable, a prohibition is again introduced which may be designated as the everything-I-prohibition. Consequence: in logic one can speak meaningfully about logical relations, etc., but not about logic (and its fundamentals) itself. The problem has not been solved as much as hidden away. Logical pronouncements about logic as such are meaningless. One can equally forbid other types or classes of pronouncements as meaningless.

(b) Another solution has already been briefly mentioned. Just as one may work with pluriform axiomatic systems, so one can do the same with multivalent logic. The beginning was understandably modest: a trivalent, at most quadrivalent logic. The end, logically and consistently, was a n-valent logic. If there are ultimately more than enough values and different possibilities, one can finally do without prohibitions and restrictive regulations.

Here too the same path was followed in principle as that taken by modern physics. Nuclear physics in particular had adopted a system of mathematical equations for indefinite but probable wave motions.

Logic followed close behind (or sometimes preceded) through the development of a similar n-valent logic notably into a probabilistic logic in which every logical pronouncement could be assigned a possibly more or less determinable probability value, lying between 0 and 1. Martin Strauss tried to build up a special quantum mechanical logic on the basis of this probability logic. Lukasiewicz is one of those who have drawn up tables of values or tables of truth for the conjunctions of certain possibilities and probabilities or impossibilities.

If one considers this course of events, it seems, in itself, not very "probable" that one could, in the final instance, completely exclude the improbable, the irrational and even the illogical from it. It is therefore not surprising that for instance Quine in 1941 could prove that, under certain conditions, no exact distinction can be made between analytical judgments true in themselves (the best example: a pure tautology) and non-analytical assertions and therefore, in principle, or in certain cases, that it is impossible to draw a complete boundary between purely logical and illogical, for instance empirical, sciences.

(c) Hilbert, for instance, took yet another direction and drew up a completely formalized system of axioms, together with Bernays, Ackermann and Pasch, which was claimed to be free of contradictions. However, he too had to admit that the tenets are not all of a logical character. Mathematics itself is consequently now limited to a kind of ever-more refined mental gymnastics with equations. This system of equations extended to the furthest limits of thought, is then, when a demonstration theory is concerned, detached from mathematics and transfered to a new science called metamathesis. This is an elegant escape attempt, with a shifting of problems which, in itself, can of course hardly be regarded as a complete solution, or even claim to be one.

Here too — as with the prohibitions or restrictions — a new set of rules, concepts, agreements, conditions, conventions, constants and definitions is concerned. In this, one can always agree not to solve the one insoluble problem and not assert the crux of uncertainty by expressly putting it out of operation or sidetracking it.

(d) In my opinion, however, the most important renewals eventuated from having forcibly to reckon with Becoming in and changing through time.

Aristotle, precisely for the same reason, had already felt the need to expand the too simple, bivalent Eleatic logic. In addition to the pronouncements true and false, he added modalities for possible and impossible, chance and necessary, potential (acorn) and actual (oak). With this the theory of absolute identity was dropped and a transition to the principle of complementarity effected: the acorn grows into an oak, from frog spawn grow tadpoles and then frogs. This is at least possible and even, in certain circumstances, probable, although not strictly necessary. Basically, the principle of the excluded middle is already rejected here. For as soon as the values

182

"chance" and "possible" are added, one leaves the bivalent scheme of true and false and trades it at least for a trivalent scheme in which there is room, for instance, for neither true nor false.

As regards time, one can reduce this expanded modality logic again to a bivalent scheme and then operate with the values now and later. However, this gives no solution for the uncertain change in time, and such a system means literally going backward.

(8) As the reader will remember, quantum physics had also already wrestled with the problem of time. The idea of the continuity of time divided into fixed points of time — as with Newton and Leibnitz — had had to be abandoned. There was no exactly definable and divisible point of time for every situation. This was due both to the established discontinuity in the leaps of electrons from one orbit to another and to the fact that as long as one wanted at least to determine their spatial location exactly, this point of time, depending on the speed and power of motion, proved uncertain. Heisenberg, Schrödinger, De Broglie and Dirac had therefore to discount the changing event in time in a mathematical calculation of probability. In addition to this, Einstein, as previously stated, was obliged to include macrocosmic time in a relatively curved, four-dimensional space-time continuum which behaved according to postulates other than those of the classical laws of motion.

(9) However, computer cybernetics and space travel also made new demands of a modernized and elastic logic of time which could digest the processes of changing in temporal events (real time processing). Thus a special computer logic and information logic were created.[8] The continued exploration of the cosmos, building on Einstein, will undoubtedly lead further into a separately refined logic of exploration and communication which will be applicable to a worldwide relay system of artificial satellites or surveyors and their increasingly deeper penetration into space and time.

(10) How the possibilities and the possible limits lie in that respect is still difficult to say, because modern logic itself, as the result of an ever-increasingly accelerated rate of technological development, is also still fully in progress and subject to change. A. M. Turing has already proved that machines working on the solution of problems can also definitely not be restricted to a simple true-false logic if they are indeed to give useful and accurate answers. However, just how this bivalent restriction can be overcome, especially in thinking machines with their still current, essentially bivalent switching logic of 0 or 1, is a more difficult question to the solution of which intelligent machines themselves, in due course, will perhaps be able to make a fruitful contribution. The answer will probably be given also with the aid of a *stochastic* logic which has modalities for chance and growth built into its system.

183

(11) Here, however, it is not necessary to go further into these already realized or probably still further extensible refinements or ramifications of logic. For our purpose, it is more than sufficient that we can already indisputably establish how greatly classical logic has already and long been surpassed and outstripped by a modern, more and more complicated logic. Or rather perhaps by pluriform logical systems of thought which demand the utmost of an extremely flexible and completely unconstrained thinking that is far removed from classical logical styles of thought and long undisputed, prevailing strict methods of thinking. The new, broader approach equals — and runs parallel to — that of modern physics. Here too the measure and scope of that broadness can only be designated by rather big words like deviation, transformation and even revolution. Big words, but not *too* big.

5. Dogmatic certainty and prognostic uncertainty

In view of the multiplicity of movement and diversification of concept-forming, with corresponding modern versions of mathematical logic or logical mathematics, it might still seem somewhat premature to draw certain conclusions. Yet I do not wish to obstain from making some provisionally concluding marginal notes on this wildly fluctuating process of motion.

As regards these repeatedly renewed efforts and shifts in *these* fields, the most striking thing to me seems to be the attachment to the heart of the best philosophical tradition, according to which *no lasting bond* with any philosophical tradition or the prejudices resulting from it is acceptable in the long run. A gratifying, anti-dogmatic attitude of mind, attended with and testifying to great freshness, freedom and independence with regard to new ideas is characteristic of this development right down the line. To this extent it is also possible to observe an unmistakable analogy and affinity with the transformation from classical into modern natural science outlined above.

One could state that a general search has been undertaken in order to find or construct a new pons asinorum for thinking so that — to keep in style — after having set foot on it, the sheep can be clearly distinguished from the goats, i.e. the free and liberal thinkers from the orthodox and all the more so from the unteachable. Only the problem is that the most liberal, too — a genius such as Wittgenstein is one of the few exceptions which confirms this rule — as soon as they think they have finally found the way, tend in turn to go over to the camp of the orthodox. Or, in other words, they begin to consider that only their own pronouncements are sensible and all others are senseless. Consequently, a new, more liberal movement will also have set those pronouncements, considered in a monopolistic, dogmatic way as exclusively valid, aside again as senseless or, at least, not exclusively sensible.

This is in fact already happening in reality. For in the comprehensive effort of reform, including the removal or an outmoded and fossilized dogmatics, two main lines gradually deviating from each other but reinforcing themselves are — if I see aright — beginning to stand out.

(1) In the one line a natural desire for the restoration of equilibrium seems to me to be the most characteristic aspect. All that existed has been demolished and an attempt made to create something new and better in its place. But for this new construction too, which is regarded by its creators as extremely successful, these creators are again seeking the best possible certainty, preferably indisputable and infallible.

(2) In the other line, the most striking thing seems to be the admission and acceptance of a certain degree of uncertainty which is after all inherent in the nature of things, in both their existing infrastructure and their dynamic structural change, and therefore inevitable. In other words, uncertainty both as a shaky starting-point and as an unavoidable change of the latter in time. Then too, almost a fortiori, a scientific code likewise changing itself urges and compels the acquisition of a perhaps no longer absolute but at least relatively maximum certainty.

Re 1. The development towards the direct acquisition of more certainty can be traced back to the search for permanent systems or methods of logical mathematical formulation and formalization. Just as Nietzsche wanted to liberate philosophy from the final tyranny, that of truth, so neo-positivism and logicism in particular want to free us from the tyranny of the word. They oppose the unclear verbalism dominating philosophy and especially noticeable in its metaphysical and ontological systems of thought. They wish to replace it by purely physical, i.e. logical systems of thought.

However, there is an invisible but dangerous snag in using the word "pure". What is pure? According to some, it means a liberation from unproven suppositions and hypotheses. According to others, it means a purging of everything that is not basically observable and provable. Let me try to demonstrate, with one striking example, how such postulates must per se lead to untenable positions. One of the first, most shrewd and influential protagonists of this neo-positivism in the second half of the 19th century was undoubtedly the Austrian physicist Ernst Mach. For instance, he emphatically condemned any atomic theory as senseless and useless. In itself, this was perfectly logical and consistent with the ideal of a physics free from hypotheses: at that time no physicist had been able to prove the hypothetical existence of atoms or even make it plausible.

This conviction was therefore fully shared during that period by a large number of prominent physicists. The direct proof of the existence of atoms (a theory which had already been held some 2500 years ago by the atomistic

185

natural philosophy of Leucippus and Democritus!) was not given until several decades later in our 20th century with the aid of the discovered X-rays and the techniques of diffraction applied to these rays. This example, however, is much more of a paradox than it might appear at first glance. For the physicists were only finally convinced of the existence of atoms when it was proved that they did *not* exist, that is, not as the last, indivisible, elementary building blocks of matter. In fact, the enforced acknowledgment was, remarkably enough, really and rightly a denial at the same time. They only started to believe in atoms when these broke down into nuclei and an ever-increasing number of subatomic particles. Precisely at the point when one begins to puzzle about the question of what, properly speaking, exists in reality or is "pure" as a mathematical formula. As so often happens, we moreover see here again too that the scientific postulate is not applied to itself: the term pure is definitely not purified from a linguistic point of view.

For the rest, neo-positivism leads pre-eminently to preceding analysis of language, its syntax and grammar, and from there to a logical, mathematical linguistics, exactly expressed in unmistakably clear symbols, signs, letters, relations, formulas and figures no longer open to misunderstanding. For linguistics as such, this analysis is certainly of great importance.

Danger threatens when thought itself, and all scientific thought models, have to be covered by its cloak. This danger comprises essentially two things. In the first place that once again it is compulsorily laid down dogmatically, and therefore once again aprioristically, apodictally and aggressively how a scientific procedure may and must occur exclusively. In the second place, there is a considerable risk with this that linguistic analysis and construction entails a reduction of reality which can then only be grasped as a cross-section or snapshot. In this case, however, it is extremely probable that the process of structural growth and transformation, the kaleidoscopically shifting pattern and the constantly renewing architecture, as the changing image of the whole, cannot be understood. In other words, in terms of my own verbalism, this lacks a synthetic view of the totality and also a perspective image of the future.

Now progressive thinkers know this of course themselves. They naturally adduce, at the same time, that the existence of different languages of thought and methods of expression also entails the relativization of corresponding linguistic logic. On the other hand, however, a continuous effort to prove that all these languages in turn exhibit some uniform and universal primordial characteristics opposes this acknowledged relativization. Thus the old dream of a "mathesis universalis" returns — blood thirsting for certainty is thicker than water. This is only imaginable in terms of one methodologically valid logic for all science, leading, therefore, to a "unity of science" supplied with one essential basic structure.

While the symbolic logic and criticism of language thus began to elucidate and unmask all kinds of profound philosophical discussions as sham problems, it is now equally in danger itself of lapsing into coercive, doctrinaire tenets. Neo-positivism, which built on the in itself fertile, renewing positivism of Comte, Mill, Mach, etc., has undoubtedly formed an indispensable transitory stage in its attack on untenable aprioristic and dogmatic ways of thought. After reaching maturity, it tends after exaggeration towards a defensive attitude of mind which proceeds to display all the signs of a renewed dogmatics and which will therefore have to be conquered and broadened itself. For it now threatens to become bogged down in its exact formulas which, insofar as they are significant and positive, are often no more than tautology. However, insofar as they are seized by a mad fear of the word, content sense and totality, such formulas may end up either in meaningless, negative pronouncements or in absolute silence and barren emptiness. They may thus in fact be "clear and obvious" according to Descartes' classic motto, but meaningless as a solution for dynamic problems.

Re 2. The other line takes an, at least originally, quite different starting-point. It recognizes that human thinking, scientific thinking included, is unavoidably associated with axioms, postulates, premises, suppositions or hypotheses no longer demonstrable in themselves, with written and unwritten rules, methods, or whatever names one wishes to give to these starting-points — also including their own initial starting-points or last bases.

His history of philosophy, or of metaphysics and ontology, has in fact always struggled, and always in vain, with these fundamental starting-points under different names. With Plato, the transcendental, perfect ideas formed the primordial source of all knowledge. With Plotinus, the One, the divine spirit or "nous" (as "causa sui", i.e. existing as an independent, primary beginning). This is the provisional end of a long philosophical road beginning with the Indeterminate (apeiron) of Anaximander, refined by Xenophanes into the eternal and only Godhead, continued to the fervently animated pneuma and the rational logos of the Stoa. Aristotle called these founding, inscrutable starting-points the first causes; Descartes innate ideas; Leibnitz primary truths (for instance finding expression in metaphysical monads); Spinoza a divine-natural substance; Kant aprioristic synthetic judgments, as with Aristotle divided into categories; Hegel a rational world spirit; Schopenhauer the will to observe; Nietzsche the will for power; Husserl the essential being; Heidegger the existential Sein zum Tode, etc., etc.[9]

We are and remain conscious that these starting-points are dependent on such mental representations as intuition, evidence, surveys of essence, speculation, etc. We can arm ourselves against them with large doses of skepticism, historico-critical insight and an undogmatic attitude. We can even look at purely speculative philosophy, such as Hegel's, for instance, which reached a spiritual climax, with appropriate distrust and reject this direction, coinciding here with the first one mentioned under 1, as completely unfounded with respect to its content of truth.

Nevertheless, on the other hand, we ought to continue to be impressed by the well-known pronouncement of a genius at renewing mathematics such as Gauss: "I have already found the definite solutions; I only have to find the proofs". The Dutch mathematician Van de Corput already proved, before the invention of thinking machines, with simple calculations, that even a rather limited human thought process is not possible without creative imagination. The number of mental actions for decisions which have to be taken is so tremendously large that even the non-existent, lightning-fast, purely logical mathematician, needing only one millionth of a second for each action, would require astronomical periods of time to answer a relatively simple question. Creative, speculative thinkers such as Gauss and Einstein, who themselves were very conscious of the value and truth of this postulate, were exceptions, however.

One gets the impression that most thinkers, even if the inherent uncertainty of the chosen starting-points is taken as given, are nevertheless ultimately deterred by the radical consequences of his boldness. How can they know if they are on the right track? What guarantee is there for scientific work and truth? Sooner or later — certainly not least under the influence of the first-mentioned direction — here too doubt is transformed into a renewed need for certainty and a strictly responsible scientific approach.

In that case, this direction is irresistibly drawn toward inductive and empirical logic. In terms of methodology, this introduces the requirement that every scientific theory must be verified in order to establish its validity as such. Such confirmation after the event sanctions the starting-point chosen in advance.

This is in itself a completely reasonable requirement which, however, can be denatured or, in its turn, absolutized. Particularly by the addition that such verification must be applied continuously and immediately as an indispensable part of any self-respecting procedure calling itself scientific.

One is then inclined to forget or neglect the fact that a fulfilment à la minute of this postulate is impossible in certain circumstances. This is an impossibility which may extend over a definite length of time or even one that is indefinite in advance.

In 1781, Herschel discovered the planet Urbanus with a home-made telescope. In 1846, Leverrier discovered the theoretical existence of a planet, Neptune, which at that time was the one most remote from the sun. He did so on the basis of systematic research into celestial mechanics and also on the strength of interferences exerted on the orbit of Uranus. Legend has it that he was in no way interested in experiments which would actually trace and observe Neptune in space. Consequently, his findings lacked verification for a considerable time. Now the question is too seldom asked whether the

188

theory was, therefore, invalid or at best in abeyance as long as this observation had not been actually made — and this was to be so for quite a long time — and crowned with success.

This phenomenon repeated itself when, again because of inexplicable interferences in the orbits of Neptune and Uranus, the existence of an even more remote, trans-Neptunian planet had to be assumed, although determination of the correct direction and position gave great difficulties. The interval of time for verification, however, was much shorter in this case and in 1930 the planet Pluto was in fact discovered.

Einstein's theory of relativity existed for quite a long time without any verification, and even seemed in flat contradiction of certain experiments of that time. Einstein himself, as stated, did not take part in the experiments appraising his renovating theory, which extended over several decades. Was his theory not valid in the meantime, was his work unscientific or not scientifically sound? No one would dare to maintain this now. Yet this conclusion is logically implied by a narrow, strictly doctrinaire interpretation of the dogma of verification.

Einstein's theory of relativity has also been of the greatest conceivable influence on astronomy and cosmology. The Dutch astronomer De Sitter has been able to make certain predictions on the basis of the Einsteinian speculative theories and calculations, predictions which have later been verified by others as being true. But precisely this field of cosmology, as previously established, is, at present, the one field pre-eminently open to new, different, sometimes very daring and always speculative theories. In connection with the principle of spectral shifts (nebular systems move away from earth at a velocity proportional to their distance) or with certain chemical and geological investigations, attempts are still being made to bring the mysteries of origin and decay, of infinite and finite, of expansion and contraction of primordial matter, of space, time, distance, speed, motion, change, etc., in the universe closer to a solution.

Needless to say, support is sought as far as possible from facts for the correctness of these highly divergent hypothetical theories. But no one in his right mind would nowadays dare to make the strict demands of an absolutely complete verification which is not at variance with a single phenomenon. Such aprioristically valid, imperative and unsparing prescriptions are naturally not applicable here at all and therefore, not at issue either. Besides, quite apart from the more searching question of what exactly constitutes fact[10], one now knows from long and mature experience that large numbers of facts can be combined into theoretically divergent interpretations. Their mutual differences are often by no means reduced by newly added factual observations, but sometimes even considerably increased. The enormous mobility, expansion and explosion of these new and repeatedly newer theoretical working and explanatory hypotheses keep in step with the events studied in the vortex of the universe itself. After the successive discoveries of gigantic interstellar nebulae of innumerable other solar and galactic systems and of various types of extragalactic nebulae, supernovae, quasars, cosmic radiations and belts, etc., and also anticipating the discoveries which will doubtless follow in this field.

Logically speaking, it is hardly possible to give a rational explanation of why that which is permitted, even as a matter of course, for something so immeasurably immense must, on the contrary, be regarded as completely forbidden, by the strictest ukase, for the development of theories on a reduced earthly scale. For that matter, in addition to the exception made for the macrocosmos, that made for the microcosmos holds good just as much. Theoretical predictions of certain behavior in nuclear physics, as well as of the hypothetical but undeniable existence of certain particles which, at that moment, are still concealing themselves from every attempt at observation, have sometimes not been verified experimentally until a considerable time later. Alternatively, they have not yet been verified, or have to be accepted as a provisionally inexplicable, possibly even unprovable, in short as a so far tenuous mirage.

The strict methodological postulate of verification, in the sense of a proof which is immediately and directly required upon the creation of a hypothetical theory, testifies to a quite alarming and astounding lack of general knowledge of the history of science, and indeed precisely of an absence of understanding of the theory of knowledge. It betrays an absolute lack of realization of the basic meaning of a requirement of predictability which is also connected with it. For, if one could prove a prediction immediately, this would be a contradiction in terms: in that case it would not be a prediction, but a purely tautological statement. The neutron predicted by Rutherford was discovered 10 years later; this could in principle have been 5, 50 or 100 years as well. Fifteen years ago, the direct linear relation between the gene structure (in accordance with the information code of DNA and RNA) and the structure of protein was predicted: this has recently been confirmed. At present, all kinds of hypothetical forms of explanation, motivation models and predictive information theories are being drawn up about the nature and the workings of the human brain with the aid of physics, neurophysiology, biochemistry, psychology, mathematics and cybernetics, etc.[11] In the next quarter of a century, we shall see it decided more exactly whether, and to what extent, this predictive material will, or can be confirmed. The same is true, mutatis mutandis, of various hypothetical methods of explanation concluded in part from synthetic experiments on the origin of life. No right-minded person will regret that the human brain or the living organism itself is now, much more intensively than ever before, becoming the object of interdisciplinary research. It would be absolute and complete nonsense to attach to that the immediate requirement of absolute and complete verification. This postulate has a function only at a point on the scale of the *future* which cannot be defined more closely. Here and now it cannot but cancel itself out or contradict itself. Future confirmation or denial is the only requirement that can be rightly made. It being understood that an explicit refutation often proves to have the greatest driving force for real progress.

I therefore feel that one must be very careful not to detach the postulate of verification which, in itself, is to be appreciated as a wise prescription, from its elastic and functional movement in time. One should be on one's guard against elevating it to the unlimited power of a dogma which always applies inexorably and from moment to moment to every scientific researcher, no matter what his field. For, in that case, one might bar the way to the theoretical reform which in retrospect may prove to be the most fruitful one, restrain or almost stop scientific progress in an intolerable fashion by a methodological whetting of knives. In that case a modern natural science would not have come into being, or at least not as it is now. Why impose this unbearable compulsion outside this science? The chance of a completely opposite effect than becomes considerably more probable. Precisely because of that, the *inferiority complex* which prompts this compulsively neurotic procedure and pre-eminently dogmatic methodology would indeed run the risk of changing into a real, almost irreparable *inferiority*.

This fault becomes all the more serious if and insofar as verification, as a law of the Medes and Persians, is also connected with the inexorable postulate of quantification. This is, for instance, expressed in the motto of Lord Kelvin: if you are able to measure what you are talking about and express it in numbers, then you know something about it. In itself, this is definitely not incorrect and it is also beneficial to much of scientific research. However, the logical principle of the excluded middle underlies this again; if you cannot measure it, and if you cannot express it in numbers, then you do not know anything about it. In adopting such an attitude, one does not worry about the fact — or one simply does not realize — that certain fields or researches are not at all (not yet or ever) tractable to measuring and calculating operations. These would therefore automatically be excluded with one stroke of the pen, pushed under the table with one wave of the arm, however important they may be in themselves, indeed urgently required for the acquisition of more knowledge. Such a prescription, which narrows the mind, is based on deplorable conceit. It is not only anti-philosophical in general (which it is often also meant to be), it is, in addition to that, also anti-natural science in a wider sense and very particularly anti-social science. As a rule, the one-sided measurement and calculation controller knows nothing of this last field, though he thus unconsciously influences it considerably and exerts great pressure on it. A pressure which is too heavy and which might discharge some time in an asocial manner, precisely because of improper abstinence from the scientific investigations which are exorcised on the strength of such a stringent prohibition.

This reprehensible attitude of mind too is unfortunately still a rudimentary dominant of an obsolete and meanwhile strongly changed natural scientific thought model. A speculatively theorizing and therefore non-dogmatic Einstein could at least represent his new, unconventional and nonconformist ideas in mathematical relations, formulae and models. This is also true on the whole of astronomy, cosmology and quantum physics, high-energy physics and molecular biology, in short, by definition, of all exact science. Not all science, however, allows itself to be squeezed into the framework of a pure exact science, even if the highest attainable degree of precision is aimed at.

This is especially true in the field of social science of many branches of modern prognostics which will come up for discussion separately. Here we are in a world which can at the very least expect capricious chance and at best assume the probability of change in time which cannot always be precisely measured or calculated in advance and which is only verifiable after the event, because not until then can it be observed.

Dogmatics and prognostics are fundamentally incompatible. For penetration into the dimension of the future a specific logic of the future and a mathematics of the future are also required in which speculation *and* verification, quality *and* quantity, intuition and consistency have in principle equal rights, which are equally indispensable and unconditionally necessary in pairs.[12]

The two logical and empirical directions of thought broadly described here are already tending too much to close themselves off for good, in order to acquire or retain certainty as the highest value. Again and again they should do as they did in the past and, by making sufficient concessions, open themselves for the future too to a visionary, renewing power of thought with a built-in minimum degree of uncertainty. Only in this way will we be able to make our future to some extent . . . *certain.*

6. To know is to predict, not to predict is not to know

But let us leave economics on one side for the moment, and psychology too. Are we then left with a sufficiently large complex of exact and other sciences that can be regarded, as in De Groot's approach,[13] as "behavioral sciences"? I think that sociology may fairly be taken as a representative pars pro toto. How does De Groot's methodology apply to this particular case? His key proposition again comes to mind: If I know something, I can predict; if I cannot predict, then I know nothing.

The first reaction to this is automatically to declare that in that case, sociology, which predicts nothing, and neither wishes nor is permitted to predict, knows nothing and is *not* a science. And yet it would surely be both unfair and incorrect to label all social science with the socratic aphorism "The only thing I know is that I know nothing". The social sciences have amassed a rich store of cognitive potential; but its application is in part absent, and in part wrong or inadequate.

The irony of history, once again, is that in its early origins sociology enthroned by Comte with considerable acclaim and seen above all as a new, urgently necessary *predictive* science which would even look down condescendingly on all other, exact, sciences; but that even if modern sociology still means anything, not a word is ever breathed now about its predictive capacity. Its thought model (cf. Chapter 8) is now a pre-eminently no-future model.

If one recalls in broad outline the historical account given earlier, it is not difficult to appreciate this fundamental change of mental attitude. For a long time it was believed that — as with the classical natural sciences — laws of social movement and development, or at least structural laws or partial formulae for particular situations, could be discovered. These would have made it possible to unfold and accurately forecast the future as a splendid panorama, in accordance with the Leibnitz-Laplace world-formula. Unfortunately, no such laws have ever been found. On the contrary, nearly everyone is now convinced that they never can be found. For the simple reason that, according to this consensus of opinion, they do not exist. That glorious sociological picture of the future has been thoroughly tarnished by sociology itself. As it happens, quite rightly too, in so far as it was exclusively tied to a dogmatic, unvarying future-model that had very little to do with the real future.

It is not simply that the cherished idea of the possibility of future forecasting based on causal-legalistic and thus determinate connections has had to be wholly renounced; this illusion has also been destroyed in other ways. For what were the findings of the empirical investigation of social reality? The realization began to gain ground that it could no longer be regarded as a systematically ordered and essentially unchanging cosmos but on the contrary had proved to be a capricious, erratically shifting mass of a well-nigh chaotic and in any event incalculable nature. If Goethe still talked of the cosmos as "der Gottheit lebendiges Kleid", this could now be regarded as no more than an aesthetic view of nature.[14] But for social developments especially, such a divine-cosmic description seemed now devoid of all validity as an empirical reflection of reality. The essential characteristic of the new social reality, and not a particularly attractive one, is continuous change instead of unchanging beauty. Social dynamics, and its often convulsive tides and violent fluctuations, affects every social researcher. The acceleration of tempo and the ever-increasing impact of social change as regards intensity, range and scale, have a disturbing effect on any research that is undertaken. How could the average investigator lay any convincing claim to socio-scientific predictability, with the ground subsiding or moving beneath his feet, leaving him no firm spot on which to stand?

And this *despite* the fact that *in other respects* he adopts the same criterion of logical empiricism.

Let us look at it again in this light. He can either try to escape the avalanche of events by constructing a timeless, logically consistent and formal-abstract theory which as such is indisputably valid. But because it says little or nothing about concrete reality, it is of course even less capable of commenting on a future that is also concrete and will presumably be very different again. Its value is only one of deaf-and-dumb certainty, not one of previsionary truth.

Alternatively, he can declare a preference for the empirical and experimental study of existing reality, for an analysis of its component parts. However, the present of the here-and-now is as a whole so full of pulsation and fluctuation, so complex, difficult to grasp and comprehend as an entity, that it can only be studied in a piecemeal and fragmentary way, by dividing it up into isolated portions and miniaturized units.

But how can the process of disintegrating the whole, of taking it out of context and reducing it to tiny individually studied portions, yield any reasonable certainty about a future development in which everything is again related to everything else and which it is assumed will be quite different?

To this must be added a factor that we should not underestimate, whose effect here is exactly the opposite of that which it has in some important areas of natural science, the time lapse between the postulation of a theory and the sufficiently comprehensive and satisfactory verification of it can sometimes be relatively, perhaps extremely, long. So long that some researchers will not live to witness it. Einstein was still alive to receive the acclaim that his intellectual innovation brought him, after decades of intensive and systematic study by many thousands of research workers in numerous adjacent fields. It may be doubted whether a number of no longer youthful astronomers and cosmologists now erecting speculative theories of the utmost profundity, will live to see them rebutted, confirmed or modified. Copernicus' revolutionary work on the revolution of the heavenly spheres appeared in the Nuremberg edition just in time to be given to the author on his death-bed (in 1543). His death saved him from the Inquisition: the book was not placed on the Index until 1616, whereupon it was immediately published in Amsterdam in 1617. At that time Galileo too, a follower of Copernicus, was already at odds with the Church about the latter's teaching. All in all, it was more than a century before Copernicus was fully confirmed (by Newton) and received posthumously the full honor that was due to him.

Cosmic time reckons in terms of hundreds of millions of light-years and more. The movement of terrestrial time, and of social reality in particular, is approached in a quite different order or magnitude, subject to an accelerated tempo of development. Even before a forecast about it — assuming it is a short-term one, since anyone who looks further ahead is not a student of social science but at best a visionary or a prophet — can be really completely checked and verified, the chances are that the future of the forecast has already passed into the present or even the past. Though it can go on being discussed afterwards (post factum), the anticipatory value has been completely eroded and devalued by the acceleration of tempo during the period in question. The most that could be said then is: "I knew something", certainly not, unconditionally: "I know something".

Now it is a fact that De Groot deals superfically with consequences of this kind, at one point only I think, in his 400-page book.[15] To illustrate them he takes two types of Gestalt theory which, mutatis mutandis, show a remarkable degree of agreement with the type-theory indicated here in connection with sociological theory formation (i.e. a concrete-present part-theory as compared to a timeless, abstract-formal general theory). He observes of theories like these that they "are better abandoned; firstly because they provide very accurate knowledge about almost nothing, and secondly because they provide excessively vague knowledge about almost everything".[16] With the latter pronouncement I most heartily agree. Only De Groot apparently fails to realize that if generalization is necessary and legitimate here — and that is my own standpoint — then he himself has delivered a mortal blow to the Achilles' heel of his whole methodology. Such linguistic metaphors, borrowed in this case from the Homeric epic, are permitted by De Groot in the first instance[17], though I fear that he will grant no more than "surplus significance" to the image I have used for figurative illustration here, or that he will dismiss it as an unscientific "interpretation scheme" (in the good company, by the way, of both the Oedipus and the inferiority complex, among others[18]). Fortunately, within the framework of a strict scientific code there are always means enough of making a person feel, if he simply will not listen, with the help of technical jargon. Nevertheless, I shall make so bold as to remark that De Groot fails to show how his methodology could ever give rise to another, *third* and more fruitful type of theory.

My criticism may appear to be resolving itself into a rather disparaging negativism. Doubly negative, as regards both this logical-empirical methodology and sociology, or the social sciences, which tend in this direction. But such is not the case. In fact, the opposite is true. I should be extremely happy to see the key feature of this methodology raised to the status of a motto for the social sciences: if I know something, I can predict: if I cannot predict, I know nothing. Conversely, though, this would inevitably entail a revolution in the special methodology of the social sciences as it has prevailed hitherto[19], since they cannot now predict anything and, partly for that reason, have no desire to. Furthermore, it would seem the abandonment of other, not unimportant parts of De Groot's methodology for the behavioral sciences which he has forged into a coherent, normative system. In reality, though, the word "predict" proves to have a much less clear meaning than it should rightly be possible to assume. In De Groot's system, the meaning of the term in fact shrinks to the emphatic repetition and confirmation of what may be presumed to be known and familiar already. In the eyes of true prognostics, that is virtually the equivalent of *not* predicting! For me, prediction means a dynamic striving towards and penetration into the realm of the not-yet-known (or the not-known-for-sure).

This is not the place in which to analyze in great detail the implications of all this. For the sake of clarity, however, a rough outline of at least some of the guiding principles will not come amiss.

Those who take as their starting-point the unity of the sciences, as expounded by a number of leading neo-positivists such as Schlick[20], Von Neurath[21] and Reichenbach[22], with whom De Groot principally associates himself[23], are rightly able to adduce certain arguments for their position. I leave unanswered the question whether *all* the earlier objections to them by thinkers like Rickert, Windelband, Dilthey, Troeltsch and Max Weber should rightly have been swept aside with one disdainful gesture.

But I must add two reservations here. Firstly, that this unity of science was wrong to look (as it still often does) for a link with the classical physical-nomothetic cognitive model; and in my view, without properly realizing the extent to which the modern thought-models of natural science have already moved away from it, with in many respects cognitively critical differences of an almost black-white degree.

In the pursuit of a scientific unity on particular points of methodology, or in a justified attempt at at least some measure of unification, this can also lead to extremely profound differences.

In the second place — and to my mind of decisive importance in this connection — the fact that an ineradicable and wholly essential difference always continues to exist between the social sciences and the natural sciences, however they are practised (classical or modern), is as a rule totally ignored. It is a fundamental difference which can leave unmistakably specific and extra-ordinarily deep marks on the practice of the social sciences too. In principle though, it need by no means stand in the way of close collaboration.

Since Francis Bacon, one view of the natural sciences has persisted almost unchanged, like a theme with variations. Thinking men are able to detect a certain order and regularity in nature. By determining and recording man is able, while himself obeying the laws of nature theoretically reconstructed or synthesized in this way, to acquire indirectly and increasing measure of power over that part of nature. The universe itself he must accept as a given reality, but by continual exploration and unraveling of its secrets he is more and more able to control and dominate it and subdue it to his own will.

7. Changefulness and changeability

Nevertheless, there is and there remains one ineradicable difference between these given natural phenomena and the existing social reality. Social science can of course try to approach nearer and nearer to the latter by means of comparable thought models and its analogously operating, theoretically regulatory devices. What I am referring to here as deviating from this concordant pattern is not the relative, if gradually and steadily growing difference from the reality of global phenomena, as regards the *changefulness* of social phenomena that has played such a great, and increasing, role in the past century and particularly in our own time. That is not the only reason why uncritical copying of successful thought models of natural science, was doomed on every occasion to dismal failure.

The fundamental difference to which I refer has to do with the possibility which exists in principle, of the *changeability* of social reality[24]; that it may be changed by man directly, not indirectly, through the application of *human power*. Not therefore, repeat *not*, by observing rigorous obedience to acquired knowledge, but rather by rebellious *dis*obedience towards vested interests. All social reality is a *man-made situation*, with forms of existence and substance that man can *transform* if he so desires.

One could philosophize about this at great length, of course. Briefly however, and greatly simplified, it comes down to the idea that the cosmos was not created by man, but is and remains a datum for him. For this reason, all cosmogonic mythologies and religions, from the most ancient times, have had to create the idea of a Creator with superior power. A quite different cosmos would be conceivable only as a divine (or natural) miracle.[25] If, for example, man uses his acquired knowledge of nature to transform matter into energy or vice versa, or changes one form of elementary matter into another, or gas into plasma; or if he brings about atomic fusion or fission, indeed even if he should succeed in destroying the planet Earth or reducing it to primeval chaos by sparking off a chain of nuclear reactions, he has still achieved only superficial, external changes. Nature and the cosmos as such have not been changed; in their most profound essence, they are not really changeable by mankind. Nor would this be the case of the human race were, for instance, to control climate and so bring rain as required to the parched deserts, or cause rain to fall only at night in the future. The same would be true in principle if, say, the whole terrestrial globe were to be moved to another point in the universe. But if at some time, e.g. in the Biblical sense (as Joshua caused the sun to stand still), men could temporarily or permanently halt the sun and the planets at will, or reduce the speed of light, which is constant everywhere in the universe, or make time run backwards, only then — philosophically speaking — could the question of changeability, in natural phenomena too, arise. Relative to the perhaps infinite and in any case unmeasurable vastness of the universe and its countless galaxies, such comparatively trivial matters as the drying or desalinization of bits of the sea, the melding of the polar ice-cap, the prevention of hurricanes and other natural calamities, or even profound alterations to the seasonal cycle, are not of the same order of magnitude.

197

For then one would still be operating *in accordance with* the principles and potentials, *within* the framework of the natural or cosmic regularities or probabilities whose existence had been discovered. These are by no means rendered inoperative. They are controlled in part and up to a certain level, but not basically overruled. In its germ-cells and in its essence, despite all the gradual changes and local transformations, even irrespective of the evolution of living organisms on earth and in the sea, or elsewhere in the universe, nature is now precisely the same as it was a million years ago, and without a doubt as it will be in a million years' time. The changes, whether "natural" ones, or explosive ones with power to create and destroy, or resulting from human action, however far-reaching they may be, make no difference. Man acts in and on the cosmos, but the cosmos is not man's, it is not his handiwork. The cosmos is, as it were, *laid out* or *laid down* for man. If he can find the appropriate keys, he can tinker with an extremely tiny part of it. He can do no more, however important it may already be — and it will undoubtedly become more and more essential — that he should. On the other hand, the social reality on earth (and soon outside it) is the *work of man*, created by the human creature who was in turn initially a subordinate ingredient of cosmic reality or substance. Culture, civilization and their history are all man-made.

The triumphs of the natural sciences have gradually disguised this fundamental difference between cosmic and social reality, or even paradoxically turned it upside-down. It is nature, on the contrary, that is often thought of as being changeable in principle, even especially so, while social actuality is only regarded as continually changeful. The first notion is wrong, the second incomplete. Not only is nature, as a Ding an sich, *not* fundamentally changeable despite all the possible ways, both potential and implemented, of transforming its elements or constituent parts. Further, the changefulness of social phenomena is in fact a secondary consequence of their primary, potential *changeability*. Only if we properly reflect on the equivocal, wholly erroneous, and — once again — essentially dogmatic way of thinking exposed here, shall we be able to break through it. This has considerable, indeed surprising and extremely far-reaching consequences for the social sciences. Much might be said about them in the framework of philosophical sociology or, if you like, social philosophy and social ethics, and of course of political sociology or concrete social politics. I will confine myself here to the intermediate region characterized by the diametrically opposed poles of dogmatics on the one hand and prognostics on the other, and offer just a couple of introductory observations.

(a) It is immediately obvious that, seen from the standpoint of the social scientist, there exist two particular facets of thought relative to the observable, man-made social reality. From a didactic point of view, both these facets are in some respects comparable to the twosome of pure and applied natural science, though they are certainly not identical. The social science, after all, is concerned with a kind of duplication of reality — the reality evidently present as the existing order, as against a quite different reality which would or could have been, and indeed, according to certain views on society, should have been or will have to be. This contraposition is related to that between "sein-müssen" and "sein-sollen", which is quite inconceivable in the case of nature and the cosmos; the antithesis between that which now exists de facto as the result of a historical development hitherto brought about by man himself and other, equally possible (but not necessarily desirable) developments. Developments which could have occurred in the past or, in view of the postulated principle of changeability, are intrinsically conceivable as a possible form of the future. This duplication can perhaps still be best expressed using the terminology of Leibnitz: on one side are *"les vérités faites"*: on the other, *"les vérités à faire"*.

(b) The human race is potentially capable of radically changing and re-creating its reality. The extent of these possibilities, and the precise limits of human power, are questions we shall leave aside for the moment. Suffice it to make the virtually unarguable assertion that while these possibilities have always existed as such, they have constantly grown and become capable of faster realization. A parallel phenomenon is that the frontiers of what once seemed impossible have repeatedly to be pushed back a long way and at an ever-greater rate to a new spiritual horizon that is continually forced to recede. All this is part of the new era of exponential acceleration and transformation that has dawned (see Chapter 15), or, to put it another way, of the impressive transition from groping *Homo Viator* to purposeful *Homo Creator*.

Thus it is that the social sciences are faced with problems quite different from those of the natural sciences. The key question is surely this: can and should human power be refined and sustained by knowledge acquired from social science, an exercise of ever-greater and more extensive scientific power? Or is this not to be allowed under any circumstances? Great methodological conflicts in the social sciences have often been attempts to resolve this key question either positively or negatively. The negative answer has been far and away predominant in a methodological dogmatism of long standing.

Here again we come up against the reversal of attitude that has been touched on already: a highly remarkable and yet, in essence, profoundly dramatic one. The natural sciences, so immoderately admired and often slavishly copied by the social sciences, now regard it as entirely self-evident that their research potential, multiplied by practically inexhaustible financial resources and manpower, not only serves directly as an instrument of endless search in the continual unraveling of the ever-mysterious universe, and so for the unlimited increase of knowledge and pure scientific truth. Unmistakably, this constant expansion of knowledge also stimulates endeavor in a quite different direction, namely the further extension of the range of human power in the future. But it is just at this crossroads that the social sciences generally, and abruptly,

199

break the close ties with natural science. In imitation of Francis Bacon (knowledge is power), this second facet of the natural sciences (including technology), whose intellectual activity has expanded on an almost inconceivable scale and in a truly stupendous way, has been gradually, indeed well-nigh predominantly, pushed to the forefront. The enlargement of natural-scientific knowledge has become virtually identical with a simultaneously postulated enlargement of man's coercive power over nature. Once acquired, such knowledge is rapidly applied over as wide as possible a range, partly by virtue of industrial laboratories and military institutes. Whether, on second thoughts, these applications are judged as proper use or misuse is in fact a question of the use of human power and characteristic human behavior and really lies outside the domain of the natural sciences; it occupies a transitional region between natural and social sciences.

Applied social science, on the other hand, is distinguished by its almost complete absence. I think I may fairly say without overstatement that in most respects and in practically every case it is non-existent.[26] What is almost incomprehensible and hard to accept is that precisely where human power is fundamental and essential, because it is faced with *changeability* and a challenge to scrutinize carefully the possibilities of *purposeful* social intervention, the social sciences — with a few exceptions — are simply in default nowadays. Hypnotized by what they rake as strict natural-scientific methodics they grind to a halt in a mid-course or even make a resolute about-turn. This occurs systematically whenever they are confronted with a prospect which applies to them particularly and concerns them directly: the extension of the natural sciences into actual implementation and the application of human power to the dynamic developments of the future. Humble admiration of their specifically future-oriented sister sciences suddenly, when this climax is reached, reverts to agnosticism and asceticism, timid silence or repressive inhibition. Although it can hardly be open to any doubt now that, as social sciences, they must be specifically concerned with the way in which human power can be exercised to change society, they go on obstinately and almost blindly opting for the wrong methodological half of the "pure" natural sciences (and that in an entirely obsolete form). Where the other, additional and for them most important part is concerned, since it relates to the whole social dynamic, they insist on an apathetic attitude of mind — and take pride in it, into the bargain![27]

As a general rule, as we have seen in previous chapters, scientific-philosophical thought, including religious and socio-ethical thought, follows an almost synchronous course that is reflected in nearly every aspect of culture. A surprising effect of contrast that becomes apparent here is that the social sciences, once caught up in the wake of the classical natural sciences, seem to have cut themselves off completely from the modern, very different development of the latter. And this at a time when the parallel could and should be sustained far more widely and more productively.

200

The social sciences could have undergone a methodological conversion to the classical scholastic principle known as "Occam's razor", which is that of achieving the greatest effect by the fewest and simplest possible means — an economic principle also found in nature itself, where it is a governing rational and cosmic principle. The present-day social sciences, however, wish to wield an extremely sharp razor in the firm resolve neither to cut themselves with it nor to hand it over to anyone else with clear instructions to that effect. For this very reason it cuts deep into their own flesh. Or, to continue the methaphor with that of Buridan, an adherent of Occam: they behave like Buridan's ass, who starved to death in an agony of indecision, immobilized between two enticing ricks of hay — the incredible advance of modern natural sciences on the one hand, and their marvellous technical applications on the other.

Let us return once again to our central point of departure: to the premise that men can themselves change and recreate social reality, that they have done so more and more throughout the history of human civilization and will surely do so on an even vaster scale in times to come. It might be illuminating to examine the whole course of human civilization, from prehistoric times up to the present, in the light of this law of the changeability of the social picture through the purposeful and effective application of human power. But it is more important for us now to realize for the future the vastly increased potential which the increase of that power offers. It can be assumed without the slightest exaggeration that we are on the threshold of the greatest social and cultural metamorphosis of all time and of all historical civilizations.

Both this changeability and, proportionally, the changefulness of social reality have gradually acquired a comparatively much greater intensity and extensiveness. All the factors which operate in the field of social dynamics (mass, energy, acceleration, cumulation, interaction, dynamism, rotation and transformation) have reached unprecedented levels of thrust and potential. In this massive and overwhelming increase of scale and proportion, the purposive application of *human* power has assumed a much more active and effective participatory role than ever before. As a result, an almost wholly new social dimension has opened up before our very eyes, though many people have not yet noticed it. As always, of course, this future-dimension again has the same bipolar appearance. On the one hand, how will socio-historical reality develop in the midst of this swirling movement? On the other, with the tremendously powerful socio-dynamic powerhouse available to us, what directional influence can, may and must we consciously exert upon it?

In this pregnant situation we are once again brought up sharp against the De Groot criterion of science: If I know something, I can predict something; if I can predict nothing, I know nothing.

But this dictum has now acquired a highly accentuated meaning. For in order to withstand the dual pressure of changeability and changefulness and

201

to understand their true significance as regards the probable "shape of things to come", we *must* in fact be able to predict. The art of social forecasting has now become a dire necessity for the very preservation at least, and for the improvement where possible, of our existence.

I could therefore wholly concur with a pronouncement which is by implication contained in this train of thought: if, under these circumstances, social science is unwilling or unable to predict, then it does not deserve the name of science.

At the same time, though, I am clearly compelled to leapfrog unceremoniously over De Groot's system; mainly because I find it still excessively attached to classical natural science, and for that and other reasons insufficiently aware of the critical predicament of our social reality as it moves swiftly towards the future.

For what is it that has to be predicted? Only what might presumably be our future lot as the result of the autonomous movements in the field of social dynamics? This is no more than the phenomenon of *changefulness*, the discovery of which, moreover, is almost synonymous with laissez-faire.

Or must we also predict how and to what extent the future can be favorably influenced in accordance with clear and deliberate choices, by particular applications of human power for the responsible determination of our own destiny? This would also cover *changeability*, advancing from a sound foundation of basic social science.

Personally, I regard the latter element as of prime importance. I count it among the most important tasks of social science to make the best contribution they can, not only to purely exploratory future-prediction but also to a normative exploration and optimum *shaping* of the future. In this last respect especially, applied social science and social technology would become more comparable with applied natural science and technology. In other words, modern natural science and modern social science would thereby come closer together again, precisely because the difference of principle which characterizes them would be taken fully into account!

PART THREE

Prognostics

The revolutionary process of development of forward-thinking
brain techniques and technical brains

Despise not prophecies. But prove all things:
hold fast that which is good.

I THESS. 5: 21,22

I Diagnostics

Turbulent process of transformation of world events and mental attitude

So schritten auch den grossen Geschichten
ihre Geister schon voran und in dem Heute
wandelt schon das Morgen.

SCHILLER

CHAPTER 10

New literature: new visions of the future

1. Thinkers penetrate into the fourth dimension

The pursuit of science and scientific research have, as everyone knows, multiplied and spread unbelievably quickly by a process of mutual cross-pollination in all the highly developed countries of the world. This is true both of the overall extent of scientific production and of the specific scientific fields, which are increasingly differentiated numerically, and studied more intensely by a constantly growing number of people. In particular, this ever-faster rate of propagation applies to publications, which exhibit an exponential growth curve in all these fields, whether in the form of books or articles, while the number of scientific journals has also multiplied with almost bewildering fertility. In short, the situation has become increasingly like the unstemmable flood which inundated all the workers despite the ever-larger army of minia-ture broomsticks set to work by the sorcerer's apprentice. Nobody can now keep pace with his field of study, no matter how specialized and continually narrowed by new fragmentations, let alone command a view of the interrelated whole. It is estimated that the best trained specialists are nowadays out of date in as little as 5 to 10 years, and then possess on average only about half the knowledge they require. There is talk of an explosion of scientific information. The beginnings of a breakdown in feedback and communication are showing. Even the device of special journals containing only abstracts can no longer bridge the widening gulf between "production" and "consumption". Maybe new forms of electronic data processing and documentation, drawing on the infinite, indefatigable and universal memories of computers and used in con-junction with the equally inexhaustible capacity of microfilm, will bring a solution nearer, or at least bring some solace to the specialists. There are those, however, who reckon that the growth curve of scientific activity can only go on rising until it comes up against its own limit and, as it were, finds itself forced to flatten out. Personally I do not believe that this process, once it has gained momentum, can be stopped by itself or anyone else. Bearing this in mind, and consequently also the possibility of a continual process of disintegra-tion, we are faced all the more inescapably with the question how synthesis and integration are going to be possible just when they will be needed more than ever. The posing of that question must make it seem as if we are definitely getting no nearer, but rather further away, from the possibility of ever meeting the requirement of a comprehensive prognostic approach.

As early as the beginning of our own century, Wells pleaded for the systematic exploration of the future. The term futurology was, as far as I can discover, first coined and circulated in the Forties by Professor Ossip Flechtheim, now a professor at the Free University of Berlin, though at the time it failed to arouse any favorable response whatever. It is significant that the different articles which he has since published in journals have only just appeared in collected form (in the English language, in Germany!); in choosing the title for the collection he has manfully, and to my knowledge for the first time in a book intended to be scientific, included the word "futurology" on the cover.[1] Manfully, in the first place because even now a separate and yet comprehensive faculty of futurology is still an offensive abomination to many minds. And because the word futurology still smells, too much in the sceptics' nostrils of soothsaying and pre-scientific astrology and thus, for an activity striving to achieve full scientific currency, may not be too happy a choice. But this is even truer of its associations with "futurism".[2]

Perhaps because of the powerful opposition with which he has to contend, Flechtheim himself has not progressed much further in recent years than a spirited plea for and an attempt at a more clear-cut definition of a comprehensive future-study along these lines. The true spiritual fathers of further expansion seem to me to be two other Europeans.

Firstly, Dr. Robert Jungk, whose "Die Zukunft hat schon begonnen", a report on America which appeared in 1952, rapidly became a best-seller in many countries and earned for him a world reputation which went beyond the bounds of journalism. He has since been a tireless campaigner, writing and launching initiatives for the establishment of a scientifically grounded study of the future. For some years now he has been the director of a small "Institut für Zukunftsfragen" in Vienna, originally subsidized by the Austrian Government.

Next to him I must place Bertrand de Jouvenel. Since the early Sixties he has managed an institute in Paris (until recently financed entirely by the Ford Foundation) where the emphasis is on methodological studies under the collective name "Futuribles". Futuribles is a contraction of "futures possibles", a borrowing from the work of the Spanish Jesuit Molina which dates from the second half of the 16th century. Its publications include a bulletin ("Sedeis"), a revue ("Analyse et Prévision") and a large number of monographs. De Jouvenel himself, who was already famous as a scholar through his writings on politicology, published one of the first fundamental books on futurology[3], which has received international attention. The years 1962, 1963, 1964 and 1965 saw De Jouvenel organizing international congresses on prognostic topics and problems, interest in which grew from one year to the next, resulting in new publications issued by his institute and contacts throughout the world.

Giving honor where it is due, it is in fact true to say that *France* has not only played a leading role in this sphere, it has also witnessed the greatest diffusion and given official recognition to this new approach. Much is owed to a French philosopher taken too soon from this world, Gaston Berger[4], who for years was director general of the French Ministry of Education, and the inspiring founder of the "Centre d'Etudes Prospectives", which also publishes its own journal, "Prospective". Also of great importance in France was the separate study group set up by the Prime Minister at the end of 1962 to investigate longer-term future development under the supervision of Pierre Massé ("Commissaire Général du Plan" until the end of 1965). Its final report, which appeared in late 1964[5], met — naturally, one might almost say — with much criticism[6], but it exerted, as a unique model, a particularly stimulating influence on future-thinkers both at home and abroad. Another influential, future-oriented and specifically French movement is that of the "Conseillers de Synthèse", highly valued in French industrial circles, to which is allied the "Centre d'Etude des Grandes Techniques Nouvelles" (C.T.N.). Other groups with similar objectives include the "Institut de la Vie" (Prof. Marois) and a fairly large public following for "Planète", which is partly mystical in character and consequently perhaps less well favored in strictly scientific circles, though its many publications do stimulate future-oriented thought in broader strata outside this narrow sector.

Finally, France also has a number of independent future-thinkers of scientific calibre, the foremost of whom are Louis Armand[7], Jean Fourastié[8], Pierre Bertaux[9] and Alfred Sauvy.

The fertilizing influence of such minds is already penetrating quite markedly at somewhat lower levels, which may be described as popular scientific and predominantly journalistic without any value-judgment being implied, because publications of this kind can make their own contribution to the shaping of public opinion. Examples are Alfred Fabre-Luce and Jean Marabini.[10]

In *Britain*, where the seeds of modernization are often sown by the generally unsensational but nevertheless high-quality work of Royal Commissions, e.g. the Buchanan Report on Traffic in Towns, the present moment does not seem to be a time of great activity. As long ago as 1952 a grandson of Darwin, Charles Galton Darwin, ventured into the field of future-research with his book "The Next Million Years", which appeared too soon and, apparently, looked too far ahead. Moreover, his pessimistic view was still too much a part of the declining anti-Utopian period.

A great deal of interest was aroused in 1964, however, by a series of articles which appeared in the "New Scientist", by some 100 leading scholars describing expected developments in their own special fields over the next 20 years.[11] A fascinating preliminary study of the same type, though this time a single-handed effort, had already appeared in 1962; it was Arthur C. Clarke's "Profiles of the Future".

Even prior to this, a series of lectures entitled "The Future of Man" (Methuen, London 1959) has been given on the B.B.C. by the subsequent Nobel

207

Prizewinner Medawar; they were overshadowed a few years later, however, by a book which shocked many people, published by an international, though predominantly Anglo-Saxon, congress on this subject held in London by the Ciba Foundation.[12] At the same time the Hungarian-born physicist Dennis Gabor, who was working in England, received international acclaim for his book "Inventing the Future". And finally, I must mention Peter Hall's "The World Cities", a study of the future of urbanization.

Must it be said that Flechtheim's pioneering work in the field of futurology has met with a comparatively weak response in *Germany* itself? My impression is that the reflex movement got under way somewhat later there, but is now beginning to build up momentum. Robert Jungk, one of the first futurists[13], is at present collaborating with H. J. Mundt on a series of books in 15 parts called "Modelle für eine neue Welt", of which I think about four have appeared to date.[14] In addition there is Richard Kaufmann's powerful repudiation of the Ciba Foundation congress report mentioned above.[15] Another book from the same period is Fritz Baade's "Der Wettlauf zum Jahre 2000".

The important writings of Karl Jaspers have set the pattern for a specific kind of futurist literature.[16] Reflections on the future also include works by Thomas Regau, Wolfgang Koeck and Robert Gerwin. And lastly, let us not forget Fritz Sternberg and his ideas on the evolution of world politics.[17]

There is of course little point in weighing up the numbers, quality and originality of various publications in different countries and balancing them against each other. I do think it relevant that academic circles in Germany are also beginning to show signs of interest in this development. And of course there may be more proof of this than I have so far encountered. An "Institut für wissenschaftliche Zukunftsforschung" in Tübingen has been opened under the direction of Professor Horst Wagenführ. A "Studiengruppe für System-forschung" is now attached to the University of Heidelberg, and the Tech-nological University at Karlsruhe has instituted a "Seminar für Zukunfts-forschung". Apparently the universities of Berlin and Hamburg are also plan-ning a new approach in this direction. Further, Dr. Lothar Schulze is head of a "Gesellschaft zur Förderung von Zukunfts- und Friedensforschung", of which I know little more at present than that it exists. Finally, the Werner Reimers-stiftung (Frankfurt), through its director (Professor Ch. Zwingmann) has ex-pressed real interest in the promotion of modern future-research both in Germany and elsewhere.

In *Russia*, the first country to launch a Sputnik into space, there is also lively interest in the future as a long-term concern. There probably is a mental link between the two bold plunges into the new dimensions (or at least newly brought within the human reach) of time and space. Moreover, interna-tional contacts with the West on questions which go beyond present-day problems, taking a mental leap into the distant future, are much freer and firmer than is the case with other matters which are considered as more topical

208

and so subject to political bias. It is the partial unreality which makes this communication so much more real. The president and a number of leading members of the Soviet Academy of Sciences, as well as other eminent scientists, have performed future-studies in a number of specialized fields. Their views have been translated into English, partly from recorded interviews, and published as a "Penguin Special".[18] Russia is much more active in this sphere than the West is aware, and the central figure in this activity seems at present to be Professor Glagolev. According to my information an institute for social prognostics has been founded in Moscow under Professor I. V. Bestuzhev. Previously it was the leading Russian philosopher Mitin whose name was best known in this context.[19] The lively interest in Russia in what is achieved elsewhere in this sphere is evidence of the weight which the Russians attach to this type of research and future-study.[20]

Before turning to the United States of America, let me mention three other separate figures who have initiated their own special kind of work on the future. The first is the *Swedish* economist Gunnar Myrdal, whose "An American Dilemma" dates from as long ago as 1944 and threw light on the whole problem of negro integration, and who has since continued to do pioneering work for the future. The second is the famous *Greek* architect C. A. Doxiadis who, once again with the help of the Ford Foundation, has founded the Research Center of Ekistics in Athens — "ekistics" is his word for the new science of human habitation which must be founded — which has published its own monthly journal of the same name, in English, for some ten years now. The great future-project (at present still a utopian one) which is the ideal of Doxiadis and his research team, and which should optimally be adapted to the development of modern technology, is called "Ecumenopolis".[21] The third is Marshall McLuhan, until recently attached to the University of Toronto in *Canada*, who, in particular, expects advances in electronic communication media to revolutionize future human life quite drastically[22], although he has himself not managed so far to make his interesting new ideas easily comprehensible to many people.

As is usual nowadays, the greater part of these rapid developments (and we know it to be such because of the virtual absence of secrecy) is taking place in the *United States of America*. Future-research in that country is not only proceeding amazingly fast, it is being pushed along on all sides — hoisted out of the ground, as it were — by vast cranes.[23] As with almost everything in America, there are two marked characteristics: the preference for teamwork and the variety of approach.

While in Europe it is mainly individual authors whose names come to mind, this tends to be the exception in America. Of these exceptions Norbert Wiener, a man of genius if somewhat eccentric, and the founder of cybernetics, has of course been a great fertilizing influence on future-research. We must also mention Lewis Mumford, a visionary in the old tradition, and Harrison Brown, one of the first specific future-researchers.[24] Further, D. S. Hallacy Jr.[25], Robert L. Heilbroner[26] and Derek J. de Solla Price, a specialist on the future of science.[27] Finally, Donald Michael on young people[28] and Theodore Gordon on technology.[29]

Much work is being done or stimulated by national institutes. The Twentieth Century Fund has had a high reputation for a long time in this field.[30] The Center for the Study of Democratic Institutions at Santa Barbara, directed by Robert Hutchins, is strongly "future-oriented". The same may be said of the National Institute for Mental Health, the Hudson Institute (Herman Kahn, author of "Thinking about the Unthinkable", inter alia) in Washington, and the Stanford Research Institute at Menlo Park. We have already mentioned the "think-tanks", partly taken up with military research; one such is the Rand Corporation at Santa Monica, whose independent, greatly expanding daughter institution the "General System Development Company", likewise in Santa Monica, also deserves a mention.

The large American foundations are also showing increasing interest. The Ford Foundation, to take only one example, which co-finances the publication of the French "Futuribles" and the Greek "Ekistics", has also financed the great work "Resources for the Future"[31] which Harvey Perloff had directed. In addition, the dynamic American universities have quickly realized the growing importance of future-research. The big universities (Columbia, Harvard, M.I.T., etc.) even compete with each other in this regard.

Mesthène of Harvard received a grant of $ 5 million from IBM to keep a team of scholars doing future-research on "Technology and Society" for 10 years. Roger Revelle of the future-oriented Centre for Population Studies is also attached to Harvard. Elise Boulding is doing research into visions of the future in the developing countries and of Mexican immigrants in America, at the University of Michigan, Ann Arbor, and the University of Colorado, Boulder. At the Southern Illinois University, Professor Buckminster Fuller and John McHale are conducting a very ambitious project, to consist of several parts[32], for a new "world design" in our scientific age. Finally, I must mention Professor Charles Osgood of the Institute of Communication Research, University of Urbana, who is working on a so-called Apollo project whereby computers reveal a variety of possible futures in accordance with decisions made by mankind to make various choices to that end.

The selection I have made is rather arbitrary and represents too small a sample of what is being currently accomplished in this field in American university circles, and of the new material that is added, so to speak, almost every semester. It is therefore not surprising that even the American Academy of Arts and Sciences, itself certainly no less venerable or solemn than its national counterparts in European countries, appointed a "Commission for the year 2000" in 1964 under the directorship of one of the protagonists of scientific future-research, the sociologist Daniel Bell of Columbian University, New

York, who is establishing his own institute for future studies there. This commission has since published five thick volumes of working-papers, reports and minutes of its interesting meetings. The eventual outcome is as yet rather hard to predict[33], but the all-round stimulating influence on and of the 50 or so leading participants and advisors in this work is, I think, an undoubted fact.

Clearly, all these projects, which are almost acquiring the nature of a new kind of industry, require considerable investments. In America of course, the flow of funds is most abundant. The IBM's total of 5 million dollars in 10 years is no exception. General Electric have established the organization Tempo (Technical Management Planning Organization) in Santa Barbara with an annual budget of 7 million dollars, to enable 200 practitioners of the exact sciences, sociologists, economists and technologists to think about the future. The U.S. Air Force spends 15 million dollars annually on the Rand Corporation in Santa Barbara, a significant part of which is likewise intended for thinking about the future. In 1966 the Ford Foundation made a fresh grant of nearly $1^1/_2$ million dollars to the "Resources for the Future" team.

Clearly, funds of this sort are not available in Europe; and, in my opinion, they are certainly not needed on such a scale. Instead of the separate future-institutes employing many hundreds of scientists, such as Olaf Helmer is now planning in America, it would be enough to have a few dozen, or even less than a dozen, staff members. Both the limited financial resources and the extreme shortage of manpower make this a reasonable approach. De Jouvenel, with the backing of the French Government, seems now to be busy converting his private project into a permanent, official futuribles institute in Paris. It is reported that Mark Abrams, the British sociologist, is progressing with the setting-up of an "Office for Forecasting" in London, financed by the British Department of Education and Science.

Now you will ask, what is the situation in my own country compared with these developments beyond its frontiers and overseas? Is *the Netherlands* backwards in this respect? In two respects at least it may even consider itself advanced: Tinberger's unique Institute for Development Planning[34], which is attached to the Netherlands School of Economics, Rotterdam, and the work done by Jac. P. Thijsse in the field of town and country planning at the Institute of Social Studies at The Hague, which has likewise attracted international attention. These two subjects have also inspired interesting work on the part of Theil, Boot and Kloek[35] and Beljon[36]. Another field, quite different but characteristic of this country, is covered by the review Toekomst zonder Gezicht[37].

It may be a gap in my own knowledge, but I should find it hard to think of other equivalent examples in Dutch university circles. The Central Planning Bureau did take some preliminary steps towards long-term planning in the Fifties, but these were not followed up. A plan for the medium-long term (until 1970) has just been published. Studies abroad often aim at the year 2000 or even beyond.

211

The Government is at least interested to some extent[38], as is evidenced for instance by the existence of an interdepartmental working party intensely concerned with the problems of the future. This working party was originally the result, I believe, of a liaison committee between the Government and the social science council (of the Royal Academy of Sciences). It is reported that it recommended to the Government and the Royal Academy in mid 1965 the setting-up of a special committee of experts for this purpose. Maybe the energetic nature of the American Academy can inspire us to make the necessary decision? Or are we once again to be floored by the old stumbling block, that familiar trio of chosen objectives, available manpower, and financial resources?

Dr. Vondeling, ex-Prime Minister appeared to go much further at the beginning of 1966, during the 20th anniversary of the (Socialist) Wiardi Beckman Foundation, when he proposed the establishment of a separate Office of Future Studies. Even so, he did not appear in the first instance to regard this as an independent Government responsibility, to say nothing of the problem of finance; furthermore, the "world of science" would apparently have raised quite a few objections. Steering such a project safely and swiftly between the cliff of Scylla and the whirlpool of Charybdis will be a difficult job. Have we a Utopia for the present then? But how can the new Council for Scientific Management function properly when future-research is consistently falling behind, since it encompasses all scientific developments in particular?

Meanwhile, we are not entirely empty-handed. Some years ago "Working Party 2000" was established on the ecumenical foundation of close collaboration between a Protestant and a Roman Catholic education centre, devoted to the problems of the future and to the dissemination of the new ideas generated in this sphere.

Furthermore, an international group of currently 500 or so scholars and thinkers from Western and Eastern Europe, North and South America and some developing countries, with a declared preference for establishment in the Netherlands, very recently founded the organization "Mankind 2000 International", whose membership is rapidly expanding throughout the world. Mankind 2000 sprang originally from an initiative of Robert Jungk and other kindred spirits.

One of the avowed aims of Mankind 2000 International is the establishment of an international research center for studies on the future. Its purpose would be to document, coordinate and integrate the research now spread over many countries and many subjects. It is conceivable that such a project, wherever initiated, could, despite very modest beginnings, later develop into a far bigger organization. Eventually, in conjunction with the United Nations and UNESCO, there should after all be room beside the World Health Organization and the Food and Agriculture Organization for an all-embracing World Future Organization.

212

But all this, however logical an extension of the present train of thought, is, if not exactly an illusion, at any rate no more than future tense. If we were to start, however, by ourselves achieving something of value, joining forces to concentrate our power, that in itself would be an important beginning. At present, we must sadly admit that the earlier question can only be answered in the affirmative: indeed, the Netherlands *is* a backward country in this respect.

Can a "Council for the Future" really give counsel? Maybe "the future" could still at some future time be included in a party political program in the Netherlands, or even form the fundamental material in the formation of a cabinet. A separate Ministry of Technology and Future Affairs would definitely not be a superfluous luxury!

2. Is integral future-vision equal to squaring the circle?

The sole aim of any survey of prominent future-problems is to bring as clearly as possible to the fore the many problems, their extent, level, weight, complexity and urgency, which will increasingly demand our full attention in the future; to show that our attention must be focussed on the forms they are likely to take, the dangers they may entail, and the possibility of a favorable outcome achieved through appropriate control.

I am quite well aware that the set-up I have adopted might have the opposite effect to that intended. The social sciences are lying in wait for their prey, or at least for an opportunity of rubbing salt into its wounds. For instance, they could very well produce just as emphatic a counter-argument along the lines of: if there are in fact so many different future-problems, each of them highly complex in itself and touching on a number of specialist fields, how could such a heterogeneous collection be scientifically amenable to unification under one common denomination? On the other hand, the only social science which has in fact significantly enlarged its scope and advanced its technique, namely economic science, could definitely claim some right to occupy a position of such a general character.

Athough the former argument is a strong reminder of the initial opposition to the new science of sociology (which has meanwhile grown into a stronghold of resistance to innovation) — and could it ever embrace or grasp all the diversification which appears in social life in the form of processes, institutions, attitudes, groupings, relations etc.? — I nevertheless want to take this objection quite seriously. All the more so because it is initially bound up with a related question which has already been mentioned and which at first seemed to present just as insurmountable an obstacle. It is the question whether, at a time of unavoidable increase in scientific differentiation and even somewhat disquieting disintegration, when even the narrow specialist is faced with the

213

greatest difficulties in mastering an immeasurable surfeit of material despite his self-imposed restrictions, a comprehensive prognostic approach is at all conceivable. Is not such an attempt as much condemned to failure as the squaring of the circle? To this question I have so far not been able or willing to give an answer, partly because this problem will be dealt with in a more detailed way later, as soon as we penetrate deeper into the material. And yet, I do not want to avoid it altogether here. Nor do I simply wish to plead — though in general it is an elementary truth — that the history of mankind to date has never produced a task, however unmanageable it may have seemed at first sight, which could not be tackled successfully sooner or later once it had been set out clearly and understood as an inescapable duty. Parents often drill into their children the idea that "there's no such word as can't", but the history of human civilization has in fact provided continuous and adequate refutation of the "non possumus" attitude. That line of thought could very well lead to the objection that the question is essentially false. The question is not whether we can do it, but that we *must* do it as soon as possible, so that the only things left to ask are *when* and *how*?

The future will of course soon form an indivisible whole, a composite network in which, with the advantage of hindsight, we shall be able to trace out the then recognizable effects of all the above problems and many others, and the connections between them. But for us today there are still various possible futures, and so various networks and interconnections. I am convinced that we must have the courage to accept the challenge contained in the question of knowledge and conscience, whether we can also construct a usable overall vision of these alternative future-forms *in advance*. If the scholars of the 16th and 17th centuries had not had the courage of their convictions to inspire them in this way, we might perhaps still be living in the Middle Ages and the antique world picture which was current in those days. But our present views and general attitudes of mind regarding the innovations of prognostics are as yet little further advanced than medieval notions. Historians in the 21st century will probably be able to fill fascinating volumes with reflections on the Copernican turn of our age, on the laborious struggle toward — and the fanatical opposition to — a world picture again in need of renovation: the creation and contemplation of a human picture of the *future*.

Merely to summarize a series of important major problems and all that is associated with them is of course very far from providing a suitable insight into the corpus of possible or probable future-configurations. On the contrary, it can do no more than provide an insight into a number of strongly active forces and tendencies, but certainly not into their possible combined outcome. The objection may be raised even more forcefully against all those fragmentary studies on the future separately drawn from various specialist fields by extremely specialized and competent scholars, however interesting they may be in themselves![39] It will never be possible to arrive at a correct basis for general decision-making and purposive action simply by lining up or pasting together a number of separate analytical studies of this kind. On the other hand, however, this proves equally well that we could not attempt, with a sufficiently extensive general knowledge founded on integrally planned pre-study, to achieve a rather more homogeneous prognostic picture. This calls for a systematic study of existing and conceivable procedures, aimed at synthesis and integration; an area at present virtually neglected precisely because the main tendency for a long time now has been towards sharper differentiation, specialization and micro-miniaturization in study and research. The versatile, universal thinkers who were famous in earlier times are now pushed into a corner. The great system-builders are out of fashion. Their associative, combinatorial and structural thought processes are now almost as strange and unfamiliar to us as the future itself. All primitive peoples, imaginative children, and the unique, classical philosophers, could illustrate the essentials of these thought processes: "bien étonnés de se trouver ensemble". The famous French "encyclopédistes" of the second half of the 18th century thus brought about one of the most revolutionary breakthroughs in current mental attitudes.[40] Why should an objective — comparable if not identical — now be ruled out of the realm of possibility?

Of course, all this is closely related to more or less theoretical questions of scientific education and research, which I must pass over for the time being.[41] But it is relevant to consider the answers or solutions which are in practice being sought or indicated. Generally speaking, there is a distinct tendency to discover or to make a sort of Ariadne's thread through the labyrinth, the overwhelming confusion of entangled and even conflicting problems. The most attractive of effective means of integration is the utmost simplification and reduction to a few comprehensive, and in any event most dynamic, tendencies, and possibly even ultimately to one main central factor. This is what is attempted in various of the leading studies from present-day literature.

For example, Dennis Gabor, who ranks as one of the main "futurologists" of the day, links his reflections on what he tellingly calls "inventing" the future to a sort of triptych. The trilemma with which he confronts us embraces what he sees as the principal and essential problem of the future — war, leisure and overpopulation. He relates many other secondary problems either loosely or closely to these, or omits them altogether. This is of course a quite possible choice of priorities; the procedure is unavoidably somewhat arbitrary.

Once one adopts this line, the temptation to find one central, unifying factor is almost irresistible. This is also a vulnerable approach, of course, since it too is to some extent arbitrary. But such systems do at least render the great service of showing that in many regards there is more homogeneity than might at first sight be supposed.

In accordance with this approach, many people today see as the central problem one which also kept Kant fully occupied towards the end of his life:

215

the burning question whether it is possible to ensure lasting peace between the peoples of the world. Other possible future conflicts and tensions are either related or subordinated to it. Coordinated peace studies on a national and international level are certainly an extremely important part of prognostic research. Of course, certain areas might, or would even have to, be omitted from it, but that is inherent in the system selected.

Many others, successors of Malthus, follow the overpopulation line; to translate it into present-day terminology, they see the question of world population as the all-embracing, or at least easily the dominant, problem of the future, which at the same time largely includes the problem of the developing countries.

There is a third category, to which I feel some affinity, which regards Marx's striking vision as still unreservedly valid in this respect, and which consequently points to the evolution of technology as the central driving force in a socio-economic, socio-cultural and socio-political scene which is of course also moved by countless smaller forces. It is relatively easy, for instance, to transform the above triology of Gabor, who incidentally is himself a technologist by profession, into a technical "monologue" with three important interrelated facets. In many cases, the problems raised by other writers about the future can be largely reduced to the motive power of technology, i.e. of applied natural science and technology. And this is not so surprising because, as scarcely anybody will deny, technology is very largely responsible for two of the most characteristic and striking features of our progress toward the future: on the one hand, the constant and continuous process of change and transformation; on the other, the increasing acceleration to which this very process of change appears to be subject. Faster change and revolution are the paranymphs of present-day technological evolution, affecting human existence both in depth and in breadth, in an ever-intenser way.[42]

Partly related to the above views on the world and on society, and partly opposed to them, there is the predominantly philosophical standpoint (Christian and/or humanistic) which takes man as its focus — either man as a person or man in relation to his fellow-man. In the first case, much attention will be paid, among other things, to the nature of the above-mentioned accelerated change processes and their effect on the individual, i.e. in particular on the resultant, continually increasing and very worrying tensions and neurotic tendencies towards psychosomatic symptoms in the second case, the problems often crystallize around those of the developing countries, or ethnic minorities, or particular social or international problems of future human society and, not least, the cardinal future problem of the "people-makers". Further, very high priority may also be given to the extremely vital problems of educational reforms, modern methods of teaching, communication, information and instruction — some of whose major concerns will be the most urgent questions and extremely responsible choices of the future.

Another view in which man is the central figure seems to have a stronger biological slant. One author in whom it is apparent is Bertaux — also analysed in greater detail later — whose opinion is that man is already undergoing a new mutation in his historical evolution, without the need of any artificial intervention. For this reason, according to him, the exploration of new future-dimensions and the design of an appropriate new strategy, of new techniques and patterns of thought, are required. And required as a matter of the greatest urgency now, because otherwise it will no longer be possible, in time to deal scientifically with the resulting masses of problems which will soon overwhelm us, or with the future-corrections which will have to be applied.

In these essentials, therefore, there is some divergence in the fundamental starting-points, or at least the axiomatic leitmotifs which determine the preference for one road or another, when the laborious pilgrimage to the future begins. It is of no special importance for us to go into greater detail on the pros and cons of the different solutions, since they alwas turn out to be roads which at times run parallel, at others intersect or eventually merge into one. The fact of setting out is in itself of greater importance than the where and the how of beginning. Many roads lead to the same goal or the same objectives. Often, although the starting-point and the bearings are different, one keeps coming across largely the same major problems concerning the future, in the already sizeable literature of prognostics, and the overlaps and interconnections are thus shown up most clearly. These striking, characteristic main problems are after all a significant pointer to the fact that the striving for synthesis is no inherently pointless task, let alone a quite hopeless one.

One of the prime functions of prognostic research is to give a closer analysis of the connections thus revealed, but also of mutual antithesis or counterforces, and even contradictions, in the overall complex of problems. Further, to elaborate in greater detail how different approaches to problems, and contrasting solutions, might also lead to alternative future possibilities which would take the form of different crystallized networks. But that is far from all. There are not only different future *possibilities*: there are also different future *desirabilities*. These latter differences are associated with conceivably divergent objectives, each of which can also be achieved or pursued with a variety of means. The conceivable objectives mostly stem from a small, aristocratic intellectual élite, a creative minority. Generally, they do not exist among the mass of the people, or not yet to the same extent. This presupposes a large-scale process of information and education. The public will have to be made future-conscious and choice-conscious, in a democratic way.[43] This too is quite definitely a task which falls in the first instance to prognostics. To this end, again, the complex whole must be reviewed in the context of its countless problems, it must be clarified and, in its collective aspects and its priorities especially, it must be popularized.

One might therefore argue *in reverse* as follows: if the number of problems were not so great and so serious, if their nature were not so distinctive, heterogeneous, complicated or even contradictory in many respects, then a comprehensive approach would not be quite so necessary — indeed, indispensable. And if many of these problems or their possible solutions were not interpedendent in numerous ways, or if this interaction did not generate whole areas of new, interconnected problems for future development, then it would perhaps be possible to go on tackling them separately and exclusively, each via its appropriate area of knowledge. In some of these areas, high towers have been erected, with highly developed radar equipment scanning their own particular futures. As a result we have not one but a fair number of separate, isolated towers, together increasing the existing confusion of tongues and affording no sight whatever of the interlocking whole of possible future structures. Nor can they make the least contribution to the future-choices ultimately required, which will have to be based on a comparative evaluation of priorities for particular, more or less highly prized, objectives, and for the preferred means of realizing or implementing them.

Prognostic research in the true sense of the word will have to try to embrace the possible future as one potential, but also preferable, whole, with the principal constituents which go to make up this totality, or there will hardly be any point in such research. Unfortunately, prognostics can in principle only choose between all and nothing. But if it is postulated that prognostics *must* attempt to "invent" one or more possible, or desirable and attainable, future-configurations as a complex whole, this still tells us absolutely nothing about the question of whether or in what way this integral goal should be effectively achieved.

Nevertheless, it is extremely significant that De Jouvenel for instance, although emphatically rejecting a science of futurology as such, sees precisely in this systematic discovery of probably, all-embracing future-configurations ("futuribles") a highly important task and one which, in his opinion, can definitely be fulfilled, regarding this as an artistic endeavor to be pursued. Such is the conclusion of the thorough fundamental investigation he has made into the subject. The more pragmatically minded pass over this preliminary reconnaissance stage, and start straightaway on the realization of a synthetic objective which is taken to be more or less self-evident.

Many people are concerned here with the need for interdisciplinary collaboration between fairly sizeable teams composed of specialists from as many as possible of the fields involved (and which of them are not?). Some — to illustrate an entirely opposite approach — think in terms of prognosticians as a new genius of specialists, to be styled generalists[44], evolving their own new field of futurology, using specialized studies as source material of course, and referring to specific experts in other fields for further information. If it is substantially this latter course which is to be followed, the future might also precipitate a revolution, or maybe counter-revolution, in certain aspects of social science.[45] As I have said, at some stage there must be a more detailed study of whether, and to what degree, such a development would be useful and necessary in attaining the results ultimately envisaged. Finally, it may very well be that a comprehensive science of prognostics, striving for purposive synthesis, will call for wholly novel methods and techniques which will then have to be rigorously tested on their usefulness and effectiveness. It seems to me that we have already advanced considerably further in this respect, than, presumably, is general knowledge as yet. Much attention will be paid to this aspect in the present volume.[46] Only when this is done will it really be possible to ascertain that the awkward question regarding the pursuit of the squared circle can and must be answered with an unconditional negative. Prognosticians are not engaged in pointless quixotry. At most, their efforts to fasten their grip on the dynamic movement toward the future may bring them to the threshold of the handicap of an almost ungraspable "perpetuum mobile". But that, and especially the attempt to cross this threshold, is an essential part of their new "invention".

My purpose in this chapter has been to introduce the matter of the book and enable my reader to take his bearings. To this end I have tried to pinpoint and illuminate three main aspects, which can be summarized as follows:

(1) In our momentous and overflowing age, it is already clearly predictable that a great many extremely difficult problems, depending on the more or less explosive nature of their further evolution, will both individually and collectively exert an enormously powerful, if not overwhelmingly revolutionary, influence on the future and its continual transformation into the present.

(2) Purposeful prognostic research, together with the required reversal of prevailing scientific attitudes to the future, should serve to measure the significance and effect of these forces which will determine and change the future, and to indicate how they may be controlled where possible and desirable: this concerns the ends and the means.

(3) However, prognostic investigation cannot fulfil this task by tackling it in a piecemeal way. It can only succeed (leaving aside for the moment the factor or factors which should be taken as central) if it can acquire a sufficiently comprehensive grasp of the structural composition and interaction of the great problem complexes and correlations which will condition the ultimate form and configuration of the future. The purpose of prognostics is precisely to anticipate and to monitor these forces: such is its only real raison d'être.

Whoever may have supposed, therefore, that prognostics had a similar task to fulfil, calling for a similar measure of insight and effort, as most other branches of science, now know that, on the contrary, the task is extremely ambitious, exceptionally comprehensive and strenuous, and positively hazardous — decidedly perilous, in fact. To my mind, indeed, it is not a matter of a logical impossibility or contradiction in terms, such as the squaring of the circle; the problem is that the aim which I have said is basically possible could in practice run up against a number of major obstacles. The greatest difficulty is indisputably expressed by the wise warning of "Qui trop embrasse mal étreint".

If you maintain that the effective fulfilment of such a task is absolutely out of the question, and consequently that prognosticians should abandon all hope as they enter the world of the future, you may possibly turn out to be right. But this, viewed "sub specie futuri", would be a scarcely hopeful, indeed a comparatively gloomy, prospect for all whose future it is to be. Cicero too thought there was nothing to be gained from knowledge of the future. It is a point of view to which scarcely anyone adheres nowadays. Almost nobody now denies its usefulness, though the real possibility of its attainment is still doubted. Prognostics, which is now in its infancy, will still have to prove that those who denied its factual possibility in advance were in fact wrong to do so. Besides, as will be evident in later chapters, prognosticians have started *work* in earnest in recent years. To begin with we should be critical, and in my opinion sceptical, of their results to date, and try to separate the wheat from the chaff. The path of scientific progress is after all paved with errors, mistakes and failures of great educational value. And the prognostic approach which seems at first to have failed may yet prove to be the most fertile for the future.

In short, we must seriously investigate whether, where and how a real, integral and interdisciplinary approach can be made now (or at any rate, in all reasonable probability, before long), enabling us to see ahead to *presumable*, *possible* futures, and to think ahead towards a *desirable*, and finally *achievable*, future.[47]

Pressed by continual change and the ever greater speed at which the present becomes the future, we are compelled to change the "terra incognita" of the future as much as possible, and at the same time to transform it into "terra cognita". Our day is the day of the great transition to a great new transformation. It will take us completely unaware and present a traumatic threat to our very existence, unless we really exert ourselves to the limit in an effort to observe it, and actively control and create it, with the help of a science which itself is in course of creation. We shall never be able — indeed be permitted — to say "tout est bien". But we shall have to try more purposefully than ever before, also with steadily perfected scientific abilities, to aim at "le meilleur des mondes possibles".

CHAPTER 11

New future-institutes: tomorrow is another day!

> It is always wise to look ahead, but dif-
> ficult to look further than you can see.
> WINSTON CHURCHILL

To describe politics as the art of the possible or the pursuit of the feasible is a commonplace. Wishes for the future have constantly to give way to what is real and expedient and, as far as the Netherlands is concerned, to what a coalition compromise can achieve. There is always a shift away from what the long term indicates as desirable towards what the short term dictates as possible. The result is a kind of irresolution of purpose, a hopping about between two ideas, or even a staggering forward on one leg. Vision and insight tend to lose out in the process. It can scarcely be denied that, like all Socialist parties, the old SDAP in Holland grew up under the star of a wide-ranging Marxist view of the future. Although the reality developed along different lines, i.e. different from those predicted by Marx and his followers, much of that vision has nonetheless been so extensively realized that the original picture of the future has been superseded by its very fulfilment. *No new vision of the future has arrived to fill the vacuum thus created.* Which again bears out the historical truth that too much success only blunts the initial spur to action: no challenge, no response.

1. Accelerating currents, global upheaval and the under-developed Netherlands

Two spectacular trends, or rather accelerations, although clearly anticipatory of the direction in which the world is now moving, have as yet largely escaped our attention.[1]

First is the fact that our future global and social relations, seen from the longer-term viewpoint, will be wholly different from the present ones. In other words, *the greatest metamorphosis of all time,* for as far as man can remember, is probably already occurring in drastic and dramatic form, as it were before our very eyes.

This other future is now coming into view for our present population, and the younger generation especially; and the speed of its approach and the effect of its arrival are far greater than any of our predecessors, even over several generations together, have ever experienced. *Present and future have almost become simultaneous.*

The *second* trend is the attention now being given in an increasing number of countries, in ever more penetrating and in some respects even revolutionary ways, to these future developments which themselves are just as revolutionary and to their potentialities and consequences. Not only are all the conceivable or alternative possibilities being studied; in addition, with a view to the possible fundamental shifts, disturbing consequences and dangers theatening the individual, the community or the balance in the world to which these possible outcomes might give rise, increasing thought is being given to strategy for regulated control and active correction, where the chance of their being applied to good effect is reckoned to be good. *If we do not shape the future, the future will shape* (or misshape) *us.*

The *first* point, that of the great new transformation processes which are occurring everywhere and are still foreseeable, scarcely needs much comment. The terms "second Industrial Revolution", "acceleration" of tempo, "explosion" of new developments (e.g. world population, scientific data, or global communications) are all-too familiar to us: clichés by now, in fact. It is, however, a curious feature of the Dutch that we are consistently inclined to go on regarding the latest technological marvels (space travel, satellites, rockets, robots, atomic warheads, artificial people with artificial organs up to and including artificial brains, possible brain transplants, walks in cosmic space, voyages to the moon or in the depths of the ocean under the polar ice or down to the very bottom of the sea, etc., etc.) mainly as the substance of science fiction, evoking romantic and sometimes fascinating visions, it is true, but not actually part of our real-life world.

That is no typically English understatement, but rather a sign that we lack a sense to record and process the new phenomenal developments now taking place, notably as a result of the rising tide of new discoveries and applications in natural science and technology, with their ever-growing radius of action and accumulatively greater potential. These headlong developments, like some strange mixture of hurricane and avalanche, some unknown, overwhelming force of nature, or even natural disaster, are about to overtake and engulf our socio-economic and individual existence, and finally transform it completely with a whole new set of structures and dimensions.

We Dutch, it seems, do not at present possess the ability to distinguish between the tentative probings of imagination and the onslaught of reality. To date we have distinguished ourselves by a wholly peculiar attitude which either denies the existence of change or rejects it as nonsense; and we are rather proud of it too. We refuse to be swept along. We are, and remain, ourselves.

Whatever the circumstances, we hold on to our established views and opinions. "It won't happen here". "It'll probably never happen". "We are only a small country". Expressions of isolationism, head-in-the sand-ism or a psychological defense mechanism which passes for worthy Dutch sobriety or discernment or cautious realism, partly because they have, for the time being at any rate, fared splendidly in comparison with the predictions of visionaries announced as prophets of doom. But the utterances themselves imply predictions. They predict that the changes here will surely not be so radical, and certainly not so rapid. This attitude of mind, however, has just as much influence on our future, albeit a *negative* one. *Doubly* negative, in fact. The changes to come are neither foreseen nor influenced. Processes of renewal are slowed down instead of being stimulated. For example, it is a matter of the utmost urgency that automation be further introduced; but corresponding, drastic Government intervention *is equally urgent a need*. On the one hand too little systematic, purposive thought is given to the new future already moving in our midst and to its foreseeable consequences and implications. On the other hand, deliberation in the *positive* sense, centered on the essential planning needed to guide these developments along the right lines, is equally lacking. And so the absolute necessity for early anticipation and for suitable course correction with the best chance of achieving the desired effect, becomes more and more pressing.

This brings us to the *second* main point stated above, viz. the noticeable and, moreover, steadily widening gap between ourselves and those countries which, particularly in recent years, have begun to evince a rapidly growing, indeed almost overwhelming interest — scientific, socio-economic and political — in the future as such. And in particular, a tremendously heightened interest in the trends and correlated outcomes of this wide-ranging, far-reaching totality of developments; trends and outcomes which, it is hoped, serious investigation and appropriate instruments will make it possible to influence at the right time in a positive way. The perfected methods of prognosis with the corresponding analysis of different future possibilities, the approach to acquiring a synthetic insight into their structural links, the discovery of any fundamental but problematic shifts in them and their systematic study, discussion of pros and cons, and deliberation of strategic intervention in these expected social transformations, are characteristic of extremely important development processes of which we, in this country, are almost entirely ignorant. They are at length beginning to take firmer shape here and there in the *scientific* sense, by concentration or collaboration in certain fields, to form a distinct and nascent branch, that of *future reconnaissance and control*.

2. *The prognostic paranymphs of future-knowledge: future-studies and future-institutes*

Our present backwardness is all the more striking because the "European

Spirit" has relaid the foundations for this recent development. Though the first Industrial Revolution began in *England*, and despite the pleading of H. G. Wells, it was not there but in *Germany* (just as with intercontinental ballistic missiles, nuclear fission and the theory of relativity) that the spiritual fathers of a new doctrine of futurology were born. The first of them was Professor Flechtheim, now almost a forgotten pioneer, and although now recognized as the founder of that science, he achieved no success in it either in Germany or later in America. Prophets are generally left to starve in their own country! And the German "economic miracle" was perhaps not the best atmosphere for him to flourish in. The fact that German-speaking Jews formerly played a very great part in future-renovating activities, investigations, discoveries and inventions (Marx, Freud, Georg Cantor, Fritz Haber, Karl Mannheim, Minkovsky, Einstein) may also serve to explain in part the present relative spiritual poverty of Germany and Austria in that regard.[2] The very important Jewish future-philosopher Ernst Bloch would perhaps have exerted a more profound influence if he had not, as a convinced Marxist, for a long time removed his place of work to East Germany.[3] The small "Institut für Zukunftsfragen" founded in Vienna by the visionary pioneer Robert Jungk and initially supported by the Austrian Government has to date achieved little by way of scientific results, its potential being limited by lack of manpower and funds. But it does represent a good look-out post behind the Iron Curtain.

Thus the honor fell to France of re-establishing on scientific and political foundations the long undervalued pioneering work of such men as Jules Verne and Paul d'Ivoi. That this development took place in France is a surprise to many people. How does this inevitably rather speculative concern with developments in the long term square with strictly rational thinking? It could be that rationalism is attracted to its own opposite. For instance, it is not commonly known that, despite official prohibitions, astrology and fortune-telling are flourishing in present-day France. Thus it may be that the strictly scientific, logical and systematic confinement to the present takes this counterpart — or even creates it — to supplement itself in a rather broader philosophical and sociological approximation.[4] Gaston Berger, recognized in his own country as a philosophical thinker and influenced by the French philosophers Bergson and Le Senne, was the founder of a center for prospective studies established in Paris in the second half of the Fifties. It has published a number of interesting studies on the future in which the Cartesian mode of clear, lucid thought and the universal, catholic approach of the encyclopedists are combined. Thus in part of Europe the term "prospectivism" found acceptance as a novel attitude of mind, specifically future-oriented and based on comprehensive, purposive exploration and anticipation of the future.[5]

After the premature death of G. Berger the leadership of this movement was taken over temporarily by the engineer/economist Pierre Massé, then commissionar-general for the French Plan, who also incorporated this approach into

224

the thinking which gave birth to a plan (more modestly called "considerations") for 1985. Once Massé had returned to the world of business, the most important scientific continuation of prospectivism as a renovating mental attitude came to rest on the shoulders of the politicologist Bertrand de Jouvenel. An erudite authority on classical antiquity and the French classics, De Jouvenel has clearly stepped out of history into the future. More important still perhaps, his preponderant interest in writers about power, government and politics (Montesquieu, Rousseau, and Voltaire) is significant for the dedication to systematic reconnaissance of the future that he expressly advocates for the *political* management of affairs. It is an interesting phenomenon to which I shall again return, in connection with developments in America.

Allow me to make one marginal note to prevent any possible misunderstanding. Some French prospectivist thinkers are said to be Gaullists, or Gaullists by inclination. The Gaston Berger-Pierre Massé circle could presumably be described in political terms as predominantly big-business conservative. In other words, prospectivism in France cannot be simply identified with a progressionism which is radical by commitment or inclination. But it is enough, I think, to be aware of the fact. It detracts in no way from the great merits of these investigations which press forward in new directions. Even less so where a man like De Jouvenel has been far more intent on finding a reliable method of prognostic research and certain appropriate new forms of institutionalization than on either the launching of intrinsically novel ideas (let alone the reshaping of structures) or the obstinate defending of established interests. Furthermore, as we shall see, once transplanted to America these new methods and institutes would in fact help to encourage the pursuit of progressive and reformist policies, and then wash back to fertilize their European parent country along the same lines, slowly but *un*surely. When once something is set in motion, however cautiously, it sooner or later starts to go its own way, unforeseen perhaps even by the original prospectivism, and undesired, finally taking on a life of its own quite independent of the initial purpose.[6]

One of De Jouvenel's proposals which has aroused great international interest is the setting-up of a "forum prévisionnel", known in America as a "look-out agency". At the root of this proposal lies the conviction that in the world of today neither the executive nor parliaments nor political parties are sufficiently capable of comprehending the problems of the future in all their aspects, dimensions and consequences or, once they have become imminent, of making optimally based decisions on them. He would also like to see different future alternatives thoroughly debated well in advance and the pros and cons of each one brought into the light by various forums of experts and authoritative figures conversant with the substance of the future and its complex of related factors. De Jouvenel wants to see as it were a kind of extraparliamentary Council for the Future, or his Committees, examining fully and in sufficient depth in public, and *in advance*, plans for the future or plans with

225

implications for the future (these implications are almost always present in the breathtakingly fast developments of today, whether we do something or omit to do it). In this way such future-problems and their significance could be impressed in reasonable time on the future-consciousness of public opinion, before being cast into the political arena. In addition, such a Council or Institute could serve as a sort of "early-warning system", giving timely warning of dangers foreseen in particular developments, or indicating in advance how events might be guided in the most desirable direction. These functions could also be summed up as making public opinion aware of, and attuned to, the future, or, to express it another way, as helping to create a mental climate favorable to a high degree of orientation to the future, which will increasingly constitute a sine qua non of our continued existence.

A very remarkable event in France was the foundation in 1958 of BIPE (Bureau d'Informations et de Prévisions Economiques), jointly run on a 50/50 basis by the French Government and a number of large industrial concerns. The intention is that this bureau will supply long-term forecasts for incorporation in the next 5-year plans drawn up for the country. It must therefore be expected of course that the prognoses, almost inevitably, will be slightly "colored".

Prospectivist thought in France has had a very fertilizing influence both on government policy and in business life, not to mention a variety of other private groupings and a growing number of individual authors (Fourastié, Sauvy, Bertaux, Cazes, etc.); and the influence has worked both ways.

But it has also influenced various European and international institutions, before crossing the Atlantic and later returning to a few other European countries.

Of the international or European organizations established in Europe, each has been concerned in its own specific field, in a relatively independent and one-sided way, with long-term planning. This is true of NATO, the Coal and Steel Community, Euratom, the EEC, the International Labour Office, UNESCO, etc. I do not think I am being unfair to any of them if I say that, at least as far as I can judge from the material available, the Organization for Economic Cooperation and Development (French influence?) has progressed furthest. I have in my possession an OECD report of nearly 500 pages produced by the economic affairs directorate, which I am not free to quote here since any copy is a confidential draft,[7] but which as a prognostic survey is of truly outstanding scientific caliber. It not only reveals a geographically extensive knowledge but also fully recognizes the enormous and rapidly increasing importance of these new developments, and so clearly points out the leads and (most important) lags among the 21 member-states.

The Council of Europe could eventually come a good second in this field; and at its last session the European Parliament issued, through its Research and Culture Committee, an important report on technological progress and

226

scientific research, the author of which, my fellow-countryman Dr. Oele, has acquitted himself most excellently. Unfortunately, wheels in Europe still tend to turn extremely slowly!

The Food and Agriculture Organization (FAO) and the World Health Organization (WHO) have been responsible for some long-term studies in their respective fields. To my knowledge the United Nations Organization has not so far, with a few valuable exceptions, made any specific contribution to the subject. Groups working on it at the United Nations include the Advisory Committee on the Application of Science and Technology to Development, the Economic Projections and Programming Center (not to be confused with the Center for Development Planning, Projections and Policies), each with its own interesting series of reports, and also the center for Industrial Development. Also affiliated to the U.N. is the ICAO (International Civil Aviation Organization), which has published some excellent long-term studies involving experimental technological prognoses. I should not be surprised, however, to see the U.N. in time pursuing this direction with much greater vigor and on a much broader front. The influence of the drastic reorientation and socio-technical renovation in the prognostic sector now pervading the United States will be felt. A trend which will be brought into the front rank of modern scientific practice under the more neutral methodological title of "forecasting" or "prediction".

3. America: scene of prognostic breakthrough and upheaval

The reorientation[8] and renewal in America are not just spectacular, they are also astonishing. For scores of years the word "planning" was a decidedly dirty word in America, standing for a typically Socialist or Communist product and placed somewhere near the top of the ideological index of "un-American activities". In recent years especially the urgent need for and the essential merits of long-term planning, coupled with "deep future research", have been universally acknowledged. They are accepted unhesitatingly and given high priority by American business as a condition of economic life, by the federal government in increasing measure in the defense sector, and by the academic world as a subject of study, research and scientific education.

All leading, world-famous American industrial firms now have their own extensive and specialized departments for fundamental and applied scientific research in the field of future developments. Many of their research reports primarily intended for internal use are also released for publication and review. There are at least 50 big concerns which are making a name in this field by attracting high-caliber research staff working in different scientific areas. They include General Electric, IBM, XEROX, RCA (Radio Corp. of

America), Am. Tel. and Tel. Corp. with the long-famous Bell Telephone Laboratories, Int. Tel. and Tel., Honeywell, Texas Instruments, Fairchild Camera; the aircraft companies Boeing, Lockheed, United Aircraft and Noravi (North American Aviation); Du Pont, General Motors, 3M (Minnesota Mining and Manufacturing), Westinghouse Electric, General Dynamics, Standard Oil of New Jersey (ESSO), Union Carbide — j'en passe des meilleurs — and finally the publishing firm of McGraw-Hill, which publishes highly reputable prognoses for 1975, 1980 and so on.

Furthermore, prognostic research plays a very considerable and possibly even decisive role in the creation of quite *new* industrial business structures in America. This phenomenon was originally termed diversification, i.e. the distribution of products and services over extremely divergent branches of industry. The existing *vertical* trend towards concentrations and mergers within one type of industrial activity is now being succeeded by the creation of new industrial empires stretching *horizontally* and concerned with literally everything that is regarded as a promising and profitable item for the *future*. This new development is not of course affected by the existing anti-trust legislation, which relates to only one specific industrial branch, only one homogeneous kind of goods and services at a time. On account of their purposely heterogeneous nature these new industrial complexes have also recently come to be known as "conglomerates". They do not constitute a monopoly in any particular line, and yet their positions of exceptional strength and the enormous (sometimes international) extent of the territory they cover (including the spiritual and cultural field) make their influence overwhelming.[9] We are not concerned with the question whether such concentration of highly influential and far-reaching power are acceptable or should be regarded as a new and objectionable tool of capitalistic expansion. The point here is that the phenomenal growth of these giant conglomerates is based on, and planned in accordance with, thorough, *long-term* prognostic research.

A number of American firms are not content with a high standard in their own *internal* R & D (research and development) departments[10], which are specializing more and more in their own spheres of activity, subdivided from the general line of research and conducting systematic studies on the *long-*term future. An increasing number of big concerns are also promoting this kind of institutionalization *externally*. General Electric, for instance, has set up a separate, very extensive Center for Advanced Studies (TEMPO: Technical Management Planning Operation) in California, which is also engaged in technical and military planning and forecasting. Likewise IBM, besides supporting its own research departments in this work, spends very considerable sums on promoting such future-studies at universities.

In government circles, the military planning of the Pentagon and the Defense Department takes precedence. The future-studies of the Institute for Defense and Analyses (IDA) are important. The army, the air force and the navy[11] each fulfil the same dual function as is observable in, and indeed largely taken over by, big business: namely, the conducting of long-term future-studies in their own high-caliber research departments and the commissioning of similar studies from separate, more or less independent scientific institutions to whom sizeable annual budgets are made available. The space program has become very important in this respect. NASA has its own long-term study division working on the highest qualitative level, and also places extensive contracts of the same sort with other carefully selected research institutes specializing in this field. In recent years such projects, executed in-house or placed outside, have become imperative for all the ministries and the whole of the public economy.

Since a short time ago, practically all departments of the civil administration have been using PPBS (the Planning-Programming-Budgeting System), which had earlier proved its usefulness in the context of the military departments. The President of the United States has his own Office of Science and Technology which also undertakes long-term studies of the future. And finally, the government's Atomic Energy Commission (AEC) is also important in this regard.

Such is, however, not complete, nor by a long way the end of the story. I have not yet discussed one very interesting phenomenon: the establishment and expansion of the "think-tanks", whose effects are once again specifically directed to the development of "deep future research" and the new techniques it demands. These specialized institutes, of a breed still quite unknown in Europe, receive commissions of the type mentioned above both from military and civil authorities, and from business firms![12] Tens of millions of dollars are spent on these investigations every year. The execution of such commissions generally starts with an extended and specially perfected "brainstorming" technique, attended by a scientific elite drawn together from all categories and grades of the arts and sciences, with specialists and generalists, abstract theorists and practical experts.

The first institute of this type, and now the most famous internationally, is the Rand Corporation, which is largely financed by the Air Force. Others are the System Development Corporation (an offshoot of Rand, now independent and much enlarged), the Hudson Institute (initially concentrating on new weapon and defense techniques under its director, the famous military expert Herman Kahn, but now active in a greater diversity of fields), the Stanford Research Institute, the Battelle Memorial Institute, the Center for the Study of Democratic Institutions, Resources for the Future, Illinois Institute of Technology (Corplan), and more besides. There are in addition a great many private business management advice bureaus, also strongly future-oriented, including Abt Associates, Diebold Group, Arthur D. Little, McKinsey, Varian Associates, the Samson Science Association and the Quarantum Science Association, etc. This characteristic development towards long term future-orientation also exerts an influence on such bodies as the American Management Association, the American Research and Development Ass., the National Planning Ass., the Engineers' Joint Council, the American Institute of Planners[13] etc.

The course of development outlined here, which has pervaded the whole of the United States, was essentially an extra-academic one. Its rapid "futurological" expansion threatened to isolate it from academic life. However, the organization of scientific education is much more flexible and more dynamic in approach than is generally the case in Europe. The big universities soon began to fill the breach. Columbia University set about establishing its own institute for future studies (Daniel Bell). The same task was undertaken at Harvard by Harvey Brooks, Donald Schon and Emmanuel Mesthene (the latter assisted by IBM). The universities of Princeton, Pennsylvania, California and others are now moving in the same direction, so that this snowball will, as usual, grow fairly quickly, at least in the higher and more evolved circles of university life. The same is happening in the technical colleges, led bij the MIT and the California Institute of Technology (Harrison Brown).

Finally, the development had its repercussions, much sooner and more directly than would have been possible anywhere in Europe, in the highest reaches of American scientific life: the National Science Foundation and the National Research Council. In 1964 the American National Academy of Sciences embarked on a series of research publications aimed at the long term, which came to be known under the name of COSPUP (Committee on Science and Public Policy). The American Academy of Arts and Sciences went even further and appointed, in addition to an already existing 1975 Committee, a separate committee for the year 2000 which has to date issued a number of detailed, if still provisional, reports. The Library of Congress now has a Science Policy Research Division, and the American Senate, not to be left behind, has created its own subcommittee on Science and Technology with special reference to the future, which has also produced some interesting reports likewise directed at the long term.

Unmistakably, future-directed studies have been raised almost to the level of a national fashion in *America* during recent years. Fashions, even at the academic level, come and go extremely quickly there, helped on their way by a declared preference for new models or experiments and by the promoting of new scientific pioneers, or even heroes. Where attempts have been made to throw or to jump too far, therefore, some degree of recoil or moderation may be expected. In a "brainstorming" session the most audacious and unorthodox ideas can be put forward and, if necessary, withdrawn again with no loss of face. Established reputations are not destroyed in the process, although there are more personal ups and downs there than in our own academic world, where the title of professor alone seems generally to offer a lifelong guarantee of unshakable knowledge and unassailable wisdom. The spirit of university enterprise, the taste for adventure and risk, are usually much greater in America, where unonthodox innovators are more highly and more generally appreciated. This rather generalized account of academic "faits et gestes" in America must certainly not be taken as deprecatory. On the contrary, the importance for the future of the new scientific work being done there, in prognostics for example, must not be underestimated. It is to a great extent this new, purposeful mentality which conditions and explains the increasing American lead.

For at the same time there has arisen a fundamental need for renovation, both in the practice of the social sciences and in the application of new social techniques which promote and refine, often in an extremely valuable way, the approach to this deliberate future-research. Since almost all this work has, so to speak, been fired aloft through a combination of great enthusiasm and team spirit over the past two to three years, from hurriedly constructed, brand-new launching sites, it is obviously still in the earliest stages of discovery and invention, experimentation and improvement, and undoubtedly the process is very far from complete. It must of course be extended and elaborated in much greater depth, but I think we may already speak of a promising new start — a first, carefully calculated, deliberate move which may confidently be expected to continue systematically in the very near future. Very considerable funds and vast resources of top-notch manpower will have to be invested. This perplexing twofold problem appears to find a much easier and quicker solution in America than elsewhere. Scientific orientation to the future fits in marvelously with the traditional and typical popular inclination for continual renewal and remodeling. Preparations are well under way for the creation of special *professorships* in futurology.[14] Separate university courses along these lines are being or have already been organized, and syllabi of the requisite interdisciplinary type have been devised. There is a dawning awareness that the subject "history" must be balanced and complemented by the subject "future". To complete the picture we must not forget in this connection that the big private American foundations are making considerable funds available to this end. In addition to the Rockefeller and Carnegie Foundations, it is notably the Ford Foundation which is internationally renowned for this, providing generous financial backing for future-research both in America and abroad.[15]

Against this tidal wave of activity and new momentum in America, the rest of the world makes a rather unsubstantial showing at present. Future-study is taught in France, at the Sorbonne; but we know that the subject is one of great interest in *Russia* as well as in some Eastern European countries. How far particular future-studies have progressed there, however, we do not know.[12] The Penguin Special "Life in the 21st Century", a collection of interviews with a number of leading Russian scholars, does not give a good picture. The interviews were given to journalists with an insufficient command of the widely divergent specialist fields, whose questions were often aimed at the short term and lacking in imagination, and who have really produced a rather romanticized, science-fictionish report.

In Britain, the DSIR (Department of Scientific and Industrial Research) started tinkering with the future in 1963. The function was taken over in 1965 by the new Ministry of Technology, in itself a highly promising initiative. It is of course concerned with both economic and military prognostication. A special "Office for Forecasting" is said to be in process of creation at the moment. The British "Social Sciences Research Council", whose president is the sociologist Michael Young, has also set up a separate "Committee for the next thirty years", likewise under Young's aegis, one of whose leading members is the sociologist Mark Abrams. This Council has also made a grant to the Tavistock Institute for Human Relations to be applied to long-term studies aimed at the year 2000.

In other European countries (Sweden[17], Italy, Germany), developments of a similar kind or purport are afoot, though tangible evidence in university or otherwise institutionalized form is still scanty.[18] Hardly any steps have yet been taken to span this cultural lag, which must sooner or later, for survival's sake, be bridged.[19]

The future is of course a subject of study in the Netherlands, especially in the big concerns (Royal Dutch, Unilever, etc.). As far as I know, the results are not published as they are in America.[20] Philips has created the big Evoluon exhibition which will in time, reputedly, be aimed more at the future than it is now. This might then mark the turning-point.

Except for some specific subjects (development programming, urbanization and physical planning) the future as such and long-term studies on it are, to my knowledge, hardly a feature of the academic world here. That the Dutch Sociological Association has taken a working group on "prospectivism" under its wing is a gratifying sign. The newly appointed Council for Scientific Policy will neither be able nor willing to avoid the future but, as far as can be ascertained, does not at present have the necessary institutional apparatus. "Mankind 2000 International", founded in the Netherlands by a wide-ranging group of international scholars and thinkers, hopes that it may in due course make some scientific contribution towards progress and promote a favorable future climate, both among the public at large and in the governmental domain.

II Prognostics

The technology of prognostics and the prognosis of technology

For I dipt into the Future
Far as human eye could see
Saw the vision of the World
And all the wonder that would be.

TENNYSON

CHAPTER 12

Four-part epic of an absolute necessity

A. 1930-1940

The profound economic depression of the Thirties, a successor to countless others, which shook the very foundations of the Western production system, also produced a revolution in economic thought, which was still predominantly set in the mould of classical liberal attitudes.[1] One was forced either to believe in the Marxist laws of movement and the resultant predictions concerning an inevitable ideological and institutional transformation such as had taken place in Russia, or to demonstrate that the existing system of private enterprise (functioning considerably better than hitherto, thanks to certain adaptations and reforms) could be made to work. The necessary modifications required in the first place the availability of an adequate prognostic technique. This would have to give timely advance warning (it is now known as an early warning system in military technology), by means of specific elementary indications, that if clearly defined lines were pursued, the explainable effects and interactions of a number of economic factors would inevitably lead to a depression or recession of a given extent and severity. In the second place it was necessary to know in advance exactly what instruments, reserved for appropriate intervention on the part of governments, could be brought into play effectively to prevent such a depression, or at least check it. That is to say, these instruments still had to be devised, their use as alternatives or in combination had to be defined, and their effect had to be calculable as exactly as possible in advance.

The first systematic theoretical framework for a so-called "anticyclical" economic policy was designed, as everyone knows, by the British economist J. M. Keynes. As regards the investigation of the nature and effect of the economic cycle and the creation of a suitable apparatus both for economic prognosis and for government intervention on the basis of prior economic planning and advice on policy, the Dutchman J. Tinbergen has rendered notable service. Starting with the mathematical economics devised by pioneers like Walras and Pareto, econometrics was elaborated in increasingly efficient ways to deal especially with the objectives stated above. This has also entailed the development of new methods and techniques for prognoses regarding changes on the principal macro-economic quantities and complexes, such as productivity and gross national product, growth curves and rates of change, and relating to deviation from or modification of established aims. Further, there was a vogue for the construction of models and systems of equations, the manipulation of trend extrapolations and input-output calculations, the measurement of preferences, the establishment of priorities, the design of programs and the prognostic evaluation of the effects of various possible government measures.

There was little or no chance of a decisive trend of strength in the years between 1930 and 1940, firstly because application was still only tentative and half-hearted, but ultimately because the war, or its dark foreshadowing, took a determining hand in things. Preparation for war and the economics of war pushed the problem of economic depressions entirely on one side for the time being — just as the enormous post-war problem of catching-up did for a long while after. It was not until the Fifties, when prognostic techniques and the economic armory were noticeably more advanced, that their practical application was able, where necessary, to demonstrate their value to the full. Meanwhile, economic planning by governments had been fairly universally accepted and the world of business too had been obliged to adopt the methods of planning and prognosis. Only, to begin with, application everywhere was confined to the relatively *short* term because this was the only approach then regarded as realistic and justified.

B. 1940-1950

Throughout the Second World War, national economies were of course wholly subordinated to the pursuit of the war which, particularly by reason of the great advances in military techniques, presented quite different and much more complicated tasks than the one of twenty-five years before. The military problems of modern strategy and tactics, of invasion or any other large-scale amphibious operation or other kinds of coordinated actions and campaigns, not forgetting the question of logistics and ballistics, made demands that could not now be met effectively or comprehensively and coherently by means of the existing, shortsighted and opportunist, modes of thought. And indeed they were not wholly met, to begin with. The Munich compromise and the betrayal of Czechoslovakia should perhaps be ascribed rather to the incredible lack of understanding on the part of the then Anglo-French political leaders than to the military advisers they consulted; in any event, it was due not only to an error of judgment on both sides but above all to a hopelessly wrong prognosis and a fatal miscalculation. The attack on Pearl Harbor was as unforeseen as the fall of Singapore or the German invasion of Russia. It was only because of an incomprehensible miscalculation on the part of the Germans that the British defenses, which had dwindled to almost nothing, just managed to avoid losing the Battle of Britain. The Maginot Line, built at great expense in accordance with an obsolete dogma, proved completely valueless to the French. The Dutch "water-line" was no line at all.

Suppose Hitler had heeded the warning prognoses of his most competent

235

generals (the ones they still dared supply him with); the advance on Stalingrad and the battle for it would not have taken place and, in the absence of this turning-point, the war on the Russian front might have followed a quite different course. The success of the invasion of Normandy depended to a not insignificant degree on the lack of opposition from German troops, kept too long in reserve elsewhere through a series of misunderstandings — a possibility the allies had not foreseen. The failure of the landing of the Allied airborne divisions near Arnhem, on the other hand, can be largely ascribed to the unknown, or even deliberately ignored, chance proximity of German reserve divisions. The outcome of the allied offensive in Italy hung in the balance for a long time, despite the predictions. The balance-sheet of most military forecasts on both sides is, generally speaking, hardly a matter for satisfaction: the influence of miscalculation and chance could have been reduced. The Russian occupation of East Germany and the division of Berlin could very probably have been avoided with a proper American prognosis paying greater attention to the Churchillian view. The way De Gaulle was treated by the Anglo-Saxons stemmed, not only from mutual arrogance, but just as much from a faulty prognosis which caused lasting damage. Had one of the most visionary statesmen, F. D. Roosevelt, already under the blurring shadow of death, not followed his own naive conviction through fatigue at the Yalta Conference, but acted instead in accordance with a well-grounded prognosis concerning Stalin's true intentions, the world would since have worn a different and maybe less problematic appearance. And this had been only a tiny bunch of aprognostic blunders gathered at random.[2]

And yet, like the economic depression of the Thirties, these harsh military and to some extent diplomatic lessons of the Forties were not entirely devoid of effect. First in Korea and subsequently for the cold war in particular, as well as in Cuba, quite new and, hopefully, gradually more effective military prognosis techniques were introduced, at any rate in America.[3]

C. 1950-1960

The first forerunners of prognostics came on the scene in the mid-Forties. By the end of the Fifties their novel, almost revolutionary methods had penetrated by force, first the military sector (which now sets the pace in this field), then the industrial sector which was always strongly influenced by the success of these applications, and finally, though warily, in the realm of American civil government.

Clearly, absolute necessity in the military sector has brought about a revolution. The continuing evolution of nuclear armaments and other quite new, largely electronic, weapon techniques has made this necessary. Radar, rocketry and space travel have given an overwhelming impetus. As regards the study of global conflict, the first, much vilified, prognostic brainboys have consistently amassed power and top-line positions.[4]

236

Of the new prognosis techniques which were now applied, the following are the most worthy of note: operations research (literally baptized by fire here), and all manner of strategic simulation and games techniques, together with information techniques and decision-making techniques. These in turn were largely based on the development of cybernetics and computers and the data processing methods, communication techniques and feedback techniques whose application this brought about. Even those who regard things military with pacifist aversion cannot deny that the experimental applications and techniques, with their novel equipment set to deal with comprehensive and far-reaching prognosis, have had a strongly fertilizing effect, or at least can and will have such an effect, on development processes for civil purposes — quite different in intent but nevertheless just as future-oriented. Purposes which are of course especially focussed on the preservation of world peace.

D. 1960-1967

The chronological division into blocks of years, as used here, is of course somewhat arbitrary, in that, needless to say, no given year can be pinpointed as the start of an incipient process of development. However, I think it fair to say that it was really not until the early Sixties that this process of mental reversal began to receive very powerful impetus on all sides and that its momentum began to build up. It was then that the new and continually renewed prognostic techniques, in America at least, began their irresistible advance on a broad front. And no longer predominantly in the military sector, nor tied to one particular social science, nor even to social science in general.

The initial non-alignment of social science will be considered separately, as I have said. But two questions arise here: why was this a phenomenon of the *Sixties*, and why was it confined, mainly, to *America*?

A satisfactory answer to the first question would really call for a separate study. If is clear, though, that at that time a number of existing relationships started to grow closer, and various distinct threads started to come together. From that network of intrinsically complex growth processes converging on one central point, I should like to take three as the main explanatory factors; they may also be regarded as having a more general significance.

(1) The phenomenal development of natural science and especially of mathematical thinking, with their separate branches.

(2) The amazingly fertile conjunction of this scientific capability with equally meteoric technological innovations. These progressive brainchildren of the natural sciences have not only scored enormous achievements for development along favorable lines, but have also been the subject of growing concern, by reason of the ensuing general problems and possible dangers for mankind.

(3) The potential of an almost endless series of new scientific-technical products, constantly multiplied, creates specific problems for the producer himself, and thus for the expanding industrial sector.

CHAPTER 13

The prognosis of prognosis: can we really know the future?

1. "Futuribles" versus futurology (De Jouvenel)

An overall comparison between thinking in America and France is not too onerous a trade, because only a few years ago, in 1964, the leader of the French "futuribles" movement, Bertrand de Jouvenel, produced a thorough and systematic survey of the then state of affairs and desirable developments, which was published in a book already cited called "L'Art de la Conjecture".

In the last chapter (page 343) De Jouvenel writes that his "Carte du Présent" will lose its value more rapidly as the acceleration of historical events increases. This is, alas, a fact now, in 1968. The book was already somewhat outdated when it appeared. But the real cause lies deeper: it lies in his fundamental view of future developments. He disclaims (p. 347) any desire to write "le manuel du parfait prévisionniste". On the contrary, he warns against facile optimism as regards the perfecting of prognostics. In the first place, as he rightly states, a number of different futures "futures possibles", or "futuribles" are possible at any one time. The very same causes which make foresight more necessary at the same time make it much more difficult, if indeed they do not make it virtually impossible, to move nearer the ultimate target — the most probable future. Most new changes or modes and phases of change in the future will therefore, according to him, continue to be unknowable, unforeseeable and even inconceivable. The most we can do — and that only with great difficulty — would be to *foresee* the *present!*

This anticlimax on which the first systematic treatment by one of the leading European prognosticians ends is itself a clear reflection of the widening gulf between modes thought in Europe and America. Let me explain that point at greater length. De Jouvenel's work is extremely valuable — but mainly as history. It is very scholarly, particularly where it deals with the Ancients and the French classics. Aristotle, the Oedipus tragedy and Thucydides are quoted, Cicero and Thomas of Aquinas are discussed in detail, as are Montesquieu, Condorcet, Rousseau and Voltaire. Bayle, Maupertuis, Quételet and Comte come in for considerable attention, as do Malthus, Marx, Darwin and other great figures in the history of motion, change and evolution. Caligula, Napoleon and even Hitler are considered.

In addition, the book contains a good survey of origins and evolution, notably those of short-term quantitative economic planning and prognosis, with special reference to the writings of Tinbergen, Schumpeter, Klein, Stone, Sauvy, Theil, Samuelson, Katona and Modigliani. For the rather longer-term questions, however, De Jouvenel scarcely goes beyond the older pioneering work of Colin Clark, the French concentration on 1985 and the English report by Professor Buchanan on traffic. With the exception of a few lines devoted to games and simulation, none of the modern, non-economic prognostic techniques are discussed.

There are two reasons for this. The book was presumably conceived at the beginning of the Sixties[1], just when the prodigious developments in America were on the point of unfolding. In the second place, there is an essentially more deeply-rooted cause for the obsolescence already referred to. Mathematics in particular still seems, to De Jouvenel, to be based mainly on the mathematics of Newton and Leibnitz, Condorcet, Maupertuis and Laplace, and the three Bernouillis. Mathematical economics and mathematical economic statistics are, to him, the achievement of Quételet, Pareto, Jevons and, above all, Walras, whom he regards as fundamental to the equation systems of econometric and macro-economic models.

Even older mathematical geniuses like Gauss and Von Riemann are entirely absent, while more recent models and methods of thought receive no mention. I cannot put this down to chance, and still less to ignorance. But De Jouvenel deliberately adopts the standpoint (p. 79) that practically all future-forecasts in history, even those made by the greatest minds and even when their learned predictions were fixed to a mathematical framework, were afterwards found to be valueless. Faulty forecasts and wrong prognoses of the past vex him sorely. To prognoses that have turned out wholly correct he seems to grant no greater value than that of chance success (in line with the old saw: "Even a clock that has stopped shows the correct time twice a day"). In De Jouvenel's eyes a science of "futurology" is a hubris, far too ambitious, consequently quite unjustified and unacceptable.[2] In his opinion, the most that can be claimed is that there is a skill involved: the skill of an acrobat balancing on the tightropes that stretch out to possible futures. His plea is for the enhancement and application of these artistic skills. He holds firm to this standpoint, irrespective of the various techniques employed in the past, of which he mentions *seven*. At his request, though, the American sociologist Daniel Bell provided a contribution to his Futuribles series No. 64 in 1963 which distinguishes between a *dozen* predictive methods already applied or considered applicable in the social sciences. These include a few which are not mentioned by De Jouvenel and whose future-exploring potential has been somewhat advanced. The article is twice cited by De Jouvenel, but not the techniques which Bell's analysis has added to his own list.

I find this detail characteristic of De Jouvenel's unsympathetic attitude to what in his opinion goes too far in the field of prognosis; he sees it as unwarranted pretension, not only naive and speculative but likely to have an

240

adverse effect on all purely prognostic effort as an artistic institution if applied in an unsound and incautious way. It is an attitude of mind that in its disapproval — or should I say prejudice? — is still shared by many respected European scholars. So as far back as 1963 there was a significant difference from one of the authoritative American futurologists, Daniel Bell, who was later to be asked by the American Academy of Arts and Sciences to chair its Commission on the year 2000[3]. Even so, as I said deliberately, Bell's interesting article in 1963 was only a little further advanced than that of De Jouvenel[4]. It has been just afterwards, in the last five years, that future-research in America has really got off the ground and that, as a variety of recent publications show, numerous new techniques have been devised and and experimentally applied to prognostic ends.

2. "Think-factories" and long-range forecasting (Jantsch)

Until recently the relevant American publications by academic researchers and special research institutes, and the results of studies done by some business concerns, were distributed far and wide. It was common knowledge that "think-factories" or "think-tanks" existed in America. But because these establishments, sometimes employing thousands of top-grade staff, were mainly working on military projects to begin with, their work usually remained largely a mystery outside the close circle of insiders. During 1964, the Scientific Affairs Directorate of the OECD in Paris set up a research program, and in 1965 commissioned one of its consultants to collect data in the 12 associated member-states and establish a survey on the relationship between technological trends and economic growth. By October 1966 Dr. Erich Jantsch's draft report was ready in the form of an internal working document, not intended for publication. In December 1966 I was president of an OECD congress on automation and, having heard tell of the document meanwhile, acquired a copy for personal perusal with a request to regard the contents as confidential. With this I complied, even while preparing the early chapters of this book. Since then I have learned that the report has been fairly widely circulated and furthermore that parts of it have already been published in scientific journals, albeit as reflecting the personal opinions of the author and not (or not yet) those of the organization which commissioned the study.

I assume that I may now permit myself the same liberty.[5] The report is entitled "Technological Forecasting in Perspective". It is nearly 500 pages long, contains a wealth of data, a detailed description of the new technological activities and of the institutes concerned in them (both in-house and through outside contracts), an assessment of the results obtained in various sectors, a unique, annotated bibliography of some 400 works, and finally a

241

survey of achievements in this area in each of the member-states. I think this must unquestionably be one of the most important, and soon probably one of the most influential, reports to have appeared since the war. Not only by virtue of its valuable documentation, which is assembled with surprising, unmistakable perspective: but principally by reason of its intensely interesting treatment of difficult material, the penetrating vision of the author and his discernment as to the present significance of new developments and their expected course. His critical but positive judgment, as a man of European scientific training and background, on the American prognostic techniques which have taken such a great lead in recent years, deserves high praise.

This report, which is in the main a success, was compiled in so remarkably short a time that it cannot bear comparison with the tight structure and systematic arrangement of a scientific treatise. The same phenomena had to be considered as different aspects under different headings. Besides inevitable repetition and overlapping, highly important considerations are sometimes found in the most inexpected places and among points of secondary rank. To arrive at the essential significance of the material, one must generally distil it from a number of widely scattered passages. From this point of view, the principal aspects and most striking points need a certain measure of re-arrangement. In discussing the document I shall reduce quotations to the absolute minimum, since otherwise they would run to some hundred. I shall therefore attempt to reproduce in my own words (and consequently on my own responsibility) what I see as the essentials of the report.

Besides the pronounced American lead on important points, these essentials lie, I think, in two main issues. The *first* concerns what, according to Jantsch, (and put together from remarks and recommendations at various places in the report) is or must be characteristic of all effective new prognostic techniques. In many respects, however, these will differ from, or even be the opposite of, techniques formerly employed. The *second* essential is Jantsch's individual examination of a number of main types or variants of these new techniques. (The complex or ponderous American nomenclature — somewhat reminiscent of the "tiefe Deutsche Unklarheit" — may be irritating or amusing on occasions, though this does not of course detract from the usefulness of the results obtained.)

Jantsch himself adds a *third* point which he finds very important: the institutional organization that exists or has been renewed, in military, business and government circles, which aims at the application of the prognostic techniques in question. I have already made reference to this in earlier chapters, and shall therefore omit further mention here.[6] It is open to doubt which approach is preferable from the didactic standpoint: first a consecutive résumé of individual techniques, followed by a consideration of their common characteristics, or the reverse approach from the general to the particular. Personally, I would opt for the latter, which Jantsch also favors, especially

242

since this book in no way sets out to be a technical manual. In the first instance, therefore, I can more or less disregard Jantsch's thorough analysis of the techniques he has investigated, and the pros and cons of their principal variants. For the reader who may be interested in more specific detail on them, however, or who is more expert in these matters, the appendix to the present book goes into somewhat greater depth on some particularly interesting and striking methods and techniques.

As for the purely technical development of the new prognostic methods, it will be enough for me to state that, *insofar as* they are quantitative in character, they are largely the product of the latest advances in mathematics, such as applications of matrix mathematics and Boolean algebra, modern extensions of stochastic probability theory and mathematical statistics. Cybernetics and computers of course play a large part too. Closely related to them are information and communication theories operating through enormously speeded-up and improved techniques of data transmission, data processing and feedback. Of great importance too is the very recent development of the theories of decision-making, together with those of games, strategy and simulation. Besides new, refined applications of the older processes of extrapolation (trends and growth curves) and analogy, use is made of the latest possibilities for the building of models, networks and family trees, and the systematic establishment of relation-complexes and functional interrelations on card systems, plotted in time. Of especially great and ever-growing importance in this context are two specialized prognostic techniques, themselves comprising a host of variants, that are usually termed "operations reseach" and "system analysis" (or "system development"). This last, ultra-modern, technique is now employed exclusively, or almost so, by separate large establishments ("think-tanks"), where its experimental development is continuously pursued.

I am well aware that this brief summary may mean relatively little to the average layman, though it will mean something to the initiated. May I refer the latter first and foremost to Jantsch's original report, soon to appear, and also — this goes for all other readers too — to the said appendix which gives further enlightenment on a number of major points. Here and there in the following pages I shall give some striking examples of a characteristic renewal of traditional attitudes, to illustrate the spectacular and revolutionary changes in the "technology of technology".

In fact, the differences and deviations from previous prognosis techniques are immediately apparent if we adopt the *three-part* division which Jantsch rightly indicates as typical of all the modern techniques he has examined. Jantsch's three types are: 1. Exploratory 2. Normative 3. Feedback interaction from 2 to 1 and vice versa.[7]

Re 1. *Exploratory*. It is almost tautological to state that prognosis techniques

243

serve to explore the future. But not that they *must* be used more and more for his purpose — in other words, that they stem from what I have earlier called an "absolute necessity". The potential of technology and technical-economic control is far higher than ever before, and its power is still growing. There is an abundance of new possibilities with which we must be acquainted before we can select them. We come up against limits, either in our existing natural resources or in our human capabilities, which must be investigated and if possible pushed back to enlarge our scope. Lastly, we are becoming aware of enormous future problems, dangers threatening the whole of humanity as the result of possible future growth processes. At the same time, these call for a growing sense of responsibility on our part for the life of generations to come, in a world which must still be habitable. But what are the possible, probable future-alternatives? And what will be our urgent needs and requirements in the future? All this belongs to explicit exploration of the future.

Re 2. *Normative.* According to Jantsch — and to my mind, this is the greatest innovation — the *two* elements of modern technological forecasting, namely the exploratory and the normative, must be regarded fundamentally as polarities, i.e. as mutually indispensible. He calls the first "opportunity-oriented" (possible), and the second "mission-oriented" (desirable). The former outlines alternative possibilities (in the sense of De Jouvenel's "futuribles"). The latter sketches ideal desirabilities for the realization of particular goals, in accordance with the guiding principles of preselected and subsequently formulated norms and values. These are deliberately used where necessary to overcome the natural inertia of the existing order and the resistance of vested interests by effective intervention and guidance (somewhat along the lines of Gabor's "inventing the future"). In his report, Jantsch uses the terms "goal", "value", "objective", "desire", "mission", "directive", "task", etc., for this *normative* kind of technical prognostics, without differentiating sharply among them. One might also say that in the familiar double expression "research and development", the stress, particularly on the "development" side, is laid on the pair of questions "Where shall we go?" and "Where *must* we go?", both of which require an answer. This last form of "future-creative" thinking and foresight is, in Jantsch's opinion, all the more vitally essential at the present time in countries (such as America, France and other Western European states) which are still predominantly founded on the system of individual initiative and private enterprise.

Jantsch repeatedly emphasizes, and to my mind quite rightly, that this second component is utterly indispensable to all new prognostic techniques. It is currently the subject of strongly growing interest in America, if not yet wholly scientifically formulated. My only comment here is that there is bound to be a head-on collision, not only between purely exploratory prognostics but, infinitely more so, between normative prognostics and the *dogmatics* of the future which still prevails, at any rate in Europe. Particularly with the dogmatics favored by the social sciences — deliberately, sometimes unwittingly, or simply accepted as traditional and uncritically reiterated. Even more than in Jantsch's work, this *conflict* is a *central theme* of the present book.

Re 3. *Feedback and interaction.* It goes without saying that there is a discrepancy, not to say antithesis, between exploratory possibilities and normative desirabilities resulting from prognoses. For the sake of a necessary sense of reality, in turn associated with a certain measure of historical continuity, regular feedback and interaction must consequently take place, with mutual adaptation and periodic shifts from one pole to the other. Only through flexible feedback coupling of this kind is it all possible for optimum "technology transfer" to evolve in the vertical and horizontal planes of a further technological explosion and its influence on social realities, of the ensuing renewal and transformation of the original social milieu.[8] In other words, these feedback techniques are operationally active in the two related dimensions of *space* (fixed, but subject to continual change) and *time* (extended to cover a definite future range of expectations and desirabilities.[9]

I have endeavored to reproduce in my own way the essentials of the three-part foundation for the general "framework for technological forecasting" encountered and clearly indicated by Jantsch.[10] However, to appreciate fully the principal, and extremely far-reaching, implications and consequences of his analysis — the most important and decidedly spectacular *new* results, in fact — involves considerably more effort. For the author has cast them in far less systematic moulds and, frequently linking them to particular prognosis techniques, distributed them throughout the entire report, or derived them from specific aspects dealt with only once and sometimes lurking in rather obscure places. Furthermore, his own condensed version of "Major Findings and Recommendations[11], given at the beginning, while it does light on a number of truly important points, certainly does not give a thorough insight into what seem to me to be the most valuable results. Trusting that I do Jantsch greater justice than he has tried to do himself (by modestly avoiding too personal an accent in his work), I shall now go my own way and make my own choice of the points which appear to me to be of the greatest significance.

CHAPTER 14

Aspects and effects of modern future-research

1. The time dimensions

Both exploratory and normative "technological prognoses" are projected forward from the present into the future. The question arises what time dimension to take into account. In many cases the normative future-projection has rather greater freedom of movement and a wider time margin. Yet Jantsch's analysis unquestionably reveals an ever-increasing time-depth in exploratory prognosis too. This phenomenon is ascribable to the acceleration of pace and the extent of the changes pointed out above. In the practical application of prognostics, the relative foreshortening of future times also apparently necessitates a continual extension of the future time period covered.

Economic prognosis, originally progressive and a front-runner for a long while, is now sometimes of a straggler, limping along on a relatively short term of one or more years and finding great difficulty in achieving the medium-long term of some 10 years or so.

The exemplary Rand Corporation long-range forecasting study, which I have quoted more than once, proceeds in four stages up to the year 2100, whence it enters a broad new perspective no longer defined by an exact number of years or period of time. Most formal applications still cover a prognostic period of 5-20 years, but a steadily growing number, although only informal guesses as yet, are bold enough to look 20-50 years ahead.[1]

In a later statement not included in his report, Jantsch has given further details of the distinctions made in America, relative to industrial policy on the future, between "drifting with the mainstream", "leading the mainstream" and "shaping the future". The two last-mentioned periods of industrial dynamism, characterized by a roughly 10-year interval around 1953-54 and 1965-66 respectively, also coincide approximately with the distinction between exploratory and normative prognostics. The visibility of the time to come is in the first place greatly enlarged by the latter, while at the same time the choices (options) to be made between different possible futures acquire a much clearer time signature. The normative "to *shape* the future" can only really and truly be a successor to the passive "to *suffer* the future". According to Jantsch, Europe with its traditional approach is on average a good ten years behind America where the exploratory approach to the future on a greatly elongated time scale has already been adopted by 90% of business, and the normative approach by at least 10%. The greater the expected increase of the latter, the greater also the continuous extension of the period of time that is broached. Only now is the real future-dimension starting to come into its own right, even in America, as an independent quantity. But, unless all the indications are deceptive, this new mental process will gain an increasingly wider hold in the years to come.

To avoid any misunderstanding I think I should add, as the most important features of pre-eminently *undogmatic* progress, (i) *that* the future is tackled and dealt with as a separate dimension and (ii) that the future *period* covered is constantly projected forward to a more distant mental horizon. Its precise length — whether 25, 50 or 100 years — while surely relevant and symptomatic, is nevertheless still somewhat secondary in relation to the first two features mentioned. It is also mainly a question of refining and extending applied techniques, an almost automatic sequel to the fundamental step of crossing the frontier into no-man's-land.

2. Quantitative and qualitative

I have repeatedly emphasized that present-day "sophisticated" prognoses concerning eventual and desirable technological growth are based in large measure on the very latest developments in higher mathematics and ultra-modern statistical theory. This is entirely correct — but only half the story. For one of the most surprising results of Jantsch's wide-reaching and up-to-date study is the existence of another half, at least as important but still virtually unknown. Jantsch states emphatically[2] that he has never been able to draw a fundamental distinction between quantitative and qualitative techniques, because in many cases *no* clear dividing line can be detected between them. On the contrary, *both* approaches can and *must* be adopted in one technique.[3] In his synoptic survey on what Americans call "the state of the art", he concludes: "Qualitative assessment, in many respects . . . has attained equal importance with quantitative techniques". As always, this holds valid — and will accordingly not be repeated again here — for exploratory as well as for normative prognosis techniques. A qualitative vision is essential where the life of future-man in a future-society is concerned.

For the sake of balance and compensation, purely quantitative methods that are intrinsically one-sided and lead directly into ultra-rationalistic argument, are still viewed with caution. It is scarcely possible to overestimate this prognostic development by which the two kinds of approach are kept in mutual equilibrium. The exclusively quantitative approach has an inherent tendency to manupulate material quantities and thus exclude an idealistic view that is not always or not immediately quantifiable. The conviction that only the application of cognition models and techniques with the exactness of natural science could guarantee scientific acceptability held sway for a long time.

A qualitative method was a priori suspect as non-scientific. Of course it does carry the risk of overshooting the target, of getting out of balance. As in everything else, though, the possibility of misuse must not deter us from any use whatever, if (as here) responsible use is indeed a strict condition of the success of the operation as a whole — not just for success in *prognostics* but, equally well, in the pursuit of *science*. Recognition in principle of the equal validity of the qualitative approach is an enormous step in the right direction.

A number of important components of this quantitative contribution can be further differentiated:

A. Intuition

Jantsch devotes no less than five sections of his report to "the application of intuitive thinking and techniques for its improvement"[4], i.e. to the improvement of the qualitative approach. In fact — and Jantsch's schematic representation has this too — every prognostic technique starts with the essential intuition which is necessary to it.[5] Incidentally, is not the flash of genius, the partly subconscious or at any rate still unproven "hunch", the pacemaker in all scientific activity? However, this inherently indispensable intuitive approach can still be improved and refined and so, as an added bonus, be made entirely respectable. The intuitive techniques are essential because they — and they alone — provide random access to all spheres and levels of human thought, or human sense and apprehension.

It is as courageous as it is useful on Jantsch's part to assign speculative intuition so fundamental a role. Since Hitler, with his alternating appeals to the will of Providence and his own divinely inspired intuition, this concept, which science — and notably social science — has avoided like leprosy or the plague, has never been able properly to free itself from this deadly embrace, this tinted association. On the contrary, the nasty smell has thickened into a cloud of noxious vapor. But we must now have the courage to say aloud what Einstein several times demonstrated quite clearly: that science and intuition are not mutually exclusive or incompatible but, on the contrary, eminently *complementary*. Intuition is a condition, no less, of all prognostics in the true sense of the word.

B. Fantasy

Fantasy is of course related to intuition, but deserves separate mention. Without fantasy, no vision, without vision, no prognosis. This undisguised assertion by Jantsch is right up my street. As long as 10 years ago I pleaded for "foresight with the help of level-headed imagination". A few years ago the American sociologist C. Wright Mills gave his book the title of "The sociological imagination", though sociology has scarcely become very imaginative since. As a rule, however, social science has stayed firmly entrenched in "pure" science (purely contemplative "theoria") — without noticing, apparently, that

350 years ago Galileo, in extending fundamental natural science forward like a telescope, paved its way to two new and extremely important branches: applied natural science and natural scientific technology. Applied social science and social technology, by contrast, have so far gone by default almost all along the line. If they had not made a virtue of necessity and set up their utter incompetence and voluntary abstinence as law in these areas, "social imagination" too would surely have been able to prove its value as an indispensable instrument of social progress.[6]

Jantsch rightly gives as one of his major findings in his Preface[7]: "A thought attempt to come to grips with technological forecasting in its many dimensions soon leads one into regions of an uncertain, even fantastic character". In its further development the report serves both to evaluate this significant discovery in a fitting way and also, rightly, to warn against the danger of being carried away by the seductive fascinations of limitless fantasy. Jantsch does not further elaborate this in so many words, but his intention is unmistakable. Without a fair measure of fantasy, prognostics cannot get even properly started. But pure or unbridled fantasy threatens to lead it along false trails. What is needed above all is a fantasy that is based as far as possible on science, or at least accompanied, held in check and balanced by a scientific spirit. This fruitful cooperation can only be achieved by a happy combination of forward-looking imagination and a scientifically critical attitude of mind. The spiritual elite available for this is very limited and would consequently have to be assigned a place of considerable eminence. But, outside America at any rate, the opposite is now the case. All fantasy is necessarily the untrustworthy product of a wild dreamer, of a speculative and therefore unscientific mind moving in the inadmissible realms of science fiction — the "science" part of which is scientifically unacceptable — a description which indeed would do him too much honor.

In the evolution of technological prognostics from its "poetic" beginnings into a specific "art" and finally, if possible, into a separate science (though De Jouvenel will not go so far), an element of speculation will, according to Jantsch, always be needed to explain what is not rationally intelligible, provided it is kept within reasonable limits.

Thus it is no wonder that Jantsch has no reservations about counting science fiction as a prognostic technique on the basis of his own experience.[8] He is certainly not unaware that, as has been indicated above, science as such has, to put it mildly, shown very little appreciation of this unworthy appendage. But, even aside from the not insignificant anticipatory powers of science fiction in general[9] (from Jules Verne and H. G. Wells to Arthur C. Clarke, Isaac Asimov, Bradbury and others), Jantsch states that he has found science fiction or science fantasy constructed for the purpose of scientific-technical prognosis to be of unquestionable value. Under certain conditions and in certain circumstances, he considers this purposive kind of fiction[10] and fantasy to be an extremely useful implement.

249

Indeed, Jantsch regards this as valuable evidence of "emancipation". The venerable domain of the natural sciences is now also — indeed outstandingly — the scene of the strangest, most astonishing events, of things that speak to the imagination. Take for instance the field of high-energy physics (to say nothing of astrophysics), where the unknown appears dramatically through "signals" and "effects" that reach us from the immeasurable void, shrouded for Pascal in endless silence. Jantsch quotes an expert as saying: "Quantum electrodynamics is today more fantastic than any vision by religious prophets.[11]

C. Creativity

Intuition and fantasy together constitute the principal conditions of scientific creativity.

Jantsch devotes several paragraphs to the special relation between "creative thinking" and "forecasting" and to desirable training techniques for systematically increasing creativity to this end.[12] Personally, I have no great faith in a scientific "education" for creativity. Either one has what Arthur Koestler, following Plato, calls this "divine spark", or one has not. To the extent that development is possible, I would place greater faith in self-discipline and the full personal deployment of those intellectual gifts one has at one's disposal. The sweeping-away of scientific obstacles and barriers to free and liberal creativity would, I think, release much that is now smothered or strangled at birth. It is therefore my firm opinion, as it is Jantsch's, that *creative future-thinking* especially has been left far behind in the headlong, future-changing development of technology.

With the normative and feedback techniques in particular the crying need is not only for "future-oriented", but also effectively "future-creative", thinking. The new prognistic techniques serve both to illuminate and to create (or re-create) a possible, and desirable, future.[13]

This is achieved by inventing the future, by formulating dynamically compelling, idealistic visions of the future[14], by drawing up blue prints for the future, and by artistically creating logically consistent sketches of the future.

It is therefore in no way surprising that, as well as defending science fiction, Jantsch also reports a marked rehabilitation of Utopia as an effective prognostic instrument.[15] The current American view of it, at least where it is expressly employed for this purpose, is as the creative product of a "scenario"[16] written for specific future needs, and to this Jantsch attaches great value.[17] The rehabilitation of *idealistic* Utopia, championed especially by Ernst Bloch, in an eminently *pragmatic* country like America, and the acknowledgment of its primary and fundamental task, is as much a matter for rejoicing as it is pre-eminently characteristic of present-day developments in prognostics.[18] I shall return to it more than once in another connection.[19]

250

D. Brainstorming

"Brainstorming" is originally another typically American product of informal and provisional scientific practice which, however, has since been refined and improved for prognostic techniques in particular. It contains, of course, the qualitative elements of intuition, fantasy and creativity. In the Fifties, however, it expanded to become a separate technique employed, for example, by a stimulating "buzz group" or "brains trust" selected from a variety of experts and aiming at "operational creativity". I agree with Jantsch that the value of these rather primitive "bull sessions" is frequently doubtful, and it may be that the technique is already coming to be thought of as a little obsolete[20] in America, having given way during the Sixties to more modern techniques like operations research and decision-making.

However, a new and vastly improved brainstorming technique has now been developed and found relatively successful; this is the "Delphi" technique, devised by researchers at the Rand Corporation. It takes place in a number of consecutive rounds, questions being put to top-level experts drawn from a variety of sectors; these experts are not in personal contact with each other but only anonymously with a central point, via computer data which is provided on all opinions given.[21] Thus they can amplify or revise their original views without any loss of face, so that their opinions can lead to common culminating points, or at least to points expressed by particular groups, via this regular exchange of ideas in some kind of controlled way.

3. Normative

In his analysis, Jantsch repeatedly emphasizes a quite novel, and indeed spectacular, discovery. It is that the original absence of a normative sense of purpose severely handicapped the prognostic techniques formely employed. From the outset, and at different places in his report, Jantsch argues that the rise of the newer prognostic techniques and their success are primarily attributable to the deliberate introduction of a sufficiently strong normative component. One of the most important of his "major findings" is, I think, the following: "The full potential of technological forecasting is realised only where exploratory and normative components are joined in an iterative or, ultimately, in a feedback cycle."[22]

On as many as four separate occasions, Jantsch devotes a number of paragraphs to the vital nature of the normative element in technical prognoses that are of value.[23] He himself regards this as probably one of the most important results of his wide-ranging investigation. He is moreover very well aware that the "technology of technology" has thus entered upon a successful phase of its development, not only, de facto, free from existing specialist fields and conventional attitudes to science, but also running quite counter to these very

251

principles, and in an unorthodox way. Precisely because Jantsch is not himself a product of the social sciences (he is, I believe, an astronomer by origin), this unwelcome experience certainly fills him with surprise, and even some bewilderment; and he is of course unable to find an independent solution to this problem which, indeed, goes far beyond the scope of his report. He does sense, quite correctly, that there is some deep-rooted, largely hidden, and utterly inflexible future-dogmatic holding the social sciences helpless in its vicelike grip. But he sees himself faced with a wall of tradition and ingrained, or calcified, prejudice which it is virtually impossible for him, as a predominantly natural scientific thinker, to overcome.

It is moreover quite clear why this development in a normative direction got under way — indeed, why in fact it *had to* happen. For what scientific purpose would have been served simply by the ability to say something about the chances of possible and desirable future developments (know-how) without the capacity to add something about other and better, therefore desirable and also attainable future phases (know-what)? The age-old problems of "quo vadis?" and "knowledge for what?" were bound to be pushed to the forefront again by the mounting pressure of increasing acceleration and actual transformation. Even if the practitioners of social science failed to meet this prodigious challenge at once, the technological forecasters felt themselves called to respond. Called, and bound, to respond: in the military sector it was vital to know the answers to questions like "Where do we want to go?", "What must and can we do?", "What goals are attainable?", "What form of guidance offers reliable information on the best means of achieving the potential targets (tasks, missions, functions etc.) set for the future?" The same was true in essence of the industrial sector and the government sector, in their component parts and in their totality. Purely from the pragmatic point of view, these solution were universally required for the pressing needs of good management, and ultimately they were found by teams of technicians.

The profound consequences of this transition from exploratory to normative prognostic methods, forced on the scene by dint of necessity, are now starting to be clearly visible in many areas of American life. For instance, in the military sector, the clear division that existed formerly between the army, the navy and the air force is now completely antiquated. Now it only makes sense to think in terms of coordinated long-term strategic and tactical plans, of joint intercontinental assault and defense techniques or civil defense on a continental scale, in terms of space travel and man-made satellites, etc. The separate government departments are also losing many features of their distinctive character and tending to unite, to form a normative "business model" embracing the whole of the administrative economy like some gigantic concern.

Most characteristic of all, however, is the change of attitude which is becoming apparent, not only in the big progressive think-tanks themselves, but equally well in the highly specialized future-research divisions of big industry.

252

They are looking for wider commercial outlets for their refined prognostic techniques and models, further and further outside their original field of activity. They no longer wait for military and civil research contracts to come along. They are increasingly setting out of their own accord to offer their services in the search for solutions to the most pressing national (or regional) and social problems. They make their top staff available for integrated forecasting and planning, which is tackled as "large system thinking" in such important and comprehensive fields as the *future*, urgently necessary, reorganization, reorientation and recreation of education, urbanization, and recreation, transport, power, food (including artificial food), communications, health, natural (planological) space and physical planning (on land, in the sea and in the sky) etc., etc.

I come back to something on which I remarked, in passing, earlier (Chapter 1, 3): the "exemplary" American models of thought and our own European attitude. On the one hand this normative development deserves our most enthusiastic acclaim, but on the other hand we cannot observe without great hesitancy, perhaps not even without a slight shudder, how, mainly as a result of the vacuum artificially created by the social and cultural sciences, the continued development — and hoped-for progress — in the social sphere threatens to become a decidedly fearsome industrial monopoly predominantly controlled by the vested interests of big business. It should be obvious by now that in the *general interest*, these prognostic think-tanks and *future-research institutes* should also be available to national governments and supranational bodies *themselves*. As a matter of necessity, ample resources should be disbursed for this purpose. Nowhere, either in America or in Europe, is this at present the case.

Yet it is self-evident that the establishment of such government foundations and super-institutes can indeed contribute to the furtherance of analytical investigations, but would necessarily grind to a halt in the normative part, i.e. the synthetic culmination. For such institutes too would need to refer to the guidelines of national, supranational and international objectives. There would have to be clarity of vision on the values and goals which they would have to adopt as the ultimate normative guiding principles of their investigations and future-projections. But on this very point there is at present a yawning hiatus of appalling proportions, because the West at least no longer possesses any such ideological, or at any rate idealistic, up-to-date images of the future.[24]

The consequences of all this are therefore very far-reaching and hard to grasp in their entirety. Even Jantsch finds himself tied up in knots, facing a battery of question-marks. Which is no wonder, since the implications not only directly concern the *practice of science* as such (see the following chapters), but also introduce *ethical* and *philosophical* viewpoints, bring *social-cultural* aspects to the forefront and, ultimately, can no longer be dissociated from a more profound, ideological, *religious* or *humanistic* conviction.

All this is contained in the term "normative". It is of course not my intention to give an exposé of this whole complex within the present frame-work of a new prognostic apparatus. I shall restrict myself here to a brief consideration of just two, inextricably related, points: that of values and that of goals.[25]

A. Values

Science, notably social science, has generally — in our century, at all events — evinced a dogmatic purism. Science was there only to make judgments on pure truth, not on greater of lesser value, or on the valuelessness of things. This is the doctrine of so-called value-free, and therefore neutral and utterly objective, science. Should the scientist succumb to the temptation to pass personal and thus subjective judgment on the object of his study, then his science would lose its characteristic of ultimate general validity, verifiable by anyone at any time — the criterion of truth. Above all, science would descend from its state of *certainty* — easily the most highly "valued" of its characteristics — to an inner disarray of personal arbitrariness, or at least preference and objective uncertainty devoid of almost all firm handholds. This meant that it behoved the scientist to confine himself to what was empirically observable and amenable to rational treatment — in short, to the positive "is", taking no account whatever of the normative "should be".

But of course, that which is to come is no longer "that which is here and now". With a little effort one could extrapolate the here-and-now of the present, trendwise forward to the future of tomorrow, as a very cautious prolongation of present time. It would be possible charitably to turn a blind eye, despite the ingrained scientific predilection for the pursuit of the timeless, i.e. the absolutely true and invariably valid — in spite of the fact that we are certainly faced with a different, more or less transformed, even radically altered, future as a result of the acceleration and intensification of dynamic social processes. But to go still further and suggest what form that future, not only could, but more particularly should, take, in order to approximate to a world valued more highly than the present one, and so alleged to be different and superior, is to sin against the scientific code by transgressing all the limits of true professional decorum. Possible and Desirable, facts and values, belong to *two* quite different, wholly distinct *worlds* that cannot be bridged in any scientific way.

But this is precisely what happens when, as Jantsch describes, a sufficiently powerful normative component is introduced as being indispensable to any useful technological prognosis. Here, he enters a region strewn with contradictions, snags and pitfalls, and although he has consulted dozens of publications he is obliged to leave the field mainly to the prevailing controversy between two poles[26], unable as he is to reach a definite verdict.

There is a conflict here, one might also say, between an obsolescent "science of science" and a renewing "technology of technology". At bottom, this conflict is itself a clash between different values and valuations.

254

First and foremost, it is once again the tremendously accelerated development of technology, with the associated fundamental shifts of social structure, that — as has been argued repeatedly — has given rise to a large number of extremely urgent socio-cultural problems. Whereas technological progress was once virtually identified with progress in the absolute sense, people are now starting to wonder where these technical developments will ultimately lead. What is the value of them; are they good or bad, or a mixture of the two? Could they hold dangers threatening the spiritual values of mankind, human dignity, Western cultural values, and the future of a human society worthy of the name? These are challenging value-problems that cry louder for a valuational answer.

How can one judge future biochemical-generic interference with the mass of human heredity? How can one judge chemical-pharmaceutical products capable of distorting the human mind (drugs, psychedelics)? What about contraception, nuclear weapons, automated production, commercialized mass media and the rest? What about the gradual elimination of human labor and the accompanying expansion of spare time?

Without value-judgments such problems cannot be discussed, still less any contribution made to their solution. An appeal is being made to science, forcing it on the defensive and obliging it to examine its own conscience. For the value of science itself is at issue here. Is science practised only for its own sake ("la science pour la science") or — this concerns the social sciences particularly — in the interests of man and society too? Can and may science remain silent where serious potential dangers connected with future developments are concerned? (danger also expresses a valuation, of feelings of disorder and disquiet). Can it not, must it not, do its best to contribute towards improved ways of influencing and guiding this future development? What degree of socio-cultural responsibility should the scientist accept for "the shape of things to come"?

At the present time, science can no longer escape this evaluative self-appraisal. The thorny problem of the funds made available for fundamental research will serve to illustrate this fact. What priorities must be applied in these matters? Must we explore further in the field of molecular biology and genetics, or biochemistry and biophysics, or nuclear physics, high-energy physics, astrophysics, electronics, cybernetics — or that of the social sciences and humanities? Must science itself take a hand in determining scientific policy?

Must science then not only plan its own future development, but also have a say in the most important comparable modern problems of government? Like assistance to weaker social minorities at home and aid to developing countries; like the future distribution of income and joint labor-management control; like the future reform of education, including university education? Like the restructuring of society that the future will demand? And above all, must it not voice its opinion on the priorities for all these things?

In this connection Jantsch makes several very "appreciative" references to the Committee on Science and Public Policy (COSPUP), jointly set up in 1964 by the National Academy of Sciences and the National Research Coucil, and now presided over by Harvey Brooks.[27] The series of reports already issued by the Committee, with the collaboration of various teams of top-level American scholars, are of very great value and cover a growing number of the value-problems mentioned above.

The development is a highly interesting one, and one which is apparently likely to be copied in Britain and elsewhere. But it is all the more interesting if we reflect that here, in the drafting of these very reports, which are undoubtedly regarded in America as being of the highest *scientific* caliber, essentially and emphatically *normative* prognosis techniques are employed. It is a scientific innovation that is permeating from the very top of the scientific pyramid to the broader strata below. Its future effect — if I may be allowed an exploratory prognosis — will probably be considerable both inside and outside America. We have perhaps tended in the past to imitate rather slavishly the exaggeratedly empirical American-type investigation of ever-smaller, and finally minuscule, areas of study. From now on we shall certainly have to pay rather more critical attention to evaluative future prognoses on the American model.

It is, however, clear from the outset that any judgment of value will require some point d'appui, something firm to go on. How must social, ethical and esthetic values be positively evaluated? How do we evaluate the negative results of technical-military and technical-industrial developments? What standards can we apply, other than the economic criterion whose sole basis is money? Is it possible to add qualitative values as indications or components in quantitative comparisons of costs and returns? This takes us into a still totally undeveloped area currently referred to as "social accounting". Here, cultural minus-values to be set on the debit side against the benefits of technical progress would include such disadvantages as the pollution of air and water, the destruction of nature (erosion) and space (recreation), the creation of slums (urbanization), the lack of living space, the shortage of school facilities, the deforming of people (drugs), unhealthy psychologenic social tendencies, discrimination, poverty, hunger, want (including the want of a chance to develop), etc., etc. All this implies a revaluation of what being a human being will mean in the future and the form human society will take. However uncertain it may be as yet, the revaluation should nevertheless be tackled as far as possible in a scientific spirit[28] (see point B).

Now the Americans would not be the practical people that they are if they had not become thoroughly aware of the risks inherent in subjective-arbitrary evaluations in their technological forecasts. Of course no future-prognosis is 100% correct — unless by pure chance there is an exact canceling-out of errors on both sides. Every prognosis contains a fairly wide margin for error which can never be reduced to zero. Every prognosis always requires periodic revision on a relatively short-term basis, especially if it is aimed at the long term. On the other hand, the Americans have invented another distinct technique for eliminating over-optimistic or over-pessimistic evaluations as far as possible from their technological forecasting.[29] It is based in part on the evaluation of a large number of case histories of statistical prognoses made in the past. These prognoses related to estimated potential economic market requirements, development costs and development times for new projects. At the same time they entailed (either explicitly or implicitly) a definite vision as regarded the changing overall situation, other technical developments and new inventions to be applied, and unforeseen historical events. Finally, this evaluative retrospective study is supplemented by a critical analysis of earlier miscalculations based on false judgments and starting-points, etc., etc.[30] Every effort will also undoubtedly be made in years to come to minimize bias and prejudice as expertly as possible in other ways.[31] Jantsch terminates his study of the accuracy of modern technological prognosis with the general conclusion[32] that "the desired results from the point of view of accuracy, awareness and long-range implications can be attained in the form of marked statistical improvement over a state of no-forecast".

To sum up, every personal assessment of future developments, even those of people who have specialized in this new, comprehensive material, includes points of sometimes great uncertainty and is never free from what are later seen as crass blunders, which may then appear ridiculous. The history of technology provides a wide selection of the most remarkable examples of this very fact. Even using the latest prognosis techniques with double checks and even computer logic, such mistakes cannot be ruled out. But they can be so reduced that their positive "values" present a reasonable, and growing, credit balance.

B. Goals

Because it is impossible to talk about socio-cultural goals without evaluative choice, science has largely declined to go beyond the study of the means by which given goals can be furthered.[33]

Now it is always a rather tricky business to decide what goals are in fact estabished. They vary with time and place. Definitions remain too abstract, imprecise and vague. In defense, the goal is the maintenance or attainment of military superiority. That of the health authorities is the health of the people, but definite values must be established as criteria of what should or should not be regarded as healthy (take drugs, for instance), and this problem of values becomes much more ticklish where mental health is concerned. The critical factors in industry are economic viability, expansion, productivity, and the public image of an indispensable and — once again — valuable service. Government is concerned with the just and effective ordering of . . . the most valuable interests of society. All this, of course, tells us nothing about the

257

scale or relative hierarchy of values, and less still about the selection of priorities among rival, even conflicting, goals. To say nothing of investing money, or raising taxes (which?), or making demands on the public (how great?), to achieve these ends.

In America, it was from the powerful military defense and strategy sector that the impetus first came for the establishment of future goals and norms in the development of concrete new weapon techniques. This was originally the main function of the research institutes and think-tanks that were created for the purpose. The creative delineation of these new objectives and of the related tasks, whose object was to invent agresssive and defensive weapon systems that would be effective in that desirable and worthwhile future, constituted the most powerful initial impetus for the designing of adequate, and so normative, forecasting techniques. These were subsequently recognized as highly valuable in the context of civil, i.e. principally industrial and governmental, target definition, where they were adopted, generalized and improved. And it was these techniques that gradually underlined the close mutual connection between the goals of industrialists on the one hand and of government departments on the other.

In fact, these prognostic techniques are being increasingly employed precisely in order to obtain more detailed material for discussion, to contribute to the solution of burning problems. Judgments vary enormously on the value and usefulness of the exceedingly costly, dollar-devouring space program, the gradual penetration of the cosmos and the occupying, or at least exploration, of other celestial bodies. Is it necessary? Is it too high or too low on the list of priorities? Should the pace be slackened, or should it be hotted up? Should an anti-missile missile system be installed, should atomic fallout shelters be built in large numbers for the civilian population? How might one resolve the controversy between the "doves" and the "hawks", both of whom are working towards the same goal — an early peace in Vietnam — either through the cessation or by escalation of the bombing? Is rapid and universal automation of industry desirable in every sector, or should there be a sharp slow-down, or even a temporary halt all-round? Where goals are wholly controversial, as in such cases, modern prognostic techniques can throw more light on consequences and implications, on main results and side-effects, on favorable and unfavorable outcomes in a great number of related areas.

Jantsch's report is also of particularly great interest because his extensive study of the prognostic techniques increasingly adopted and developed by the big American industrial concerns has taken on a dual character as regards its aims. No good *industrial management* is now possible unless full account is taken of future developments. Indeed, the *main emphasis* has clearly *shifted* from the *present* to the *future*. But what does this future mean? What products will it be possible to manufacture profitably? Of course, this continues to be

258

a goal. But the "product-oriented" goal of the large concern is shifting, by degrees towards a "function-oriented" or "mission-oriented" one.[34] This means a broadening or deepening, in two senses.

In the *first* place, there was a move — reflected throughout industrial organization as a whole — towards more purposive research and the prescribing with priorities allocated, of specified new inventions, fitting into the general framework of future developments anticipated as possible and desirable. In the *second* place — this follows automatically from the first point, but forms a quite new, particularly noteworthy and "valuable" addition — it began to be realized what a dominant role was going to be played in these general future developments by the *social* goals established (mainly national ones) and by *international* objectives which could be expected or encouraged in the future (economic and political in character).

As a result, normative prognostic techniques for concrete industrial purposes began increasingly to take account of general human values and social goals which, it was assumed, must necessarily exert a heightened, purposeful influence on future development.[35]

This again, of course, led to an intense mutual interaction with the ever-larger government sector; in particular, with the modern prognostic techniques adopted and applied by the various departments (or by way of departmental contracts with academic or independent institutes), notably the widespread Planning-Programming-Budgeting System (PPBS)[36], alone or in combination with analogous techniques such as those of COSPUP mentioned earlier.[37] In other words, the social and international goals of government are again used as "input" for the prognostic and feedback techniques of industry. Conversely, these normative industrial prognoses and the impact of their technical realization on the social scene provide important data for the normative prognoses of government, which may correspond or which may, as regards goals, be divergent, corrective or adaptational.[38] How and to what extent this can and must lead to improved integration of technical development and the future interests of the community, is a question that will be dealt with separately.

At all events, the fact is now beginning to penetrate, slowly but surely — even to parliamentarians and politicians, and the executive agencies — that modern government is today no longer practicable unless unequivocal positions are taken up vis-à-vis a future that is rushing towards us at breakneck pace and changing everything in its path. "Gouverner, c'est prévoir" is a phrase that has been piously mouthed for as long as anyone can remember, but it has seldom been anything but an "empty box". What provision (the word suggests pre-vision) must now be made for the future preservation and protection of nature (space, air, water), for the preservation of human personality and privacy in mass-structures, for worthwhile leisure activity in a workless world where all wants are satisfied? How can the younger generation be prepared (education, training) for these new, changeable social structures;

how can they be made to participate in the continued workings of democracy? What other standards will apply for the other future-people in another future society? Where is scientific-technical-economic development leading and in what way can we and must we try to reshape where necessary, by purposive intervention, these reforming development processes themselves?

"Future-creative" planning, accompanied by normative prognosis techniques, is absolutely essential for this. One of the prerequisites is careful political preparation. This, according to Jantsch,[39] is why De Jouvenel's idea for the establishment of a pilot "look-out institution", where all sorts of standards, objectives, tasks and plans for the future could be thoroughly debated on a high level (pre-parliamentary), has been well received in future-oriented circles in America.

Furthermore, the idea is beginning to take root that the desired manipulations and transformations might be assisted by the setting-up of information and data banks and model banks, on the lines of blood banks, offering facilities in accordance with changing situations and requirements. It is of course realized that normative prognosis techniques are only an instrumental auxiliary. The persuasion is growing that to protect our present-day goals as it were from back to front, i.e. towards the future, is no longer adequate and that on the contrary, with new future-values established at the outset, the process should be one of thinking back to the here and now. But there are many scholars, notably in Europe, who regard this as "complete nonsense" or equate such arrogance with that of the sorcerer's apprentice.

According to some progressive American thinkers who are deeply conscious of their social responsibility, mostly attached to the Rand Corporation[40] and its offshoot the System Development Corporation[41] (now far larger than its parent institution), these techniques that revive the old attempts at "social engineering" should be subordinated to a new "social technology"[42]. This would thus come to stand on a level with applied natural science, which has soared so high in our own time. Here too, the crux of socio-cultural and national-ethical objectives remains unchanged.

Looking back on the field of values and goals, the conclusion is inescapable that reflection on the future of culture, and social ethics, while as yet almost virgin territory[43], is a matter of pressing need if prognostics is to achieve any valuable progress.

4. Interdisciplinary

We have so far considered in turn three surprisingly new aspects of modern technological prognostic techniques. First, the constant shifting and extension of the future dimension towards a more distant period of time (though it is always thought to be closer); secondly, the qualitative nature of quantitative

260

prognoses (intuition, fantasy, creativity, spontaneous brainstorming); and thirdly, their essential normative character (with the values and goals this implies). In each case I have broken off the discussion at a point where the question of the practice of science as such can no longer be excluded from the debate. We too are faced with the same problem in discussing this fourth aspect: where does technology end and science begin? This particular knot can only be cut with some degree of arbitrariness, and an attempt must then be made to tie the ends together again.

Here too, on the now essentially interdisciplinary nature of modern technological prognosis methods, Jantsch's report is a rich mine of information. He also expressly highlights this fundamental characteristic.[44] Indeed, logical reflection shows that to try to explore a number of possible (desirable) futures in their overall complexity, i.e. as an integral totality, is quite simply the only reasonable approach. All kinds of separate, fragmentary portions of the jigsaw puzzle are of little avail unless they are fitted together in the best possible way to form an image of the future depicting a number of main areas of development — and thus the scientific branches and technical specialities relating to them. One cannot hope to survey all the lines in the development, to "invent" *the* future, from one single field, however important it may be in itself.

This explains why Jantsch himself expresses in a variety of slightly different ways this idea of an inextricable interwearing of the multifarious threads in the development, using as many different terms which in fact mean the same thing. It is really so self-evident that a more precise definition is almost entirely superfluous. It is enough to know that the vital need is to acquire as firm and complete a grip as possible on a future complex, totality, aggregate, structure, pattern or system. Each prognostic technique of the kind described here therefore strives, by definition, to be comprehensive, integral and synthetic. Progressive scientific circles in America have already come very close to the "Declaration of Interdependence" that is now required.

The names of many of these prognosis techniques (mentioned in Appendix) bear emphatic and eloquent witness to the essential feature of comprehensiveness. They sometimes appear to be rather daunting names, striving frantically to be different, but serving virtually one and the same purpose. On the other hand, the many variants give an instructive insight into the central theme.

The following are some of these integration-directed techniques, which are also used in various combinations. (Most of them are separately described by Jantsch; see also Appendix).

Profile outlining; Envelope curves or cycles; Networks; Multi-level approach; Aggregated level approach; Morphological research; Communalities research; Feedback loops; Transformation methods; Integrated decision methods; Systems analysis, systems development and systems engineering; Integral models; Contextual mapping; Integrated relevance tree techniques; Comprehensive (vertical and horizontal) programming; n-dimensional matrix analysis; Synoptic scenarios; Simultaneous, iterative time series and sequences; Multistage probability chain processes; etc., etc.

The ambition in each case to catch and embrace the whole of the future is evident, irrespective of the merits of the various techniques, whose usefulness is assessed individually by Jantsch.[45] There are however important consequences for the organizational structure of the future-research departments of big concerns, for the institutional methods of leading consultancy bureaus and think-tanks, and lastly for the methods of scientific practice itself. Jantsch has reported very extensively on the first two points[46], complete with the computed results of, and estimated investment for, longterm forecasting procedures organized in this way. In American industrial practice, it appears, the interdisciplinary approach roughly resolves into a 50/50 split between scientific-technical and economic staff.[47] In the case of the private institutes this is harder to judge because it can vary enormously from one study to another. A total of 82 persons worked on the oft-quoted long-range report of the Rand Corporation, of whom 35 were permanent staff there and 7 were employed freelance. Of the 82, 56 were on the natural science/technical side, 12 were economists, 9 social scientists and 5 had literary backgrounds. At the Stanford Research Institute, a pioneer in the field of technological forecasting and the most interdisciplinary-minded of all the institutes (to judge from its regular Long Range Planning Reports), about 40% of the output is generated by permanent staff and about 60% by collaborators taken on for particular projects.

On one point Jantsch is content simply to refer to Helmer.[48] This is presumably one of the few things the extreme importance of which has to some extent escaped him, unless he regarded it as self-evident. Because future prognoses *must* be interdisciplinary, a new type of expert, the *generalist,* is being formed. The Rand Corporation has experimented with them in its Delphi technique. This kind of expert can be asked to comment on one point (symmetrical), or panels of different experts can be set up to advise on different aspects of one problem (asymmetrical). Lastly, teams of specialists, generalists and various combinations can be formed.[49]

In Europe, the generalist with no particular specialty is decidedly not "in".[50] But neither are the modern interdisciplinary prognostic techniques; and last of all, the intuitive-imaginative-normative attitude of mind which is a part of them.

5. Operational

For the American research methods chiefly described by Jantsch, this element is in fact so obvious that he has very little to say explicitly about it.

Indirectly, he says a lot. Whenever he speaks of these new techniques as modern management techniques, his meaning is quite plain. What they enable leaders (military, industrial and governmental) to do unmistakably *better* than before is the decisive factor. These techniques always entail an inherent obligation on the management concerned to apply operational, i.e. demonstrably more effective, decision-making. Operations research and decision-making are the midwives of these development processes. The quality, the scope and, we trust, the wisdom of the decisions taken, whose influence on future events will be profound, must be served and supported by these techniques.

These techniques reveal the connection between the policy decisions taken in separate sectors. They also show the connection between the development of science, technology and management. They are only of "value" operationally in the sense that they are able to analyze and at the same time integrate these connections.

In view of the continual growth of applications in America, it may be assumed that the new technical aids have already given decisive proof of their untility. Apart from their application to military and industrial ends, which has already received separate mention, they are employed in the fields of medicine and education, to solve problems of recreation, urbanization, transport, and traffic, communications, planology, food, power and raw materials, for development programs and, last but not least, in many kinds and functions of research itself.

We may also infer from Jantsch's report, though he does not say it in so many words, that the term "operational" is starting to acquire a changed meaning as a result of the application of these techniques. For the characteristically rather impatient, dynamic, restless American for whom everything has to work right now, or better still yesterday, it means a slow but sure shift towards what is going to turn out well in the *future*. There is in Jantsch a still almost imperceptible but highly significant, gradual identification of the concepts "operational" and "mission-oriented". Properly to execute the mission of the future, as yet unknown but explored and invented at the expense of valuable time, money and energy, and linked indissolubly to the policy decisions of here and now, that *is* the right operational method.

A single example will suffice. When Wilhelm Fucks, a well-known professor of plasma physics at Aachen, publishes a book now widely acclaimed in Germany,[51] containing a far-reaching prognosis of global politics, the question arises whether it can be considered operational from the standpoint of policy. For his forecast on the future patterns of political power he uses only three parameters — population growth, steel production and energy consumption. His global formula runs: Power is equal to the sum of steel production plus the product of energy consumption and the square root of population growth. According to his calculations, China will, in terms of industrial-political-military strength, outstrip Russia in 1970, America plus Western Europe in

1980, and both blocs together in 1985. Of course, no sane person doubts that the power of China will grow in time. But this exact future-prognosis, which in fact bears a closer resemblance to prediction and prophecy, seems to me personally to be neither interdisciplinary nor operational, but simply nonsense. If such a prognosis had any sort of real predictive value, it would not be on the basis of such a simple, narrow and to my mind pseudo-exact formula, but through the convergence of a large number of other factors.

Which goes to show that not every specialist scientist who steps outside his own narrow field of study may, for this reason alone, lay claim to the epithet "generalist" — which should surely be closer to the notion of the "uomo universale". Perhaps it is precisely the old-fashioned, one-sided, quantitative approach and the complete absence of a *qualitative* vision that will deny such work the highly sought-after quality of "operationality" — at any rate, outside Germany and China, presumably.

In conclusion, I must add that I do not mean that all the American prognosis techniques touched on here are already faultless and fully operational. I have described a development which, after a rather hesitant start, has only been powerfully (albeit still experimentally) evolved over the last 5-7 years. Needless to say, we should approach these experiments with an open and thoroughly critical mind, and make constructive contributions where we can. In times to come, some of them will prove unable to stand up to reasonable criticism, while others will need much improvement and amplification. The ultimate criterion continues to be the measure and the manner in which these techniques, once amended and perfected, are eventually capable of meeting the specifications. They are required to give more and better insight into future developments, to act as a usable instrument for the purposive, effective guidance and control of potentially conceivable, or even probable, processes of transformation in social dynamics, to the extent that this is possible with human assistance, and wherever it is desirable and justifiable from the socio-humanistic point of view.

It is also, or indeed primarily, the function of prognostics to keep the future *open* for continual improvements in the design and application of prognostic techniques.

PART FOUR

Counter-prognostics and continuous prognostics

I Agnostics

Frigidity and sterility versus social-scientific creativity and procreation

Thou shalt not answer questionnaires
or quizzes upon world affairs
nor with compliance
take any test. Thou shalt not sit
with statisticians nor commit
a social science.

W. H. AUDEN[1])

[1] A Reactionary Tract for the Times,
quoted from the Jantsch Report, p. 44.

CHAPTER 15

Exponential acceleration, explosive dynamics and fundamental reconstruction

We have so far advanced on a variety of fronts to a position from which, in the following series, a concentrated attack can be made on the Great Wall. For the social sciences, this is the Wailing Wall, behind which lies the sacred, heavily fortified bastion of the holy temple of Solomon. Its toga-clad high priests, though equipped with the most antique and somewhat rusty weapons left over from the romantic age of dragons and knights-in-armor, nevertheless guard it effectively. These weapons consist mainly of sacred initiation rites, ideological formulas, magical incantations, esoteric chants, herbs and medicines sometimes dulling the senses, sometimes arousing ecstasy, and last but not least, ascetic rules of abstinence. In other words, and more to the point, everything is done (or not done!) according to the dogmas of *tradition* and *authority*.

To begin with, we discussed[1] a great number of urgent world problems of the highest priority. We then considered a number of the most important works of national, and ultimately international authors who clearly reveal how much the future of mankind has come to depend on a timely and satisfactory solution to these demanding future problems. Thanks to this new change in our thinking about the future, which was brought about out of sheer necessity, we have seen the establishment and development of specific institutions of various kinds in a number of countries (the most spectacular of these being the American think-tanks). They offer a "new grip on the future". They represent a modernized, institutionalized form of "human dignity" which, during the Renaissance as typical determination of one's own destiny had breached the then accepted permanent and pre-ordained order of the Middle Ages with the power of new knowledge.

In subsequent observations[2] we pointed to an extensive series of new techniques used by the above-mentioned thinkers and think-tanks. These have been created and refined, and tested experimentally, to get a grip on the interrelated development trends and on the interaction of technical and mental forces in the field of the socio-cultural dynamics of today. For it is from this cocoon that a winged-future of multi-colored splendor will emerge which, if we are not prepared in time, may blind us with its surprising, unexpected glare. It may even, like Father Time, reveal a tendency gluttenously to devour its own children — the coming generations.

Through all the chapters which we have recapitulated here, there runs one continuous thread of thought. This is the thread which, as we previously mentioned, can be seen where the period of the Renaissance wriggled out of the irksome constricting whalebone corset of the Middle Ages. Likewise, this thread is seen where the French Revolution breaks the bonds of the "ancien régime" and crumbles the pillars of aristocracy and bourgeoisie. Again, we find the same thread when Marxist-Leninist Socialism, inspiring the Russian Revolution, dissolves the framework of oppressive Czarist rule and breaks the claims of the exploited proletariat. The same thread — the thread of radical revolutionary development — leads from the first Industrial Revolution over $1^1/_2$ centuries ago to the second Industrial Revolution (really a socio-economic, socio-political, socio-cultural revolution) which is occurring with impetuous, unbridled, irresistible power, *now*, in the second half of our very own century.

What has been successively described in the form of new, accumulating, possibly over-powering world problems, drastic future developments and radical shifts towards new future-institutions and adequate new future prognosis techniques are only facets of and reactions to one and the same theme (with variations). All of these observations relate to the same outstanding and explosive happening. This is an historical (at present, ultra-dynamic) happening which I have attempted to clarify by using the term "changeability": changeability in the use of human power. It is basically identical with the history of Renaissance and Revolution, but now drastically compressed in time so that it develops in our own age with a highly increased power factor and an enormous accumulation of far-reaching consequences. We are confronted with a steep, high-rising curve soaring up with amazing rapidity; a kaleidoscopic telescoping of our existing social system and its traditionally styled cultural patterns.

In other words, with regard to energy, speed, wide range of action, intensity, impact and substances, this is another completely different and separate happening. In short, one in which unprecedented quantitative excess and abundance could easily develop into a particular, special *quality*. The transformation processes caused by this may write the future-history of a revolution sui generis. Even if we try to keep usual contemporary over-estimations in check as much as possible, such a revolution still seems capable of exploding the historical frames of thought. Via previous, smaller-scale revolution, we have been prepared for this impending *"revolution of revolutions"*, which will be identified, judged and provided with suitable comparatives and superlatives only by later generations of historians[3]. We only hope that future historians will be able to mention in their chronicles that in our days, for the first time, a systematic effort was made to control this more steeply rising curve of development as much as possible and, where necessary, to intervene and bend it in a more favorable direction. Without this well-planned and firmly held control, future history might run completely amok.

It has been attempted, over and over again, by means of contemporarily comprehensible terminology, to give a reasonably thorough account of this unique process of development which is occurring right before our sightless immobility. But the onrushing waves of the future are destined to destroy all previous historical frames of reference as if they were no more than mere outlines traced with a stick in wet sand. It is a symptom that many well-known prognosticians must resort to the use of expressions which are in many ways too weak, rather exaggerated and definitely over-exuberant, such as *exponential growth,* violent *acceleration,* dynamite-like *explosion, structural* reconstruction, *revolutionary* renewal and even *mutation.* Anyway, these are tempestuous developments that may culminate in a chaos of disintegration which would have disastrous, perhaps even fatal, consequences for human society as we know it. And in spite of such pretentious words, this vision is not founded on an intentional cultural pessimism as much as it is the simple result of an entirely dispassionate, pro-eminently realistic prognosis.[4]

Precisely and solely because an unfavorable course of events can be avoided by wise prediction and purposeful action, and because we could achieve a *better* society for ourselves in the future by our intentional efforts to this end, *all* our attention is focussed on incipient developments of the present time. This is as it were the prefabrication of a future which is either promising or disastrous.

Which is happening *now!* The acceleration and revolving motion leading up to an explosion, the starting-points of revolution and transformation, the decision between chaos and order, the shape of things to come — all this is inherent in what, according to the accepted policies of our time is decided, done or left undone. In other words, our future depends almost entirely on the methods and measure of predictions that are being developed now and translated into actual, purposeful activities. Not only does the future-dimension appear as a separate entity with an obvious breach in time, but also, and seen from a completely objective point of view, the future dramatically appears as nothing less than a probably striking metamorphosis.

Thus far, I have not, in an effort to gain moral and intellectual support for my radical opinions, quoted many like-minded thinkers. Now, however, having reached this strategic position where decisive steps must be taken, diametrically opposed to what has so far been accepted, traditional and — consequently — only too easy, some friendly support would be very welcome. I would, therefore, like to offer at this point two characteristic illustrations which are of American origin. Although I do not subscribe to them without qualification, since they appear to see everything a little too rosily, or at least their predictions of a golden future era are somewhat over-optimistic. These two prominent American scientists have tried to make clear to a scientific committee of the House of Representatives, in plain and simple language, that human cultural history is, at this very moment, at a very important cross-

269

Accelerated acceleration and transformation

HOMO PROSPECTANS
1968 – prognostics
1965 – biogenetics
1960 – lasers
1957 – space travel, miniaturization
1948 – transistors
1947 – automation (Wiener)
1942 – atomic fission (Fermi, Teller)
1930 – television
1920 – talking motion pictures
1910 – radio

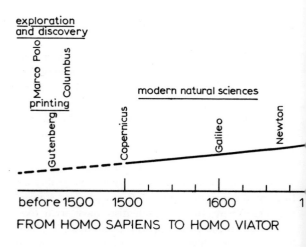

FROM HOMO SAPIENS TO HOMO VIATOR

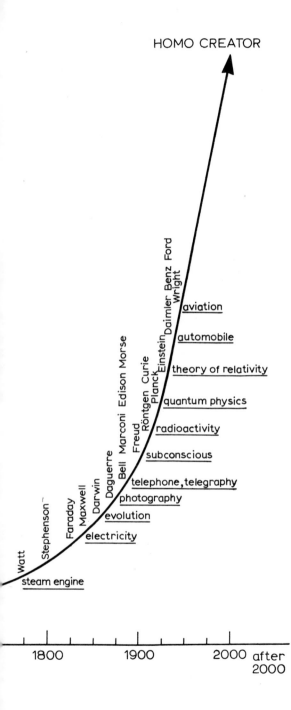

HOMO CREATOR

Watt
Stephenson
Faraday
Maxwell
Darwin
Daguerre
Bell Marconi Edison Morse
Freud
Röntgen Curie
Planck
Einstein
Daimler Benz Ford
Wright

aviation

automobile

theory of relativity

quantum physics

radioactivity

subconscious

telephone, telegraphy

photography

evolution

electricity

steam engine

1800   1900   2000 after
                                  2000

271

roads.[5] Recognizing the enormity of the task of convincing skeptical, usually opportunistic politicians, Dr. Thomas Malone drew them the following broad picture. Imagine, he told them, that we were to compress the 5,000,000,000 years of the existence of the planet earth into 80 days — that is, one day equal to 62,500,000 years! Then, on the basis of this time-scale, we can chart the following historical events:

The first signs of primordial life appeared about 60 days ago and the first ancestors of man about 1 hour ago. Modern man, however, came on the scene less than one minute ago.

Agriculture was developed 15 seconds ago, the iron age 10 seconds ago, and the money economy is only ¾ seconds old.

The First Industrial Revolution started 3/10 of a second ago; the revolution in physics 1/10 of a second ago; and the equally revolutionary invention of the electronic computer less than 1/50 of a second ago.

Malone went on to say that: "The lesson in this little exercise is that while technological change has been with man for tens of thousands of years, its character and its pace — and hence its impact — have changed dramatically in relatively recent time. The industrial revolution ... marked the beginning ... The scientific revolution, by strengthening man's mastery over matter, is explosively expanding ... The computer revolution, now just getting underway, by extending the capacity of man's mind, is certain to open up entirely new dimensions ..."

Before the same committee, another famous scientist, Roger Revelle, put his comments this way: "We are dealing with the greatest force that has ever existed in the long history of the human species — the dynamic force of science. This is too often taken for granted and too often misunderstood. Within the last 300 years, greater changes have happened in the life of man than in the entire 500,000 years of his previous existence. During these past 300 years, man's new-found ability ... has literally revolutionized the world ... We can be fairly sure that under the impact of science far greater changes will occur in the next hundred years than took place during the last 300".

Personally, I would even dare to shorten Revelle's forecast in some of its important implications from 100 to 50 or even 35 years. On the other hand such revolutionary future dimensions might just as well be extended over the next 500 years. Such differences are only a matter of degree, however, compared with the fundamental agreement among the majority of prognosticians regarding the phenomenons of acceleration, explosion, revolution and dimensial transformation. The main point which shows explicitly in both the above quotations is that the accent is placed on the influence of the development of (natural) science and technology. In both views, the necessity of a scientifically based perspective is a *central category* of modern *thinking* and *doing* for the sake of organized survival and qualitative future livability of human society. Therefore, the future will require *disciplines* with *new dimensions,* the contours of which are already dimly visible.

272

But according to the general consensus there is an almost total lack of understanding of the future dynamic, social and cultural trends. Understanding, which should especially be fostered by those sciences, the social and cultural sciences (the behavioral sciences, the humanities or whatever one thinks fit to call them) which have chosen precisely the human community and its social dynamics as the subjects of scientific investigation. This is all the more remarkable since a continued existence worthy of man and the formulation of a code of social behavior acceptable in the future are among the factors deciding whether there will be any purposeful continued existence, and deciding whether these human-oriented and behavioral sciences will be able to operate effectively.

If we are now on the eve of the most complete development of human dignity, of the introduction of Homo Creator, in the far and away greatest, unprecedented range and scope, it is becoming high time that *science, all* science, is at the greatest possible service of this purposeful future-determining functions.

CHAPTER 16

Sociology as a science of crisis, and the crisis of the social sciences

As a consolation for the failure of the social sciences to come to grips with today's almost overwhelming, ultradynamic, highly charged problems, the following excuse is often made: modern natural science is already some 350 years old[1], but sociology in fact no more than 40 to 50 years. This statement is only partly true of the social sciences, and unacceptable as an explanation of their shortcomings.

Let us not get side-tracked into a discussion of terminology. Modern sociology did of course start to expand in Europe about the term of the century, and in America mainly after the First World War. But its previous history is far from insignificant.[2] It is, I think, fair to say that as long ago as Plato, social science was at least as advanced as mathematics and natural science, and possibly even more so. For a long time no precise dividing-line could be drawn between philosophy, ethics, historical and social science, nor later between economics and social science. The idealistic Utopists and social reformers were early precursors of the sociologists. Vico's "scienza nuova" in 1725 was undoubtedly, in large measure, also a sociological essay in the broader sense. When sociology was baptized by Comte, the French Revolution was only just over, the Industrial Revolution had not progressed far and the 19th century was still young.

My point is not so much that sociology, in this narrower sense, is at least 150 years old, but rather that this dual process of social transformation did at any rate provide it with its great chance to develop. The existence of society as a quantity deserving study in its own right had definitely been discovered. The fact that both revolutions had brought about, and would continue to promote, a crisis of change, functional shifts and modified ways of life in that society also impressed upon the new sociology the stamp of crisis-science. Understandably, sociology felt called upon to solve this crisis, i.e. to contribute as best it could to responsible and respectable social reforms.

The older sociologists, driven by their awareness of this responsibility, were idealistic and Utopistic social reformers by profession (perhaps, in view of Plato and his predecessors, this is the oldest profession in the world!). When the pendulum swung too far — beginning with Comte's own derivative of metaphysical religion (the so-called positivistic school) — a reaction was bound to come. While Weber and Durkheim were still only moderate revolutionaries in this regard, before long (e.g. W. G. Sumner: "The Absurd Effort to Make the World Over") every scientific attempt at reform came to be condemned out of hand as unscientific.

The influence of Karl Mannheim, who pointed to the facts of social dynamics, the ensuing structural reconstruction and the urgent need for a time-diagnosis with "social awareness"[3] together with a matching, purposeful attempt at effective reform, proved in retrospect to be of limited value in this very regard. The voice of Lynd ("Knowledge for What?") has so far, since 1939 in America, been that of one crying in the wilderness. The same fate has befallen Gunnar Myrdal's "An American Dilemma" (1944), and others. Pure-abstract theory was founded there and spread abroad by Talcott Parsons and Robert Merton. Somewhat different points of view were expounded by Clyde Kluckhohn, Shils, Lipset, Bell, Max Lerner and a few others, though one could not class them as a school in this respect.

The only great American figure of the post-war period is, unquestionably, C. Wright Mills, who raised sociological imagination to a position of eminence.[4] After his death a collection of his writings was published in token of his "posthumous respectability"[5]. But a glance at the work of the younger generation — for instance, the smoothly written "Invitation to Sociology" of Peter Berger — reveals not the slightest trace of Mills' influence now, while Max Weber and Durkheim continue to set the tone. As a "human science", sociology is again being banished with some embarrassed skepticism, or else moved outside and beyond the bounds of science.

In Europe there are some exceptions that in themselves are not without significance: the "critical" sociology of Horkheimer and Adorno's Frankfurt Institute, plus some German advocates of a more "zeitnahe" sociology, individuals like Raymond Aron in France, Thoenes in Holland, Michael Young, Bottomore and a number of younger sociologists in Britain who are beginning tentatively to find their own sociological directions. However, the situation in Europe is on the whole very similar to that in America, still dominated by standpoints which originally derive from older European thinking. The difference is that in America today powerful influences are at work under the surface, pushing and thrusting in a different direction.

At present, sociology is certainly no longer a science of crisis, precisely at a time when, according to a great many people, human society is threatened by a new crisis much more serious than ever before. My personal conviction is that, for this very reason, the social sciences are getting into a dangerously critical situation; and by "for this very reason" I also mean that the situation is partly of their own creating.

Here, I think, lies the cardinal difference between the social and the natural science. It is *not* a difference in time of, say, 150 as opposed to 300 years. It is a difference in time, but in a totally different sense. The point is that the natural sciences and technology have moved with the times, with the changing image of time and the new world picture for which they themselves are largely

275

responsible. The revolution in natural science has completely revolutionized the course of time. But at the same time and at the same pace, in at least proportional range and degree, with the opening-up of new dimensions, a continuous circular development has also revolutionized the practice of natural science, technology, mathematics and logic.[6] Atomic physics, high-energy physics, astrophysics, molecular biology, and biochemistry, radio-astronomy, micro-electronics, computer technology and cybernetics, information and communication theory, decision-making and games and simulation strategy, are some of their youngest, most progressive progeny.

Among the social sciences, however, sociology has scarcely changed at all with the changing society that is the object of its study. Certainly, with the mobilization of the emergent nations, any non-Western sociology is rejected as some sort of "foreign body". Cultural anthropology and ethnology have become increasingly independent. But sociology, which is essentially static, has hardly progressed beyond Columbus' voyages of discovery. It does study "alienation" as a sociological phenomenon, but has itself become more and more alienated from society as such. It has become petrified into something which, with the best will in the world, euphemistic terminology is now scarcely able to conceal. Frankly stated, it is the victim of a methodological ideology and orthodoxy, of a Freudian purity fixation, of scholastic dogma and sterile casuistry, and of positivically cramped objectivity. It has shut itself off in a cocoon, away from the bustle of the outside world. It has largely turned its back on human life and the social scene in a mood of isolation. Perhaps it has been inspired by nuclear physics to look at particular experimental investigations, to examine the tiniest separate particles which are split and splintered off from the macrosocial whole by the bombardments of social dynamics that increase in violence and impetus every day. But unlike nuclear physics, no single social science can relate these separate, disintegrated fragments in any meaningful way to the social nucleus or to the constantly shifting, basically transformed and repeatedly reshuffled picture of the social totality. This totality — an active dynamic of the first order — is still at best an alien, intolerable "happening" in the eyes of sociology. As scientific sociology, it claims an ability to discover all underlying factors, to relativize all standpoints, and to pry all thinking loose from its social ties. In reality, however, this holds only for the underlying factors, standpoints and thinking of all the *other* sciences, never for its own scientific attitudes and abstentions, which are taken as absolute.

Social change in time is in accordance neither with the theoretical, timeless approach which sociology aims at, nor with the neatly fenced and demarcated front gardens of the here-and-now which it cultivates. In an age of turbulence and transformation, it remains the "spectateur impassible". Thus in spite of itself, it confirms the status quo. It conforms timidly, amid a troubled and drifting plurality, to existing values. It collects masses of facts and figures translated into symbols and technical jargon. Of the present, it seizes only what is already past. With its characteristically conventional approach and play-safe caution, it ignores the accelerated pace of the second Industrial Revolution, automation, the expansion of the macrocosmos through space travel and penetration of the universe with its magnetic fields and radiation; the domination of the nuclear microcosmos and control of atomic energy through fusion and fission, the population explosion, etc., etc. The most shocking worldproblems and social dislocations are a closed book to it. The future of human society is an unknown and unknowable dimension, a "Jenseits".

Is this picture overdrawn? Yes, of course. It is a grossly exaggerated caricature. But is it a reasonably useful "ideal type" of the sociology of knowledge, so that, armed with an original invention of Max Weber, the whole of present-day sociology itself can be critically assessed with a ready-made instrument of research? Indeed it is! And in my account of the present state of affairs I have not even mentioned the most gaping and spectacular hiatus of all. After chaining itself to a classical natural scientific thought model[7] and stubbornly refusing in vain for a long time to move with any other it has entirely failed to notice that the modern natural sciences, mathematics, logics and technology have generally developed along quite new lines which have often been methodologically opposed to the old ones. It has forgotten practically nothing, and learnt almost nothing either, from these developments.

Of course the social sciences have not been oblivious to the incredibly rapid advances in modern natural science and technology, particularly since the Second World War. They have decided that this is largely a consequence of privilege: privilege in virtually unlimited finance for extremely costly research projects, with not only the best equipment but also the most outstanding personnel acquired or engaged for them; this privilege has ensured their advance by leaps and bounds. Behold the Wailing Wall!

But that is only half the story. The other half which may in fact be much more important in the context of these highly successful developments, is a matter of mental approach and intellectual flexibility. These exact sciences have constantly conceived, proved and improved new ideas, hypotheses, experiments, methods and techniques. They have broken new ground; explored new, and sometimes fantastic, possibilities; systematically erected new auxiliary sciences; welcomed new and different views, sometimes with skepticism, but always, with serious discussion and even enthusiasm. In short, newcomers with vision and imagination have not normally been banished into the desert as lunatics or excluded from the distinguished society of scholars: they have been regarded as pioneers, albeit provisionally speculative seekers after other and better starting-points or more fundamental questions. As a rule, they have been allowed to operate as the potential discoverers and inventors of new values, as the indispensable forerunners of new tasks and applications.

The stupendous dynamism, the restless creativity, the acceleration and explosion of modern natural science, mathematics and technology, are precisely those of the age which they themselves have helped to create. In comparison, the stagnant attitudes of the social sciences, and of sociology in particular — with a few favorable exceptions — almost surpass the immobility (often only apparent, it is true), the preordained rigidity and social quietism of the "dark" Middle Ages. Their resultant anachronism could really shine only as an antique museum-piece in a survey of the unduly neglected history of science, and yet it forms one of the greatest obstacles and dilemmas in the present situation.

CHAPTER 17

The gaps behind the technological gap and the sociology of sociology

Much earnest discussion in recent years has centered around the "technological gap" which has opened up between Europe and America and is said to be gaping ever wider at a constantly growing rate. Europe used to be possessed of a superiority complex which dictated that any and every fundamental scientific renewal must inevitably spring from the "European mind"; and furthermore that its technical elaboration and application and subsequent mass implementation, though occurring on the other side of the great fishpond, would themselves be largely the achievement of European immigrants there. Gnawing doubts are beginning to arise about this assumption. Is it not true that the whole of technical development, from the initial fundamentals to the applied edifice, is increasingly, and soon to be almost entirely, dominated by the pushing power of the United States? Is not the end-result of all this that American science and scientific research are taking over[1], that American concerns are increasingly influencing or even assuming control of large European industrial firms, including their research laboratories and institutes? And is this not one and the same result of the super-capitalistic build-up of resources of a great power? Of super-intelligent manpower (which can also be bought from the European pool) and an insatiably profit-conscious commercial drive? Indeed, is not Europe itself financing the methods by which it may be taken over, through an ingenious system of Euro-dollars?[2] In short, is not this course of development the outcome of an urge to which the American Creed gives top priority, towards pragmatic and ingenious, not to say brilliant, technical progress, equated with progress itself, a mentality which must be spread throughout the world by a policy of purposeful exporting and power-conscious expansionism?

In other words, must Europe not see that this technological gap is largely the result of the well-nigh inexhaustible abundance of American capital, accumulated through the desire for greater and greater profit, constantly multiplied, because to an American, higher dollar returns are the measure of greater personal achievement and success? Is there now any prospect of resisting, let alone closing, this exponentially growing gulf, this ever-vaster distance, between America and a Europe which is slowly becoming a technical colony or at best a sea of dollars, its industry more and more dependent on the United States? To say nothing of a renewed initiative on the part of Europe to match the first Industrial Revolution — an originally British and European phenomenon.

279

The anxiety is understandable. The elements of this analysis are not misplaced. The present situation is one that we cannot ignore. Something of all this is undoubtedly true; and yet the explanation given for it is one-sided and incomplete.

The fact is that the notorious "technological gap" conceals a number of other gaps which tend to disguise the essential root causes of this unmistakably growing imbalance. The brain drain — the creaming-off of the best of Europe's minds by the lure of better financial regards — is not the only explanation of the present American dominance. For this is less a cause in its own right than the effect of a considerable difference in mentality. But this is not primarily ascribable to what is regarded as American materialism, though this does of course play a part. In the first place, we need also to consider that these bright boys are offered much more attractive opportunities (as in Russia) for intellectual stimulation and experimental project work. They are often allowed to let their imaginations run riot, or at any rate to try out their absurd brainwaves and uninhibited ideas. Indeed, there is a remarkable, if somewhat reserved, respect for the odd or mysterious schemes of apparent crackpots and phoneys. This brings us close to a significant, *qualitatively* very different, *undogmatic* mentality. In contact with it, one would be in touch with an almost entirely different mental and scientific climate, which is also one of the godfathers of the technological gap that *has been* disclosed.[3]

But even then, one is still on the outside, a superficial observer of the conditions that have indeed worked in favor of the current trend. The phases, procedures, components and methods of this trend itself, however, cannot be left out of account, since they are specific contributory factors. Generally speaking, the indisputably phenomenal pace of this development is due to the fact that this very process of development has itself been made the subject of intensive analytical study. Comparatively speaking, this is done in roughly the same way as industrial efficiency and productivity used to be accurately plotted in time-and-motion studies, in order to discover the mechanisms and growth curves at work in them and to promote their systematic, calculated rise. In other words, the fascinating problems of "the research of research", "the technology of technology", "the management of management", "the education of education", "the development of development", and "the science of science" have gradually become objects of minute attention and broad-based, penetrating study. Study and organization.

In America, research into "the technology of technology" has reaped a particularly rich harvest in one special field which is still regarded as pointless in Europe, on account of a hopelessly obsolete idée fixe, and thus is normally excluded entirely from scientific study. I refer to the pursuit of "invention of invention" or, to put it another way, "long-range technological forecasting", with a specifically future-oriented management and research policy included.[4] As will be recalled, the prognostic technique evolved for this purpose is twofold: not just exploratory (the probable — what is expected), but also, and especially, normative (the conscious objective — what is positively desired). In Europe — if I may be allowed this repetition — it is still customary to contend that to predict a future invention is the same thing as to invent it at the same time, and thus to perform the logically impossible. It would mean assuming that something in the future, which is by definition unknown, is in fact known or knowable here and now with a reasonable degree of certainty. That is precisely what they are now trying to do, on a large scale, in America, where it is one of the mainsprings of their breakneck progress in technological achievements and successes. As we have seen, as much as possible is simply decided in advance: the direction, the objectives, the priorities applicable to inventions, the effective organization and the allocation of funds, the technical and intellectual manpower required, the pace and the phasing of progress towards the objectives that are set in advance and thus ultimately attainable.

This interesting, new and quite consciously organizational approach to technology needs no further illustration here; but even this is in itself only a *part* of a greater whole with various branches and novel features. It has rapidly become apparent that, as far as industrial goals are concerned, this technological forecasting cannot be considered as an independent creature. The same was true, in the first place, of the very techniques of this forecasting. Technological prognosis was preceded, of course, by forecasting in macro-economic, military, actuarial, demographic, medical and meteorological fields. Social, cultural, business, stock market and political prognoses were conceived, and indeed applied, years before. What did all these older and newer prognosos-techniques have in common? Was it advisable — it must have been wondered — to encourage "prognostics" to develop into an independent scientific discipline?

Four our present considerations however, what is primarily important is the growing realization in America that there not only existed an instructive relation between the various prognostic techniques as practised in widely divergent fields, but also — a decisive step forward — that practically no sound prognosis was really possible in any isolated field unless at the same time it was related, for the purposes of forward-looking insight, to connected overall developments in *all* fields. After all, the present situation is an entity composed of inter-related, mutually affective forces. But the same holds true, naturally, for the future: no less, and perhaps even more so. And the ultimate shape which the future will assume at any point in time again constitutes such a totality, the composition of which will in all probability be even more complicated than that of the existing reality. The road toward the future is certainly determined in part by at least two laws of exponential increase: those of *acceleration* and *complexity*.

If this *total* future-vision that is now gaining ground is again related to technological forecasting in particular, another equally important aspect of

281

its successful application as regards technical development, resulting in an American lead, is highlighted. It implies, as if self-evident, a heightened tendency to switch to a new type of prognosis aimed at grappling with this totality. It involves such techniques as the construction of comprehensive models, multi-branched schematics and multiple-circuit networks. For the same purpose of total integration, many kinds of expertise have been called upon to devise, among others, the so-called Delphi method and the all-embracing technique of systems analysis.

This change too has had far-reaching scientific consequences. If the connections, interrelations and interactions — the "interdependence" emphasized by Mannheim in fact — had to be taken into account, then quite novel scientific ground would have to be broken. The simplest, and in America most thoroughly proved, approach has of course been the closer interdisciplinary collaboration and teamwork between specialists in all these different fields. This was bound, inevitably, to lead to a separate study of the nature, essence and workings of such interdisciplinary combinations. But this was a matter of creating proper interdisciplinary links, as much as a separate, and extremely important, object of study. Finally, with the discovery that many specialists were so over-specialized that they were unable to understand each other in their Tower of Babel, and that there was more opposition and overlapping than collaboration, the wisdom of taking a pace or two backwards was recognized. True, the earlier ideal of the "uomo universale" or encyclopedist was no longer within reach, as a result of the explosion of exponentially expanding scientific information and differentiation, but "generalists" were required nevertheless: generalists who were still capable of seeing the overall picture and could play an essential part in a synthesis and integration which would make it possible to approach the inevitably and consciously sought totality of connections in the best, or at any rate in a better, way. So behind the technological gap lies technological forecasting. Behind that again, though, is another *creative mentality* and a different kind of *industrial* and *academic management* to provide a deeper, broader and stronger channel for this wildly rising flood of technological prognoses, and to channel it into more effective, integrated, courses.

Once this point was reached and these new intellectual currents were in motion, the question could be asked whether, and to what degree, the strict division of scientific activity was still sensible or tenable. Was it still possible, in this traditional way, to acquire real insight, first into the ungraspable situation of the present, but above all into the exceptionally complicated picture of the future? Seen in this light, could sharp distinctions continue to be drawn between such subjects as philosophy, history, psychology, educational science, politics and the like? It was a question that demanded an answer even more insistently in those branches of science bearing the prefix "socio-", like socio-economic, socio-cultural, socio-psychological, socio-pedagogic and socio-political.

282

The logical consequence of this ever-more probing argument was of course the question whether — for these prognostic aims at any rate — the absolute distinction, indeed the eventual clear-cut contrast, between the natural and the social sciences, was still really justified. It is an important question that quite certainly deserves a discussion of its own. But one point can already be made. I have already remarked in an earlier context, drawing on the authority of Jantsch's extensive experimental research, that the most progressive American prognostic techniques have been obliged to adopt the principle of considering quantitative and qualitative contributions as equivalent.[5] The unbridgeable gulf between exact and inexact sciences is in practice bridged here, without any profound theoretical heartsearching and without much ado. Here too, the motto is "the possible can be arranged at once, the impossible takes a bit longer". Characteristically though, this "longer" is being progressively shortened. Behind the visible technological gap lies this nearly invisible but undeniable fact that, technologically speaking, the impossible has almost ceased to exist. If all the axiomatic, dogmatic assumptions are cleared away, the impossible can be transformed into the possible, in the form of the eminently desirable and humanly attainable.

In order to account for these new possibilities, however, various progressive American analyses — again connected with technological prognosis and in continual refinement of it — focus attention on one aspect in particular, and rightly, I believe. In doing so, they follow the guidelines first mapped out by Norbert Wiener, the spiritual father of cybernetics. For this technical development which is specific to the natural sciences has also ushered in a whole new phase for the social sciences, which have always had to contend both with a shortage of significant, up-to-date information and with the difficulty of incorporating this as completely as possible in a meaningfully ordered system. Thanks to the new electronic methods of data handling, not only is material available in abundance, it can be processed quickly and reliably by computer and communication techniques, including those of games and simulation. These can be manipulated at will to provide information on the interaction of different factors or on the alternative systems to which they lead. At long last, the social sciences too are now able to conduct experiments in a test tube (in vitro), as it were, and to investigate how different choices and variously influenced forces yield a wide spectrum of mutually divergent results or dissimilarly constituted social patterns.

Now this man-machine symbiosis, for the acquisition of insight into future social development potentials, is currently becoming widespread in America. It does not simply mean that the technological gap (now fused into a dual, "socio-technological" gap) is widened by the novel addition of this social dimension. It might also lead before long to a modernization of the social sciences in America alongside the existing, and relatively increasing, obsolescence of their European counterparts. In this way a new American lead, a new "gap" could be born of the "technological gap".[6]

283

This does not exhaust the specific causes of the technological gap, nor its scientific implications, which are also, pre-eminently, socio-scientific. I have already said that technological forecasting involves the explicit statement of technological goals and objectives, and of the inventions which are to be pursued and financed in order of priority. In other words, while America already enjoys an enormous lead in "know-how", there is a surprising shift of emphasis towards the "know-what". Technological prognosis has become more and more goal-oriented, or "mission-oriented", "function-oriented", "task-oriented", call it what you will. I readily admit that this new development is extremely paradoxical. The history of Western culture has always, from the oldest times, seen Europe at the spiritual summit, and at the same time as the firm foundation, of critical assessment and reasoned elaboration of socio-cultural objectives. Under the influence mainly of Max Weber and his adherents, we have grown hesitant. In the social sciences as evolved in America since their inheritance from this last European phase, the study of such objectives was declared absolutely taboo and entirely abandoned. We in Europe have slavishly submitted to that thought model. European sociology was converted, almost to the last man, to experimental American sociology, *devoid of models for the future*. And now from America, precisely because of the experimental prognostic techniques that have arisen there, comes the call for a thorough and deliberate, future-oriented incorporation of *social goals*!

Here too, the first American steps in a direction which was European in origin were followed almost automatically by other, consciously bolder advances that were in fact logically unpreventable once this barrier had been demolished. To put it in simple terms, it was realized that as soon as the ultimate, normatively established objectives began to form part of these technological forecasts, one was faced with the selected future in its totality. There was an unavoidable confrontation with close connections and interactions between *all* plans and endeavors, but above all between deliberate tasks and objectives for the future. Suppose that a powerful industrial concern, engaged in a technological forecast in the narrower sense, had an intrinsic preference for deliberate research aimed at achieving a radical invention X, for later commercial exploitation. But suppose this were to conflict entirely with the equally deliberate plans for the future devised by the government and having international or socio-cultural elements (e.g. development aid to emergent nations or achievement of the "Great Society" at home). To avoid such foreseeable future conflicts where possible, the independent, specifically technological forecast would have to be enlarged. A factor which may be referred to as "social goals" is being increasingly taken into account.

A marvelous idea, but what are "social goals"? The social sciences were not able to say. Their practitioners had been forbidden to give them their attention for upwards of half a century, on pain of banishment for intolerable infringement of the social scientific code. The courageous warning voiced by the sociologist Lynd, "Knowledge for What?", was boycotted. Sociologists were not social reformers; they dismissed out of hand any treatment of social goals, which necessarily carries the stigma of subjectivity. The "know-why" of what had happened was within bounds, provided it was split up into tiny portions. The "know-what" of the "where to?" was out of bounds (and terra incognita too) and the social ethic of "ought" and "preferably" ran counter to the scientific ethic, at the same time far exceeding the limits of science and professional decorum. Result: in the first place, a few progressively-minded American technological forecasters started, by dint of necessity, to steep themselves in, and tinker with, this new material. They were forced by the prevailing situation to fill this vacuum as best they could; if possible, with the help of authoritative generalists — who are, by nature, frontier-crossers.

Looking back in the other direction, people now began to wonder, understandably, how comprehensive a good "technological forecast" really needed to be. Since the demand for this kind of valuable forecast, and consequently for these all-round forecasters, was rapidly growing, this fact not only influenced scientific practice itself but also had a distinct, double effect of broader impact. It affected both scientific education at high levels and top management appointments in industrial and governmental posts. It was there, after all, that these prognoses would have to be properly stimulated in the right direction. These too were the people who would have to be able to interpret these forecasts correctly, in the interests of the ultimate business of decision-making for the long-term future policies.

From the moment when technological forecasting came to be a subject of intensive study in the upper reaches of academic, business and governmental circles, it acquired a status and assumed a function in America which alone are able fully to clarify the extent of the technological gap between Europe and America. In fact, one obstacle only — though a major one — remains to be surmounted in America, for the wings to be spread even wider. For even there, the social sciences still have a lot of catching up to do. The areas are now beginning to be clearly felt. The storm-clouds are starting to gather.

Strangely enough, it is in the world of natural science and technology that the first real anxieties were being expressed about the ground that was being lost. Naturally enough, many scientists are frightened by the effect or the possible consequences of their own new inventions and revolutionizing applications. The silence and the passive, sterile approach so peculiar to their colleagues in the social sciences are, to them, quite incomprehensible and also decidedly reprehensible. The contrast between "hard" and "soft" sciences often drawn in America nowadays is essentially not very flattering, but it is in any case significant.

The purism and abstinence which the social sciences continue to regard as unquestionably admirable modes of conduct and eminently laudible virtues repeatedly seduce notable natural scientists and technologists into giving their

285

own views on what ought to happen in the socio-cultural and socio-political arenas. For want of adequate social and socio-economic schooling, their solutions are generally naive, sometimes harmful and almost invariably useless. The technological forecasters from mainly natural scientific backgrounds are finding themselves compelled, as I have said, to move into this field. One of the most brilliant minds of the Rand Corporation, Olaf Helmer, has himself published a study along these lines.[7] He has been followed by a leading systems analyst of the Systems Development Corp., Hasan Ozbekhan.[8]

Do we really need a "sociology of sociology" in order to *predict* with a high measure of certainty that the social sciences, and notably sociology or particular branches of it, are coming increasingly under the pressure of a "better late than never" situation? They will have the choice of either submitting without delay to a position of absolute necessity (but then their boldness must entail complete devotion), or of persisting in their resignation and defeatism, with the satisfaction at least of going down with their record unsullied. Other branches of science will then gradually have to take over their still unfulfilled tasks at short notice and learn by trial and error how to discharge them. Whatever name the eventual association goes by, the development of natural science and technology and their driving urge continually to perfect their technological forecasting, must, for the sake of human society and in the interests of its advancement, be offered a socio-cultural counterpart of at least equivalent value, and one that is unashamedly goal-oriented. Scientific participation to this end, of whatever kind, and a specifically future-creative contribution, will be required.

CHAPTER 18

Antithesis, analogy, synthesis and coexistence

At this half-way stage in our analysis, it may be worthwhile to postulate a number of essential points by way of propositions.

(1) The natural sciences (including technology) have expanded much faster and much further than the social sciences, especially in the last fifty years.

(2) The social sciences have evidenced a love-hate relationship with the natural sciences. They began by a long-pursued attempt at full-scale imitation, cost what it might, followed by frustration, at least partial aversion, accompanied by jealousy, guilt and aggressiveness. Besides these there was still the irresistible, impulsive urge to prove their ability to stand comparison with the natural sciences in another area of their work.

(3) The natural sciences (read: natural scientists) no longer conceal their feelings of astonishment and indignation about the failure and total lack of interest of the social sciences (read: their spokesmen) to help repair the damage already done to the social whole, or prevent the damage which will presumably yet be done through the hasty, blind application of the successive inventions of natural science and technology.

(4) The antithesis — and mutual antipathy — between natural and social sciences are rapidly growing into acute tension and discord on the "globus intellectualis".

(5) Everyone who has any reputation, idealistic vision or sober realistic sense agrees that this disharmony must be resolved as soon as possible; but nobody suggests a way.

(6) For the first time in the 20 billion years or so that the known part of our galaxy has existed, it contains a living being capable of comprehending the world and itself, yet apprehending the world more and more and itself less and less: mankind, in the context of society on earth.

(7) Never before in the course of human civilization have the individual and collective possibilities of determining one's own destiny been so abundantly plentiful: in terms of natural science and technology, mankind can not achieve, within relatively wide limits, practically everything it wishes and pursues with determination and discrimination. By contrast, never have the systematically ordered capacities of discovering and deciding what people ought to want and to create (the determination of socio-cultural choices and objectives) left so small and saddening an inheritance — a real "testimonium paupertatis" — for posterity.

(8) Our proud scientific age has taken us not one step forward: no further

than the folly of Erasmus, or of the primitive, legendary figure in one of Grimm's grimmest fairy tales who could not even pronounce three wise wishes for the future, though the fairy promised in advance that they would come true.

La critique est aisée, l'art est difficile. No, even criticism is difficult enough, and not always fair either. The practitioners of science (of whatever kind) who adopt particular positions in particular periods and situations, proclaim particular visions and, indeed, attribute absolute and general validity to them, do not of course do so from blind stupidity or arrogant conceit, not even from asinine stubbornness. They do what they do and act as they do in accordance with what serious study and conscientious appraisal show them to be optimal and wholly justified in a conscious and definite way (we shall not consider the unconscious twinges of doubt) — in short, they give what seems to them to be the highest and purest intellectual product of which they are capable with complete integrity.

I have only one complaint, but it is a weighty one and is aimed especially at the practitioners of the social sciences, notably sociology. The eventual genesis of sociology developed at least *three* elementary components: "social dynamics" (with its perhaps revolutionary and in any case structural shifts), the "role theory" (closely allied to social psychology[1], the most important aspect being the changing roles that men play in space and time), and, last but not least, "sociology of knowledge".

At the present time, one which many people are convinced is the most dynamically radical and revolutionary in human memory, social dynamics has been pushed, politely but surely, into the background. The almost total transformation of existing social patterns that may certainly be expected in the future is generally granted no more than grudging and cursory lipservice. One is mostly content to record clearly apparent changes that are already nearly complete, and then usually restricted to tiny areas, as neatly divided up as possible.[2] This serious omission is one of the strongest points in an unprejudiced case for the prosecution. But since it has been dealt with already, the prosecution rests for the time being.

The case of the "role theory" is just as remarkable. All the social roles of all social actors or theater groups are, rightly, examined in a shrewd, critical, skeptical and sometimes ruthless way and so revealed in their true shape and significance beneath the mask. A similar "debunking" technique is also applied as a standard and justifiable socio-scientific procedure, with regard to ethical or religious "roles" in society that are played at set times by particular persons or groups. Max Weber, in his brilliant study of the roles of the Protestant ethic and the growth of capitalism in relation to it, showed the existence of a fundamental link between them. But in spite of this, Max Weber's views on the professional role of the sociologist can be revealed as no more than an image

288

of temporary validity. Little serious thought has been given since to the theoretical "role" of the social scientists and sociologists in society, however. With a few exceptions there is a sacrosanct and unassailable reverence for one's own vocation, one that is determined once and for all. For fear of forgetting lines which have been recited unchanged for half a century, the tendency is to stick to a heavily veiled, much less sharply defined or relativized role.

What seems most paradoxical of all, however, is the complete negation of one of the most outstanding achievements and traditions of a recognized branch of sociology, precisely where application to itself is concerned. The specific sociology of knowledge, developed in Europe by a succession of thinkers including Marx, Scheler, Weber, Mannheim, Von Schelting and Werner Stark, was adopted for American sociology by Merton and others (incidentally, following mainly in the orthodox footsteps of Parsons). The sociology of knowledge offers an analytical conceptual apparatus that enables particular theoretical thoughtmodels and cognition schemes to be imputed to the historical situations of social groupings and to socio-historically (if you like, space-time) or ideologically linked worlds of the imagination. Thus it recognizes related image-complexes, prejudices, endeavors, valuations and social philosophies in particular stances, a particular social milieu or position, class or grouping, or even in periodically varying social experiences and stratifications. It goes without saying that the practice of social science, or sociology, should also — indeed, above all else — be approached from the same point of view and in the same spirit and be repeatedly *interpreted afresh* in time and space and so, where necessary, *reoriented* and *restructured*. But who is to hold up to the sociologists the mirror of their real knowledge; who is to tear off their beautiful but bogus masks, as they themselves are only too keen to do to others?[3]

Although from the point of view of the sociology of knowledge it is quite possible to understand the stubborn resistance, the ultraconservative and sometimes aggressive opposition of sociology to this critical self-analysis, the "noli me tangere" attitude is extremely hard to appreciate. For it is here, if anywhere, that mankind and society could and should be best served by such consistent, relative thought. And yet here we find the warning sign with its life-size capital letters reading NO ENTRY for Unauthorized Persons (including sociologists of knowledge), on pain of expulsion for extremely harmful asocial behavior, and if necessary by force, from the sacrosanct reserve of the social sciences. It is not even a wild-life reserve, but only one for tame functionaries trained to a peak of self-discipline. They are for ever the same circus performers, always walking cautiously along the same tightrope stretched across a void, well trained so as to keep their balance, just but do not think they are daredevils, for the safety net is there to safeguard them against any unpleasant contact with the never-changing, familiar circle of reality in the enclosed arena below.

All this sounds rather spiteful, hostile almost — as I am only too well aware — but perhaps it is because I feel myself to be a sociologist body and soul, and am tempted to hide my shamed embarrassment in trenchant language. And even Ortega y Gasset does not mince his words when denouncing specialists as "civilized semi-barbarians", by which he means the social scientists as well as the natural scientists. His ardent appeal too, of course, was aimed at building a bridge between the two approaches. But the gulf has only grown deeper since then. As I have said, the urge to close the gap has come mainly from the side of the natural sciences during recent decades (Haldane, Bernal, etc.), and has met with scant response from the social scientists. And not long ago, C. P. Snow (doubly qualified, as a researcher in natural science and as a man of letters, and combining British courtesy and devastating irony) restated his great alarm about the dangerously widening hiatus between "the two cultures".

To perceive the problem is certainly a quite different thing from fully understanding it, not to mention solving it. Sermonizing has yielded precious little to date. The problem is too comprehensive to hope that it might be settled in a few paragraphs here. On the other hand, it touches the core of this book so directly on a few points that I cannot ignore it entirely.

I trust I shall not be suspected of a subversive inclination to annex the social sciences after all with the natural sciences. I have indeed clearly demonstrated that the social scientists, in their frantic endeavors to amass vast piles of facts and figures for the tiniest areas of microsociological detective work, are often out of touch with the massive advances in the natural sciences, technology, mathematics, logics etc. of today.

Even the complete outsider, the layman, is constantly struck by these developments and made to wonder: why should it be possible there, but not here? Of course, analogies between different branches of science are nearly always misleading. The history of science has proved that to transplant concepts (e.g. from mechanics or biology to history) is almost always to court disaster; and the complete construction of a science of social physics was an abortive project.

Personally, I am less interested by the full details of processes and techniques of other sciences than by the fundamental thinking that underlies them. To take a simple example, still from the classical period from Descartes to Newton: there is no doubt whatever that the elaboration of mathematical differential and integral calculus has brought about an enormous advance. Maybe it sounds like a childish play on words, but I wonder whether, and if so why, the social sciences generally employ only one part (the differentiation process), but not its counterpart, the integration process.

Is the analogy the result of an accidental or arbitrary association of phonetically similar names? Let me stick my neck out a little further. The Riemann-Einstein era taught us to work with unorthodox systems of axioms and non-Euclidean geometry. Has the thought even received tolerant consideration — even by way of supposition — that perhaps, for certain space-time situations, a novel and fruitful approach might be tried now and then with other postulates, such as non-Weberian or non-Durkheimian sociology? The acquisition of the theory of aggregates has assumed enormous importance in modern mathematics. Its central essence consists — if I may be allowed to express it so — of a built-in thought-instrumentation for the carrying-out of justified transformations. In studying social dynamics, high priority should be placed on the mastering of structural transformations. I am not of course saying that the theory of aggregates offers a mathematical tool for this purpose; far from it. But I do wonder why the concept "transformation" has to go on being regarded as a more or less dirty word in the social sciences.

To take another fairly recent mathematical innovation, equally important and difficult to grasp: topology. Seeing its apparently very weird, distorted, misshapen and deformed constructions, the layman is inevitably reminded of the various ridiculous pictures of the human form provided by distorting mirrors at amusements parks. The social scientist should, however, fully realize that precisely the same process has been used from time immemorial by Utopists and cultural philosophers. Comparisons with satirical visions of the future or imagined pictures in time and space like Plato's Atlantis and other fantastic island-worlds, Robinson Crusoe adventures and fictitious journeys to the moon, or even Persian (Montesquieu) and Chinese (Quesnay) pictures of the imagination, made it possible to focus attention more shaply on the short-comings of the real societies of the present. At the same time, however, they were an important aid in driving the ideal desirability of particular social reforms home to a wide audience. Thus even then their function was twofold: exploratory and normative.

We need not confine our attention to mathematics either. Is it not, for instance, just as significant, in contrast to the predominantly static and timeless nature of sociology, that present-day computer logic is, and had to be, capable of "real time processing"? Have not biology and genetics labored long and hard to arrive at a single numerical code, from which the whole future development of a human life could be deduced in all its minute detail, including the type and color of the hair? Does not all natural science in fact strive to unravel the complete structure of a totality? No matter if that totality, as with an atom, breaks down into an ever-greater number of less easily identifiable components which finally seem to have no physical magnitude at all; or if the totality comprises the whole known universe, with various sciences diligently searching for a beginning and an end, for growth and decay for relationships in (or of) time and space.

It seems to me that in all their specialized studies of minute areas, the natural sciences never lose sight of this totality because, as with the theory of relativity for instance, every particular theory must ultimately fit into a general theory that is somehow constantly renewed.

291

Human society is such a universal totality. Not everyone, of course, can concern himself with this totality. Whatever their talents, not all social researchers have the gift of synthesis and integration. But it is just as absurd for all researchers to be able, or even forced by its complexity and variability, to take no account of the shifting, changing and transmuted whole. This fundamental neglect of the essential object of knowledge is simply unthinkable in the natural sciences. Yet the lesson needs hammering home rather hard. Without strenuous efforts at synthesis — and at alternative syntheses above all — there is precious little value in large numbers of part-analyses, however much empirical and statistical material they comprise; furthermore, the changing, onward march of time renders them extremely transitory.

If we now draw up a balance-sheet, we may perhaps perceive that a certain degree of progress has been achieved or can be achieved in the meanwhile. We must not forget that any real approach between the two antithetically opposed schools of natural and social sciences can only come in the long run through generations educated to this end (the educators of educators included). This has of course been fully appreciated by thinkers like Ortega y Gasset and kindred spirits.

The fact remains nonetheless that besides this royal road, which cannot be short-cut, there are side-roads that offer a practical solution. One of these, one which I regard as highly important and which lies at the heart of this book, involves the proper application of modern prognostic techniques — though that in itself is no panacea.

I think the National Academy of Sciences, for instance, has realized this very clearly. Its original series of so-called COSPUP reports, which have already received passing mention, are the result of close collaboration between top-class natural and social scientists. The Commission on the Year 2000 of the American Academy of Arts and Sciences (whose president is the sociologist Daniel Bell) works basically on the same lines, though its approach is not so much subject-centered as in the former case but rather directed at the totality, and so — not to put too fine a point on it — has yielded fewer concrete results to date.

The famous American think-tanks also work with different combinations of qualified natural and social scientists. It is true that the accent is usually placed overwhelmingly on the former, which may be, and has been, grounds for criticism. But — again for the sake of fairness — it must be admitted that good representatives of the second category are still very thin on the ground, and are sometimes hard to discover even with a powerful magnifying glass.

The close cooperation of the two groups for one and the same purpose seems to me to be of fundamental importance, both in the interest of better mutual understanding and also for a knowledge of each other's attitudes and methods. Ideally, the future will call for two further changes. In the first place, it would have to be possible eventually to reverse the ratio in the composition of the research teams. After all, we are concerned with channeling the autonomous evolution of natural science and technology — years ago they talked of its "innere Dämonie" — and with moulding it, as far as possible, into a socio-ethically acceptable form of the future.

In the second place, the "hard" and "soft" sciences — assuming we wish to preserve that distinction — will need to assume something of each other's characteristics. The "hard" sciences will have to take increasingly greater account of "soft" socio-cultural objectives in their technical forecasts. The "soft" sciences will likewise have to take the measure of "hard" methodics if they wish to acquire the authority, influence and firm control without which the scorching pace of social dynamics cannot possibly be steered into the desired direction.

I have done no more than state a few basic introductory principles and indicate some of the main lines of general renewal. The five chapters that follow attempt to elaborate this vision in somewhat more concrete detail, with particular reference to purposive social prognostics.

II Syngnostics

Caesarian section for uncrowned social sciences

Honest to the Gods of Social Science
(freely adapted from John A. T. Robinson)

CHAPTER 19

The concept of time and dimensions of the future

From the beginning of human civilization, thinkers, philosophers, artists and scholars have continually occupied their minds with the nature and phenomena of time. It is surely no exaggeration to state that the concept of time has always been a central one in all philosophy and that, conversely, every philosophy can be recognized and characterized by the concept of time which it employs. A brief summary of a few main points will serve to illustrate this assertion. Throughout the centuries, the philosophical stage has been continually occupied by two primary, contrasting thematic attitudes — with innumerable variants and modifications, of course.[1] Even in the oldest traditions of Greek philosophical thought (from the 6th and 5th centuries B.C.) a sharp contrast between two conflicting schools is apparent. One of these — led by the philosopher Parmenides — expounded the doctrine of "Being" as the only true reality. This reality had neither beginning nor end, it was immovable and immutable. Any movement or change in time was only apparent.

From the angle of the "sociology of knowledge" it is extremely interesting to discover why this doctrine has continued to attract so many thinkers so very powerfully, despite the fact that it runs completely counter to much apparently irrefutable observations. Clearly, by restricting oneself to the firm consistency of "Being" and by rejecting all variations and all variables as non-essential, the essential could be mastered much sooner and more thoroughly. Anything which did not fit into theory could then be disposed of as an apparent deviation, and left out of account. The changing reality was unreal, the unchanging "Being", somewhat abstracted and reduced to its essentials, was the only truth, and thus generally valid, universal and eternal.

One of Parmenides' disciples, Zeno of Elea (hence the name Eleatic school) pursued this view through to its most absurd and paradoxical conclusions. But even then there existed an unshakable confidence in the absurd, a "credo quia absurdum". The best-known paradoxes are those that contradict "in concreto" the passage of time, e.g. the proposition that the fleet-footed Achilles could never overtake the slowest-moving thing, namely the tortoise, or that an arrow shot from a bow, cleaving the air at tremendous speed, was really permanently stationary. The greatest thinkers of much more recent times have continued to rack their brains on such riddles.

Against the school of Parmenides and Zeno stands a diametrically opposed view of which the principal representative known to us is Heraclitus of

295

Ephesus. This school saw "Becoming" rather than "Being" as the most essential reality. Heraclitus is known to us through such pregnant pronouncements as "everything is in a state of flux" (panta rhei), whence, quite literally, that other wide remark "Nobody can bathe in the same stream twice" (for the stream could never be the same again, as a result of changing time). Heraclitus sees this "Becoming" as constantly generated and propelled by tension, strife and conflict ("strife is the father of everything"), and this is a further attempt at an explanation which we shall see again later in Hegel and Marx.

Both views can be found in Plato, with no definitive choice made between them. As a political adviser, of course, he could not deny the fact of relative movement and change in things; this is evident from his remarks about Socrates and his own attempt to design an ideal Republic which he hoped would no longer be subject to historical decline in, and as a result of, time. On the other hand, his classical "ideas" (the true, the beautiful, the just, the good, etc.) undoubtedly represent the absolute "Being", with its perfection and timelessness.

In Aristotle we find a pragmatic idea of time as a continuous and quantitative transition from earlier to later. It scarcely need saying that quantitative time measurements were the fons et origo of astrology and thus the midwives of all exact science. The regularity of time's motion in nature was certainly the prime mover in the birth and development of the natural sciences.

Later philosophy was influenced, however, not only by these natural sciences but also by the religious attitudes of history. These religious attitudes have been related primarily to four aspects of time: life and death, fertility, natural alternations (day and night, ebb and flow, summer and winter), and a hereafter. Christian thinkers (from St. Paul to St. Augustine and Aquinas) again laid especial emphasis on "Being" — not "Being here and now" but the eternity of life after death in the Kingdom of God. Against these eschatological views of the future, the Utopists and social reformers projected their own idealistic visions of another, better society on earth in time to come.[2] In Teilhard de Chardin we have a modern attempt to fuse the "Becomes" of earthly evolution, from start to finish, with the attainment of the eternal "Being".

While Spinoza, for instance, was still preoccupied with a well-thought-out course of development towards the essence of eternal necessity as an infinite extension of God, Kant actually put an end to this absolute metaphysics of an essentially existing eternal-divine order by bringing it down to a product of our own minds. Time is only a "form of observation" employed by man, together with reason, to arrive at an ordered projection of the idea of a timeless transcendence lying entirely outside the experience given to man. If the timeless "Being" was thus relegated to some extent, the "Becoming" in time seemed to have been promoted again to the rank of Leitmotiv in Hegel's thought. This might be inferred from his suggestion of a "world reason" moving through the course of history in accordance with the dialectical set-up of thesis, antithesis, synthesis, thesis and so forth. Nevertheless, even with Hegel this dialectical historical "Becoming" passes through change and mutation to reach a destination in time (his own time) and place (Prussia), after which the eternal "Being" is given a definite chance again.

It is well known that Marx did transform Hegel's idealistic thought model into a historical-materialistic dialectic in determining his laws of motion, but in his vision too the final change (to the classless society and the rule of the worker's proletariat for ever) was to preclude all further movement in principle and usher in the timeless epoch.

This need cause no great surprise, because the natural sciences had meanwhile moved into their classical phase of timeless natural laws, which provided strong inspiration for both Marx and Comte (founder of positive philosophy or sociology, the crowning glory of the five exact sciences).

Naturally, there was philosophical rebellion either against the religious concepts of eternity or against timelessness obedient to natural laws. Dilthey was one of the first to return to historical "Becoming" and the influence exerted on it by men's outlook on life and the world. Husserl equipped his phenomenological system with essential qualitative time-differences. Bergson introduced a qualitative "Becoming" in time as duration ("durée"). Heidegger, in his major work "Sein und Zeit", brought "Being" within the confines of time, traced out by the "Becoming" human existence. His pupil Sartre, finally, set human existence against all metaphysical essence as individual and exclusive "Becoming" ("Sein zum Tode") in earthly time, which termination could never be succeeded by a better time on earth or another time of an eternally-existing hereafter — no life after death.

I have of course touched on only a few different ideas of time which have appeared through the centuries; but they are characteristic ones. My sole intention was to indicate once again the continual interchanging of these notions and the two extremes of the time scale: that which is, unchangingly, and that which becomes, the changeful. One further important point still remains.

Generally speaking, one might say that the protagonists of the absolutely unchanging and eternally-being can also be regarded as *existential optimists*. The platonic ideas are idealistic-optimistic projections of the most highly exalted ethos. The motion of the eventual coming of an eternal life of bliss in a hereafter is that of a return to paradise on earth for mankind, living or languishing since the fall in an evil world. The dialectical ideas of Hegel and Marx likewise move with inexorable inevitability towards this existentially optimistic final state here on earth.

In comparison to this, the vision of a "becoming" condition in the midst of constant strife and change seems very much like *existential pessimism*.

The perpetual cycle of history conceived by Greek thinkers, reinforced by a conviction about the evident existence of a fatal and ineluctable tragic destiny, the gloom of Ecclesiastes and the "eternal return" discovered by Nietzsche, seem to confirm this pessimism. The existential process of becoming after the Sartrean model, terminating in a futile and hopeless world of changeless, intense meanness, bad faith and vile deceit, with no escape except death, equivalent to Nothingness to which it is the door, appears to be the incarnation of such existential pessimism, as the final identification of this earthly "Becoming" with all "Being".

Yet it would be wrong to conclude that this is the final pronouncement of philosophy. For that would be to ignore entirely, and unjustly, one extremely weighty time-factor in respect of the historical "Becoming" — the unfolding of human *volitional optimism*.

This volitional optimism manifests itself in two seemingly quite distinct places.

Firstly, in the application of acquired knowledge in natural science and technology, on the basis of Francis Bacon's volitionally activistic dictum "knowledge is power" or "rule nature by obeying her laws".

Secondly, among the social reformers, whose ranks often include artists.

It is doubly tragic that not only has there been a violent head-on collision between these two forces of volitional activism; in addition, the social sciences — which were the tail that wagged the dog — eventually traded their volitionally optimistic powers of active intervention in the historic "becoming" for an apathetic existential optimism. They adopted a quietistic passivism in fact not very different from an icy "après nous le déluge", but which was formally disguised by an appeal to that very same natural scientific knowledge by which human power was so vastly multiplied.

After the dramatic failure of the agrarian reform advocated by the Gracchus brothers in Roman times, probably one of the first markedly medieval, pre-revolutionary social reformers was the anonymous author of the popular couplet:

"When Adam delved, and Eve span,
Who was then the gentleman?"

The Renaissance rediscovered the idea of human self-determination as the mainstay of human dignity. The influence of Utopists, science-fiction writers, enlightened thinkers and artists on social reforms and transformations is immeasurable. But volitional optimism again turned into existential optimism in the 18th and 19th centuries when, on the authority of the classical natural sciences, faith began to be placed in progress as automatic and even irresistible because obedient to natural laws, even in socio-economic and socio-cultural things.

Disappointment and disillusion were bound to follow. In the arts as well. At the turn of the century, the mood was typically one of "fin de siècle", in the sense of the end of the world being at hand. Camille Flammarion even gave one of his books the title of "La Fin du Monde" (1895). In "The Picture of Dorian Grey", Oscar Wilde likewise made the degeneration of his hero coincide with that of the world as a whole (1891). Even that primeval optimist of natural scientific and technological inclination, H. G. Wells, who had been concerned throughout his life with the concept of time ("The Time Machine", 1895), and with the achievement of progress in time, came at the end of his life, in his last book, to the bitter conclusion that this was a hopeless and impossible task ("Mind at the End of its Tether", 1945).

In a more indirect way — by an exclusive concern with the past — Proust gave clear evidence of his lack of interest in the time to come ("A la recherche du temps perdu"). In many modern novels, present and past mingle with each other in an undivided "stream of consciousness"[4], but the technique of flashbacks is not balanced by "flashes-forward". Present-day futuristic novels and works of science fiction, on the other hand, tend to look forward. From the Thirties onward, these futuristic novels have nearly all carried the stamp of counter-Utopia, and science fiction too has generally been volitionally pessimistic or existentially pessimistic in its approach to the abilities or skills of the human race to escape from monstrous and calamitous future developments, notably in technological things.

How have the social sciences stood in relation to time? There is no need for me to deal with the subject at great length in this present framework, but I shall give a few revealing examples.

Historical science contains the whole gamut of fine distinctions and admixtures[5]: existentially optimistic phase-theories of Vico and Turgot, the same in Condorcet and Comte, but linked with volitionally optimistic social reform. Existential pessimism, later in Spengler and largely adopted by Toynbee, albeit in a volitionally optimistic context that is not always wholly clear ("challenge and response"), but which obviously fails repeatedly.

In the field of psychology and psychiatric analysis, Freud introduced a strongly regressive tendency by his preference for reaching back into the traumatic experiences of infancy. In experimental psychology, on the other hand, much effort has been put into arriving at reliable forecasts of human character and behavior, especially through test and selection methods. I am not competent to pass judgment on the rather widely divergent assessments of their efficacy, besides which recent years have seen a surge of development in this particular branch of knowledge.

The really original and independent lines towards volitionally active "human self-determination" during recent decades have been those pursued by economics, neo-classical and quantitative in character. An economic depression like that of the Thirties has become unthinkable today; poverty and unemployment are combated, economic growth and monetary stability are pursued. The great problems have shifted on to the international plane, with overpopulated developing countries, and the generation in time of the necessary concern among the industrialized countries to resolve these painful consequences of a historical process of development.

We are left with the social sciences, which for our present purposes are sociology and its various specialized offshoots. As has been said repeatedly, sociologists as a rule were originally progressively-minded social reformers. Their endeavors were directed towards the future. That being so, their theoretical foundations were often rather unsubstantial, and their scientific approach not always wholly objective.

That a later generation of sociologists looked on the phenomenal achievements of the natural sciences with awe and envy need be grounds neither for surprise nor for rebuke. The miracles they were bringing about were truly incredible. They succeeded first in devising timeless theories with firm, universally and eternally valid laws, and then in putting these theories into practice in historical time, and even completely revolutionizing the course of history through this application. In content and tenor, this same theory was permeated by or directed towards an eternal "Being"; and yet, transformed into technology, it then proved capable of, as it were, reshaping nature itself, and assumed profound significance for the "becoming" of history. The age-old choice between "is" and "becomes" was thus made to seem outdated and superfluous. To be for ever was to become for the future.

And so, though this is to put it too simply and straightforwardly, of course, the sociologists had found an ideal and a model. The attempt to establish a science of "social physics" took on a number of different forms, but the mental background to it is now more clearly understood. Two developments that have already been mentioned, however, cut across this original scheme. One of them became all-too apparent to sociologists after a while, but the other remained largely obscure and its enormous importance was consequently unrecognized.

In the first place, it appeared that the erection of a social physics was definitely not a practical proposition. In the second place, a number of important new developments were taking place meanwhile in the natural sciences. It was found that the absolute, originally timeless and exceptionless view of the classical natural laws could be relinguished, that particular regularities or irregularities, or deviations in defined circumstances, were sufficient, and that this much more uncertain basis of existence nonetheless afforded just as good, and in some cases even better, weapons with which effectively to face the future. In other words, although (or because) there was no precise, detailed, absolutely valid basis, nevertheless there was increasing scope for venturing to look forward with less than complete knowledge, and for radical intervention with the help of the probably reliable foresight thus obtained.

However, once social physics had come to grief, sociology was forced to desist from the groundless mimicry of so seductive a model and virtually turned its back on the natural sciences; but it clung nonetheless, and perhaps even more than ever, to the single feature of the acquisition of incontestable *certainty*, which itself had just lost much of its value as a strict criterion for the natural sciences.

Certainly, sociological theory is no longer reminiscent of a natural-scientific cognitive model. But sociological theory does normally still strive — for the sake of theory — after that one most highly prized attribute, the element of timelessness, which guarantees assured and unchallenged validity.

This is the point to which I must repeatedly return and on which I must insist: such a time-concept of "Being", in the spirit of Zeno, is utterly impossible in a modern science of society. Today, in our ultra-dynamic and revolutionizing era, it is either aimed at a Heraclitic "Becoming", or it is *nothing*.

I must go even further. For "Becoming", as such, has now become too vague, pale and tenuous, too abstract perhaps. Even "zeitnahe" sociology, which was of course a great advance on "timeless" sociology, seems to me to be falling back again. It will always be predominantly rooted in the present, though at its best it takes some interest in the trends and tendencies of a changing society.

But that is *now* no longer enough. This orientation is already obsolete. Sociology must now set its sights much more deliberately on the alternative social patterns of the future. Furthermore, it will have to contribute to a study of these radical measures that would be needed if we wish to select the best possible route towards the future and be able to work towards it in a volitionally active way.

This means not only the discarding of a concept of time now completely outdated, though still very current. It also involves something extra, something else.

In the previous chapter I took a few examples to illustrate the view that the social sciences could learn something from the underlying concepts — besides the factual or technical content — of the modern exact natural sciences. Now on the other hand, as far as the concept of time in particular is concerned, I contend that the social sciences must evolve their *own* vision, which will *differ* in this respect.

Two examples will suffice for now. At one time, classical natural science achieved a great step forward by proving the constancy of the rate at which the rate of change itself changes.

After what I have said, it scarcely needs arguing that we must renounce such a rule in regard to future development possibilities in the social field. On the contrary, we must try to secure a foothold in a violently, turbulently swirling development process, in a pace of acceleration that may even break through the high-tension model that already exists. We already talk in terms

301

of explosions — though we dare not yet use such expressions as "the big bang" — and may be prepared for vast unavoidable transformations and violent structural shifts. We can no longer make do with a colorless symbol "t" in an arbitrary mathematical equation. We must peel off this acceleration as a separate entity with its own means of self-propulsion. Then we must use coupling and feedback to create the functional duality of acceleration and foresight.

Let us take another example. Einstein initiated a new and spectacular leap forward by incorporating what is usually called "the fourth dimension". He so to speak hitched the dimension of time on to the three existing dimensions. of space in a time-space continuum of his own design. Here too, I think, the social sciences must go further on their own initiative. It is surely not unfair to say that Einstein in fact, for his purpose, introduced time as a fourth spatial coordinate, i.e. spatialized time.

It seems to me that for the present-day social sciences, this practice would not go far enough. They do of course operate inside the space of society and the human community. But again, now that the social dynamics is so quantitatively intensified, it is assuming a different quality. For Einstein it was enough to be able to work with different spaces, or time-spaces. Sociology must learn to work with *alternative, possible and desirable future-times.*

For the new sociology, working with the *future* as its proper dimension, now indeed rightly called the *fourth dimension,* will be essential. Conversely, space, *future space* that is, then becomes as it were a *coordinate of time.* The existing time-concept of sociology will be renewed by the creation of its *own* kind of *relativity theory* for the future potential possibilities of human society. For the future potential possibilities, but also *desirabilities* and the associated radical or flexible *provisions* for the future. For future *spontaneous Becoming* and future *desire for something different,* with their respective variants and alternatives. Social research thus comprises two essentials: *exploration* of the time to come and indication of how, where necessary and practicable, the social shape of the future can be *recreated.*

CHAPTER 20

Futurography and futopology

This chapter contains the essentials of *both main components* of a *modern prognostic science*. As far as the content is concerned, therefore, its conception and elaboration are very important. Nevertheless, as far as the form is concerned this chapter is no more than a relatively brief interlude, reflecting what precedes and foreshadowing what follows. For it scarcely seems necessary again to define prognostics itself as the science of future-thinking and future-research, involving novel techniques of future-exploration and future-control.

Unlike a great number of people, including my decidedly progressive spiritual cousin De Jouvenel, I believe that the future-needs of humanity at this time have been better assessed, and thus more visionary foresight has been shown, by some of Flechtheim's followers. The pressing need for scientifically grounded anticipation of future developments is going to increase continually and at an ever-faster pace in numerous fields. It is consequently a foregone conclusion that — unless an existing social science stirs itself now to make the necessary preparation at the eleventh hour — scientific inquiry into the future, including the techniques and methods evolved in the process, will shortly acquire a status of its own, and thus its own clear outline and appropriate name.

This would have happened long since, had it simply and solely been a question of a new specialist branch leaving the existing, familiar trunk and claiming separate attention. For such subdivisions and micro-miniaturizations of scientific fields into ever-smaller bits and pieces are taking place all the time: they are the order of the day. We are quite accustomed to them, and for this reason the scientific code is nowadays, as it were, a loose-leaf binder into which new sections can always be slipped. New professorial chairs of such studies and investigations, covering less and less territory but covering it more and more intensively, are springing up like mushrooms, with the irresistible trend towards deliberate division (divide et impera!) and almost infinite differentiation. Now and then a voice is raised in anxious protest against this continuous process of disintegration in the work on the "globus scientiarum", but the bacon-slicer turns happily on, the Congress of science keeps on dancing with more and more dancers bearing their own glossy, gilt-edged calling cards and stamped admission tickets in almost overwhelming numbers. The usefulness of one's own little branch of science is devaluated in scope and range like one of the many pieces of a mosaic whose outlines are becoming blurred. But this kind of fragmentation is entirely absent from prognostics. On the contrary, the avowed claim is to be *general and all-embracing*, and cannot in principle be otherwise. Its character is broad, almost encyclopedic and universal, if not speculative to boot. Its aim is the exploration of the unknown, and that in its totality. It therefore cuts right across present-day socio-scientific etiquette and the code of conduct considered proper and acceptable.

As will be recalled, the name "futurology" was suggested by Flechtheim a score or more years ago. The term has caught on with a number of people in recent years — albeit sometimes corrupted into "futurism" — but has been firmly rejected by others.[1]

Although the desire to incorporate the word "future" in the name of a new science of the future is understandable, I should personally still prefer a term that left no doubt as to the essentials of the matter in question. The aim is to be able in fact to *say* something about that future with the help of particular procedures. As I see it, *communication* with that pre-observed future and *transfer of knowledge* about it, are fundamental. That is why, after lengthy weighing-up of the pros and cons, I have settled for the term "*prognostica*" (prognostics) as used in this book.

I hope too that this novel terminology will convey the psychological impression that the original "futurology", and ancient astrology, have now really outgrown their primitive pseudo-scientific, or at any rate pre-scientific, stage as far as prediction of things to come is concerned. The pace is no longer set by heated, emotional wishes for inspired, if occult, predictions about the future, nor by esoteric arts or paranormal powers. We now have at our disposal *prognosis techniques* that are adequately tested in preparatory experiments, based on the most up-to-date methods and, although still open to extension and improvement, nevertheless already valuable and reasonably reliable.

Let me correct myself at once. I spoke of "transfer of knowledge about the pre-observed future". But we should not really go on using the simple concept "future" in a scientific framework. De Jouvenel was fully justified in reintroducing Molina's notion of "futuribles" ("futures possibles"). The future does indeed contain different conceivable, alternative and potential possibilities, divergent shapes, thematic variations, diverse aspects, consequences, situations, configurations, etc., etc.

Not unnaturally, De Jouvenel sees the revelation of these "futuribles" *not* as a scientific occupation but as an artistic, elastic, changing game. These possible futures can be shaped aesthetically and artistically and literally set out in different socio-cultural, kaleidoscopically changing configurations. Thus there always remains a variety of futures, one of which — perhaps one that is again surprisingly different from any of the pencilled outlines — will eventually stand out in historical reality and present itself to the contemporary generation as the future which has become their present.

304

This idea of "futuribles" is in itself a definite advance on old-fashioned notions about "the" future. Yet it does not satisfy me entirely. In explaining my reasons for this, I am fully conscious that I may again to some extent be undermining the still very hesitant and naturally unconfirmed faith in a science of "prognostics". But it is a matter which I regard as fundamental to my ideas that the risk cannot and must not be dodged. *Future* and *uncertainty* go together, after all.

So far, the literature that has been published in recent years, has generally speaking made little distinction, or at any rate not a very clearly expressed one, between what might be *possible* in the future and what would be unquestionably *desirable* for that future. The essential choice here is not as in the previous chapter between "be" and "become", but between "be" (or rather, become) and must. We are no longer playing an *aesthetically* fascinating game with different outcomes, but making a choice that must be *ethically* very sound, of a final outcome that is regarded as optimal and so *desirable*, towards which every nerve and muscle must be strained so that this "*must*" can be achieved.

This last choice, of course, involves not only (1) the various pre-scanned *possibilities* but also (2) the various *desirabilities* which exist with regard to future developments and, last but not least (3) those desirabilities which remain after a careful process of elimination and may also be considered as potentially *realizable* through the effective application of human power.

A thorough consideration of the implications of these three principal distinctions with regard to the future must surely convince one that "futuribles" is a concept still far too vague and ill-defined for scientific use. In justice to De Jouvenel, I must add that his "forum prévisionnel" is in fact intended to complement it. But while the political and sociologically expert discussion is welcome and heartening in itself, it nevertheless lacks the highly necessary element of scientific preparation which should embrace not only future possibilities but also the desirabilities, possible or otherwise, of the future.

I would even go a step further in clarification of this point. What essential purpose is served by the erection and elaboration of a science of prognostics? It is certainly not a case of "la science pour la science". The principal premise is unvarying: social dynamics and evolution must not only be made comprehensible; for the sake of human society it must also be possible to guide them as effectively as possible towards particular ultimate goals of the future. Man has so far progressively tightened his control over nature, but as for determining his own destiny and steering communal society on earth along effective lines, he has achieved little or nothing. The frightening idea of chaotic self-destruction is now more current than that of confident, constructive movement towards the future. Posterity — if any — will find this impotent behavior-pattern not only utterly absurd and antiquated; they will also, just as rightly, see it as an entirely unnecessary seal of incompetence and a reason for bitter reproach in the future.

305

For this reason I believe prognostics will have to be further divided into two main parts. One part will be concerned with charting as fully as possible those alternative, autonomous developments which are likely to occur without human intervention, and tracing clearer and firmer future-outlines of them. This part could be called *futurography*.

The second part of prognostics, also quite indispensable, would require another name. I suggest that it be called *futopology*, a word that may seem rather complex at first sight. The name is really an amalgam of two distinct but closely related components. It contains a deliberately chosen double meaning, and therefore can and must be interpreted in two ways: on the one hand as *f-utopo-logy* and on the other as *fu-topology*.

As we have said, scientific-prognostic research must cover not only possible futures but also, necessarily, desirable ones. Now at long last we shall *have* to answer that haunting question: *where to?*

Immanuel Kant — if I may be allowed to repeat this once again — in his inimitable, precise and penetrating manner formulated the threefold nucleus of the human problem thus: "Was kann ich wissen?" (What can I know?), "Was darf ich glauben?" (What may I believe?), "Was soll ich tun?" (What must I do?). These essential, anthropological questions of existence can be posed collectively as well as individually.

Our present subject concerns *all three* questions, but most of all the weightiest, or at least decisive, third one.

To the first question, which for our purposes becomes "Can we know anything (enough) about the future?", the answer given in this book has been emphatically affirmative.

The second question, regarding pious hope or future-expectation, is approached here not as a specifically religious question but rather as an ecumenical and especially socio-ethical and humanistic one. My own answer would be: as a hoped-for future prospect we can believe that, irrespective of our views on life and the world but in a single unifying type of social philosophy, it is indeed possible to bring about another, better society on earth that will be worthy of mankind[2] (and, thinking further ahead, outside and above the earth in the galactic "heavenly spheres").

The third, and ultimately critical, question "What must we do?" has gone almost entirely unanswered to date, especially in scientific circles. Scientific thinking and responsible scientific action, social theory and practice, unfortunately appear to be separated by an unbridgeable gulf that does not exist between natural science and technology. The gulf is growing wider as far as the future is concerned. There is no scientific theory of the future. Human volitionally activistic belief in the future is not normally accepted either by social science or by Christian theology. Scientifically-based future-action is a contradiction in terms. Those who have striven all along for a satisfactory answer have been mainly the prophetically inspired, the socio-

306

cultural philosophers, the Utopists, the socio-religious and socio-ethical reformers (including the sociologists originally) and the Marxist or revisionist
socialists. In our scientific era they have simply been condemned to silence.
It will be obvious from my earlier work[3] that I attribute exceptional value
to the establishment of idealistic-optimistic images of the future which arouse
intellectual activity and enthusiasm on a broad front, since they are a determining factor in the force field of social dynamics. Utopia — on the classical pattern of Plato (the Republic and Atlantis) and Thomas More — has
fulfilled this function of pioneer and precursor for centuries. Its social significance is only now beginning to gain recognition and appreciation in
America, where in fact the "American Dream" has performed a similar role,
strongly progress — oriented, inspiring and stimulating, for a long time.[4]
This is of course very closely connected, both directly and indirectly, with
the simultaneous strengthening and development of prognostics in America.

Without stated objectives, without direction and course, without directives
and standards, prognostics operates in a kind of vacuum. For proper technological forecasting, it is not enough to indicate a limited, purely technical goal,
and there is a growing appreciation of this fact. The "where to" constitutes a
multifariously branched, comprehensive totality that seems at first sight to
defy analysis. The "where to" does not unfold in an endlessly prolonged present, in a timeless time.[5] The way to the "where to" requires a careful arrangement of routes, stopovers and signposts and a sheaf of possibly desired
final destinations. It is true that the requisite discussion regarding these sometimes takes place on a socio-ethical plane, but this must be fitted into the
framework of prognostic analyses and models. The usual, Hollywood-style and
rather over-popular name for such models now used in America is "scenarios". It is only regrettable that scenarios of this kind are no longer devised
by cultural philosophers or socio-scientifically trained thinkers, but predominantly by minds oriented towards the natural sciences and technology.
At least this is something; perhaps something wrong, in part, but at any rate
not enough. For to my mind, these scenarios are, essentially, rehabilitated
and, of course, modernized Utopias. These Utopias should constitute a part
of the particularly important field of investigation of the scholars of social
science. Their lines should now be carried through from the future of the past
to the future of the present. Hence my proposal for the scientific analysis
and clarification designated f-*utopo*-logical prognostics. But this is only half
(or rather two-thirds) of all the work that scientific prognostics has to perform. To spell out Utopistic and socio-ethical future-alternatives in a logically
consistent way and project them as a coherent whole is given to very few
(partly because of a complete failure of education in this sense). It calls for
the powers of vision and imagination needed to step out of the present into
a non-existent, wholly unreal future situation[6]. A future that is not only
quite *different*, but also and above all, according to explicitly adopted cri-

307

teria, is essentially *better* and so preferable to the existing social circumstances of the present time. And preferable not only for ourselves but in particular for the generations who will come *after* us, since we must do all in our power to enter into their future thoughts and wishes. The task is by no means impossible, but it must be honestly admitted that it is extremely arduous if all the parts of this all-embracing projection of the future are to be soundly and properly interrelated.

But, as I have said, in addition, the scientific *coping-stone* is still missing. Older Utopias lacked it too, for the simple reason that the technical instruments needed for its laying were not available. Indeed, the great number of old Utopian worlds of the imagination that have nevertheless subsequently become reality is cause for immense surprise and wonderment. Looking back at the great future-visions of the past, the predictive value of their intuitive insight into the possibilities of realizing fantasies which must have appeared completely nonsensical is nothing less than astonishing.[7] In this connection let me recall just two, over-familiar, sayings. One is "The Utopia of yesterday is the dream of the present and the reality of tomorrow".[8] The other is the characteristically Jewish Utopia: "He who does not believe in miracles is no realist". But, however much reliance we have to continue to place on intuition and imagination, we can no longer get by with the techniques of Utopian projection usually employed in earlier times. They indicated only the final goal; for the rest, they had an admirable faith, which generally proved justified eventually, in a realization that would manifest itself one day almost like manna from heaven. They did not normally make any mention of the path towards that goal or the effective possibilities for its eventual attainment.

We no longer need to work in that way, because we now have at our disposal special prognostic techniques which shuttle to and fro between supposed future possibilities and stated future desires. The potential, i.e. possible realization, of these preferred socio-ethical desires into humanistic full-scale self-determination, also merits scientific investigation which must likewise be included in the specialist field of prognostics.

For the sake of clarity, the difference could be expressed somewhat more simply, as follows. The writing of modern Utopias (scenarios) for a socio-ethically desired future-creation can still be seen as a predominantly *qualitative* activity, at least as far as the starting-points go (although, naturally, the logically consistent coherence of such a future-projection does make scientific demands of another kind). On the other hand, the retroaction of these selected and projected desirable future alternatives and their confrontation with the future possibilities originally indicated as probable is a largely *quantitative* activity, of analysis and measurement by a kind of radioscopy

For this reason I think that the term *fu-topology* could be profitably used in this specific regard. I do not mean — let me hasten to add — that this would be a process wholly analogous to that used in mathematical topology.

I am anxious to prevent the sort of misunderstanding caused by, for instance, Kurt Lewin, who also saw his sociometric efforts (not very successful ones, in my opinion) as a kind of psychological topology in the narrower sense (with analogous concepts of living space, psychological field, locomotion, action space, paths between these spaces, etc.). Whether intentionally or not, the generally erroneous impression is given of a wholly objective and in this case realizable agreement with the mathematical concepts and theorems of topology.

What I do mean to say is that we must indeed use specific *mathematical* techniques to move from purely ideal desirabilities to desired and really attainable possibilities. To put it another way, to move step by step in the time phenomenon from u-topia (never-never land) to eu-topia (the good land); from a local indeterminateness to the future "topos" of human society, desired in terms of time and space, explored as effectively as possible, and indicated on the time-scale as accurately as possible. It is no longer simply a question of adding a desired future-dimension, but above all of exploring the variable and optimal combinations in the future time-complex of desirabilities and possibilities. We must know not only where we should *like* to steer our course but also how, whither and within what limits we *could* steer it from time to time. In the unfolding reality, the ideal always has tangible, measurable and foreseeable, if constantly shifting, changing and changeable limitations or openings. Orientation within the limits of these areas, however, has only been brought within our compass by the deliberate application of computers, by systems analysis and operations research, by the use of feedback and loop techniques, which presuppose highly advanced mathematical knowledge. Not until this third, fu-topological stage is reached can we talk of pertinent choice from among all the options and optical prospects, and of critical decision-making.

That is, in my view, how the three-part operation of a science of prognostics should proceed. Whether it would be regarded as a science in its own right or as an auxiliary science, or perhaps as a new component of the social sciences, is a question I leave unanswered. The main thing is and remains *that* something positive be done at the right time; *where* and *by whom*, or under *what* auspices or titles, is secondary. The ripening of insight into the crying need for the most adequate definition of the task for the future which now presents social consciense and awareness with a most powerful and worthy challenge, may be the sole motivation for striving towards scientific preparation and advanced development.

Whether prognostics is integrated in the framework of the social sciences or placed outside is in itself not a matter of overwhelming importance. What is vitally important, however, is the unconditional need to reform the social sciences and to build a bridge between them and the natural sciences.

309

CHAPTER 21

Renaissance of the social sciences

1. Evaluation

Imagine that there were a world government and that the present-day practice of sociology were abolished on pain of death. What would happen? Sad to say, nothing at all. Who would miss it? Nobody except the professors of sociology. Would its absence bring anything to a standstill, like a strike of liftboys or transport workers in the pre-automation days? Would the birth rate suddenly jump nine months afterwards, as it did in New York after the temporary failure of the power supply? Would society see any change at all as a result? No! Suppose — as a variant of Bradbury's "Fahrenheit 451" — that all books on sociology ever published were ordered to be burnt without exception, so that none of the next generation had any recollection of its existence; would their absence be felt anywhere? Is it not shameful that we should even have to ask such a question and wonder how it might be answered?

Now imagine the same ban imposed, for instance, on chemistry or economics. It could certainly not be maintained for long, because these sciences have become indispensable to our modern society. They have acquired a high utility value. But even philosophy and astronomy — both spiritual antecedents of all modern scientific practice — would eventually re-establish themselves, ban or no ban. Even if they have no immediate utility value, they fertilize thinking in the long term. The future, at every turn, is in part dependent on their fundamental vision and development. They cannot be willed away.

We have to thank sociology for a better insight into certain social phenomena, processes and groupings. We now know about social stratification — layers, classes, levels, or minorities and races. We also know about some of the links between social situations on the one hand and knowledge, religion, culture, art etc. on the other. At the same time we have gained an understanding of certain relationships between the individual and particular collective entities such as bureaucracy, government, industry, trade unions and military authorities, or between individuals and groups amongst themselves, or between the individual and "the others".

The principles of this knowledge have been set out in the work of such people as Simmel, Max Weber, Durkheim and Pareto. Karl Mannheim was a potential renewer; his move to a professorship of education in England, and his premature death, hampers that potential. Sociology had meanwhile become an

American science, only aware of its older European foundations, when it was still the fashion for American students to study in Europe or to learn their skills from European immigrants.[1] For want of ideas and methods of its own, however, American sociology has become rigid and sterile sociologism, or run aground on the irrelevant sandbank of enthroned but fossilized empiricism. Fresh contributions of a contrasting nature from such people as Lynd, and later from Mills and Horowitz, enjoyed some short-lived "succès d'estime" and then went largely unheeded. This is not to say that no interesting or original publications were to appear in America, right up to our own day, on sub-areas of sociology more or less distinct from the general theory.[2] It indicates only that what they call "the state of the art" – i.e. to the extent that it is possible to deal with the subject as a coherent whole — which we can still regard as being represented by the esoteric Parsons-Merton school, shows clear signs of mummification and mutual adoration, and by and large the younger generation are no exception. Any deviation, let alone contradiction, was viewed for a long time, and until very recently, as sacrilege and damnable heresy.

To sum up, the irony of history has resulted in two paradoxical effects. Firstly, while sociology was originally European, and was progressive and fairly well advanced in its origins, it has since been modeled exclusively on the American pattern which was borrowed from Europe in the first place. Furthermore, it has accepted newly ordained models and derivatives with uncritical idolatry, swallowing them all hook, line and sinker. Then, with the invariably much more zealous and intransigent religious fervor of the convert, it has in its turn exalted these thought models into an orthodox dogma of sole validity and accordingly renounced its own experience and skills where they conflicted with this dogma, swearing eternal love and loyalty in a "declaration of dependence".

The second paradox to which this leads is possibly more grisly still. It is, as has been repeatedly explained, the identification with a matching but totally obsolete original model of natural scientific cognitive theory which the present-day natural sciences themselves have long since abandoned, or adapted and modified in a number of ways. As a result of all this, I see an almost tragi-comic figure appearing — that of a science clinging in desperation, like a drowning man, to the rigid, frigid American sociological model outlined above, one which was, indeed, chosen as the only road to salvation: this in spite of the fact that at this very moment in the social sciences in America, a perceptive observer will note something stirring — some clear, if as yet timid, counter-forces finally moving away, it seems, from the cribbed and cabined confines of the present fixation.

Indeed, it was inevitable that the practical (perhaps sometimes even over-pragmatic) Americans would see the light sooner or later. Particularly when their candid colleagues in the natural sciences held up the mirror to them,

311

or tore off the venerable masks of the sociologists with scant concern for politeness or for the prettiness of their words. What are you actually doing, what have you achieved, what use are your results, how can you help with our social problems (or the problems created by our own work)? What is your view on future development, what type and measure of social control can you apply to the socio-cultural dynamic which, left to itself, is marching on unimpeded on a wider and wider front? What have you to say about the "where to" or "know-what"? What equipment have you available to tell us exactly what is happening, to what dangers human society is exposed, how we must act and what method of intervention offers the best prospects of success? In short, what must be done to guide our future, threatened as it is by unchecked development, suitably and in good time on to the best possible lines?

The moment of truth is upon us. The social sciences, and notably sociology and its multifarious subdivisions and specializations, can provide no satisfactory answers to any of these questions. Nor can "applied sociology", whatever that may be. Sociology has applied the absolute rules strictly and confined itself to a little cautious digging and hoeing in small plots of the present, cut off by a sturdy wall from both past and future, away from the great links with the totality outside, from the upsets of earthquakes, tremors, changes and social transformations. Faithful to the Voltairian motto of "cultivons notre jardin", it has to show for its digging and hoeing a tidy, neat little front garden with a single, rather lost-looking but flourishing, plant. Having adhered to the strict code of defined methods, models and statistical collections of facts and figures, it points proudly to the fruits of its labors: a heap of loose earth and some stony rubble. Sociology has been fragmented into disconnected specialties, it has decayed into administrative accountancy and bureaucratic or clerical sociocracy. It gives off the smell of the alms-house, of self-pity born of misjudgment, but whose real cause is a gradual atrophy.

This is of course *not* fair to the serious effort, the honest endeavor, the maintenance of scientific objectivity and the large amount of good work done by a great many sociologists in spite of these awesome obstacles. But if we look at the problem from the opposite side, noting the breath-constricting corset, the purposely ill-fitting footwear which hurts and mutilates the feet and literally hampers any attempt at real progress — and all because of unnatural considerations of scientific prettiness that have been discarded everywhere else — then we shall not want to talk, as Derek Price does, of "educated idiots" but our feelings must be those of wonderment and pleasure that, in the face of such obstacles and handicaps at every turn, the results are not devoid of all value.

And yet, there is a third paradox — perhaps the most astonishing of all — which, as I see it, must make the ultimate balance unfavorable in the final account, when all the active and passive items are assessed, and yield a deficit that is both unjustifiably and frighteningly large. For sociology, this same sociology, had at its disposal the fruits of some splendid earlier work in the form of *all* the requisite scientific equipment, analytical concepts, instruments, procedures and methods with which to achieve considerably better results. That is, if it had taken the trouble and shown an honest willingness to take these acquisitions and methods, this apparatus, this extensive diagnostic equipment with which to illuminate, measure and dissect parts, symptoms and processes in the whole, and *direct them to itself* with the same thoroughness and objectivity. If, therefore, it had approached its own techniques, usages and conventions, its operational utility and applicability, its own shape, aspect and dignity with equal shrewdness and penetration. In fact, sociology did not need to turn elsewhere for psychoanalysis probing right down to the deepest stirrings of its subconscious: it had built up its own comprehensive arsenal, which was available — *for others*. The religion, ethics, knowledge, culture, etc., of others were already covered by similar analysis in their own religious and moral sociology, their own cognitive and scientific sociology, their own artistic and cultural sociology, and so forth.

While the initiated will need few examples of this process of self-obscuration, an adequate explanation for the uninitiated would call for more space than can be spared here. And this is not a prosecution, requiring detailed and incontrovertible proof, nor a funeral oration, though there are grounds for sorrow, but only a characteristic transition to my succeeding argument concerning a revolt that has become inevitable and a resurrection that I hope will occur.

Since Max Weber and sometimes in excess of his precepts, sociology has in general adhered to a strict ideology of objective value-freedom (i.e. the scientist as such is strictly forbidden to express any personal value judgment about anything). Nevertheless, all social science too, and all sociological practice, inevitably pursue certain values of their own. Yet there is an almost complete absence of any critical testing, any self-reflection on the intrinsic value or valuelessness to the community of the science of sociology itself. That scientific value is at this very moment being questioned as highly disputable; even in its own circles, increasing doubt is being cast on its human-social significance.

Sociologists have conducted interesting experiments on such subjects as alienation, status, status symbols, role-fulfilment and role-unmasking. Sociology describes itself as skeptical, relativistic, disenchanting and revealing vis-à-vis every social ideology, regardless of whether it is conservative and anxious to preserve the status quo, or revolutionary. Indeed, it acts to greatest effect in its antirevolutionary character, by puncturing in time the bubble of high-flown expectations for the future and by destroying illusions that are not recognized as such.[3] Finally, thanks to its conceptional apparatus of the sociology of knowledge, it is always able to indicate precisely to what degree particular religious, cultural, humanistic or ethical ideals or opinions are simply tied to special temporary socio-historical situations; to show that they are not always to be taken seriously or scrupulously at their face value, and that their image, embellished by deceit, unreality and untruth, is thus transparent.

But none of these disclosures is applied by sociological writers so completely, thoroughly, consistently and ruthlessly to the practice of sociology itself. That this sociology, for instance, is almost totally estranged from its social object remains — unconsciously, I assume — hidden. An interesting and revealing study could no doubt be written about the status, the status symbols, the masked roles and the profile of the sociologist at the present time[4]. As for ideology, in all sociological relativization of its outside world, sociology clings tenaciously and dogmatically to its own outdated inside world as fixed by its absolute code. Its ideology is indeed overwhelmingly conservative and in principle anti-revolutionary, also with regard to itself. Yet this socioscientific ideology, together with its own scientific ideals, is not punctured in a manner appropriate to the sociology of knowledge. That its own future-expectations are wholly present-bound and futureless is not analyzed and tested as illusory and misleading, but accepted as a matter of course and pursued as self-evident.

But what if sociology itself had effectively been made the object of its own extensive dissecting apparatus, if it had been stretched out motionless on the operating table, shackled in its own chains so that — all right, under anesthetic — the effects of its own surgery could be investigated when applied to remove tumors festering in its own body or to release its own clots and obstructions; what a course of rejuvenation would then have been possible!

Perhaps then it would at least look back, though not in anger, and watch full of interest what is happening elsewhere in the world of science. For since the grand opening from Kepler to Newton, the natural sciences have renewed and rejuvenated themselves afresh in their massive onward march, themselves relativizing their own accumulated knowledge, adding to themselves, changing, sunmitting where necessary to a complete change of face, assuming totally different roles, and finally accepting with enthusiasm as definite progress new Copernical ideas which they first viewed with suspicion.

It so happens that there are no Nobel Prizes for sociology. If there were, to what scientific innovators could they have been awarded? They themselves have placed the highest value on a virtually unchanging, externally and internally uneventful classicism. The sociological innovator is a priori suspect and abject as a messenger with a new message of salvation, an illusionist with a new vision of the future, a would-be revolutionary, in other words a demagogic agitator who upsets the scientific order and must therefore

314

be harshly suppressed by all the means of legal authority. Sociology is quite willing to study revolutionary movements of the past. It refuses to acknowledge that its own field is being drastically revolutionized before its very eyes. The last thing it intends to do is to tolerate a revolution, or even a relatively mild protest, within its own scientific circle, and every time it resolutely and directly smothers any germ or douses any spark of modernism, it dies a little further.

Where in social science are the rebellious heretics like Copernicus or Galileo? The indefatigable struggles with recalcitrant material like Cantor, Riemann or Gödel? The giants like the Curies, Planck, Heisenberg or Schrödinger? Where are its revolutionary independent spirits like Einstein or Robert Oppenheimer, eccentric geniuses like Wiener, profound speculative minds like Eddington, Jeans or Fred Hoyle? Where — to come nearer home — are the unorthodox reformers like Keynes, Beveridge and Tinbergen? Where the thinkers teetering on the line between wisdom and madness like Nietzsche, the great idealists like Plato, Joachim, Condorcet, Proudhon and Lessing, the progressive Utopists like Francis Bacon, Thomas More and Theodor Herzl? Where can it show such skeptical and critical innovators as Bayle, Montaigne, Hume and Voltaire, or pioneers of new sciences like Machiavelli, Montesquieu and Vico? Where the exuberantly audacious, grandiose system-builders like Hegel, Spengler and Toynbee, and where a new spiritual father like Comte? Where in the realms of sociology are total renewers, grossly misunderstood and even accursed, but ultimately triumphant, like Kant, Darwin and Freud?

It is true: in the beginning was Marx. It was seen that his creation — of three successive world-states — was not good. And that was the end of it. Nevermore a sociological relevation of the future. If he reappeared now, he would certainly not be offered a chair of sociology anywhere in the Western world. He would be unmasked at once as a Marxist "avant la lettre". He might have followers, and his role — to use the current jargon — would pass from the latent to the manifest. But where is sociology going, with the chance, albeit minimum, of another Manifesto?

2. Revolution

Sociology is dead. Long live sociology! Alas, it is not that simple. There is no heir apparent. There has been no struggle for power among the Diadochi. No crown princes or rivals have been removed. For, outside America, there are no ruling princes; at most there are some who have had themselves proclaimed pope. Weber and Durkheim rule from their graves. They act as our household gods. There are a few understudies in the part, whose authority as such is recognized and who ensure that the sacred traditions and the standard ritual are preserved. Part of this ritual is that Isaac himself is not actually sacrified at the last moment; at most, the people are trampled to death by the social dynamic forces. Provided that they conform in advance to any compromise, so that Jacob — not to be confused with a Jacobite! — should have scientific approval to acquire his birthright for a mess of pottage, which is distributed freely among all the socially needy, though it is far from adequate to appease everybody's hunger. The only disturbing element in this oasis of peace and quiet is the stealthy placing of a number of exceedingly explosive timebombs among the solid citizenry by a few panicky and provocative troublemakers. The established interest of the irenic social sciences might also, in the long run, be equally undermined by such behavior.

I shall desist from all this ironic imagery. Without a generally renovatory, drastic and, where necessary, radically upsetting transformation and extension of social scientific practice, there is no chance whatever of a purposeful, deliberate approach to social developments in the manner and to the extent that are now starting to become extremely urgent. This book, however, is certainly not a new manual of social science. In this particular section I must restrict myself to a very brief indication that may serve to illustrate and clarify my purpose.

All serious, critical reflection must start with a fresh appraisal of fundamental starting-points. Might it not be profitable here too to adopt quite different sets of axioms? Can it be that we have taken as an inviolable, absolutely valid axiom what in fact is no more than a convention, an agreed definition which is nevertheless open to change? Must we not also investigate whether what is regarded as the object of the social sciences is really still the same object, and whether it is still the same society, to be known through the same science? Is not sociology now, as Kant said of philosophy in his time, "in a dogmatic slumber" from which — partly for the sake of its own preservation — it ought to be aroused?

All these are questions without exact, concrete answers. What is meant by an "undogmatic" attitude? That everything previously counted as a deadly sin and so strictly forbidden on pain of scientific execution, life imprisonment or banishment, is now possible and permissible? Must all the standards and safeguards of objectivity and unprejudiced neutrality be simply jettisoned? The difficulty, of course, is to draw justified demarcation lines between what is still permissible and what is not. A number of taboos will indeed have to be discarded, and a number of excessive prohibitions will have to be withdrawn. Above all, the clear-cut frontiers will themselves first have to be critically examined under the microscope.

Sociology blossomed methodologically, so to speak, with the drawing of a great many sharply defined frontiers within which it was free to move but outside which it must not venture a single tentative step.

Frontiers between facts and values, between "is" and "should be", between constants and variables, between quantity and quality, between verification

316

and unreal speculation, between reason and intuition. Frontiers drawn between disciplined observation and fanciful imagination, between exact validation and creative vision, between unequivocal relations and multilateral networks, between workable, pegged-out sections or chipped-off flakes of the immediate environment and the inextricable complex of the social totality. In short, a clear and decisive distinction between piecemeal, limited, knowable bits of the here-and-now and an unknown, unknowable future.

A difference will of course continue to exist between most of these categories of opposites, but an absolute division can no longer be maintained "à tout prix". Over-narrow frontiers will have to be widened. Frontier-crossing will generally be not only permissible but unquestionably necessary for the proper practice of a modern social science.

We have already discovered with some surprise that, especially with modern prognosis techniques (cf. Chapter 14), a good qualitative contribution is thought of as just as valuable as purely quantitative factors. We have also been struck by the important place that is allotted to products of the intellect that are systematically eliminated from the social scientific scene, like fantasy, vision, intuition, creativity, subjective expertise or opinion, ethical and humanistic disposition, normative appreciation and aims, utopian and unreal imagination, etc., etc.

For the sociologists then, such frontier-widening would imply venturing into regions now virtually unlimited and so inconceivable. It would mean, for instance, that social science, where necessary, could also embrace, encompass and deal with: the non-factual (e.g. the possible or desirable), the non-observable (the speculative, fictitious or imaginary), the non-verifiable (the assumed, presumable, plausible); the non-unequivocal (the alternative, variable simultaneous); the non-objective (a fluid material partly changed by the researcher himself), the non-essential (exchanged for the existentially growing), and even the non-present (different from the here-and-now existing). Also, quite certainly, the non-static (social dynamics), the not-yet-historical (the unwritten history of the future), the not-given (the future reality that is by definition unknown), etc., etc.

Essentially, this expansive movement is no less (and no more) than the establishment of new methods which will try to indicate more precisely where, when, in what way, to what extent and for how long the frontiers may be crossed in a scientifically responsible way. This will gradually lead to a new system of frontier traffic control that in time will be thought of as orthodox and dogmatic and will set up new official stamps and barriers and issue limited passports for the newly defined and probably equally narrow crossing-points it is willing to tolerate.

If the limits of the cognitional object itself are to be readjusted, then corresponding methodological changes must occur.

One of them fulfils a major function in this book. It is the clear-cut division in the time-object of social science. The present now constitutes a particularly clear limitation which is also the boundary of all empirical research, just as in the history of sociology of course. The past generally plays no more than a minor, literally transient, part. The future is necessarily excluded. Future-visions of past and present receive only scant attention from sociologists. The powerful influences that shape the future, such as those now embodied in the "revolution of rising expectations" in the emergent countries, are not included in the corpus of general theory.

De Jouvenel is one of Europe's most progressive thinkers about the future. Yet even he continues to base his entire work on the distinction between "facta" (facts) and "futura" (events to come) which he has borrowed from Cicero. It is possible to get to know the former through attentive, accurate study; but the latter, the non-facts or not-yet-facts, never alas with any chance of certainty. Though there is the possibility of guessing right.

With social studies enlarged to include the future, all trace of unequivocal interpretation vanishes. De Jouvenel deserves great credit for emphasizing this very differentiation in his "futuribles". There are countless future development forces and potentials, and thought therefore can and must be given to alternative future possibilities. The reader will recall that even this goes only part of the way to the future. Besides the conceivably possible futures there stands an assortment of conceivably desirable futures, and all these are mutually related in complex ways, to which I shall not return here.

I think it only right to pay explicit tribute once again to the sociological forerunners in the field of future-thinking who deserve it. I would mention in particular Karl Mannheim, who had already made it clear that the "social awareness" which he thought indispensable to all sociologists definitely extended *beyond* the "order of the day", beyond the opportunistic tasks of the immediate present.[5] Some years later, as we know, a powerful elaboration of this theme came from C. Wright Mills in his evocation of the "sociological imagination" that he regarded as essential. Needless to say, this sociological imagination would have to relate also, indeed especially, to *future* developments.

Another dimensional frontier-widening, not so much towards that which is still to come as towards the full scope of what exists, has already been championed passionately but in vain by Mannheim. He emphasized the social interdependence and structural relationship between fundamental changes. It is evident that the shortcomings in the study of society as an existing and altering totality avenge themselves quite markedly in any future-research, which can afford insight only to the extent that it is able to reproduce future situations in the synthetic context of consistent and coherent images of the future. We have already seen that a number of prognosis techniques do indeed reflect this endeavor along a variety of lines and under a variety of names, e.g. morphological, "multilevel" and "relevance-tree" techniques, networks, models, systems, scenarios and so forth (cf. also Appendix).

318

On the level of social scientific practice, the reaction of this attempt at prognostic renewal means that it is no longer the timeless abstraction but, on the contrary, the contemplation and treatment of reality as a concrete and dynamic whole that is of prime importance. But this changed mentality brings other consequences in its wake. The main one is the fact that another article of dogma on separation viz. the sharp division of scientific labor, comes under great pressure. This applies both to over-specialization within one branch of science and to over-stringent lines of demarcation between a number of different sciences all of which, after all, are concerned with aspects of human society (history, economics, psychology, philosophy, etc.). The division of labor cannot be the decisive factor then: life and society as a totality must be. Neglected border regions must get more attention. *Interdisciplinary* collaboration can and must try to explore the common ground more thoroughly. Even that one-time honored and latterly much devalued figure, the *generalist,* can make a comeback and try to regain his last authority and a new respect for his vision, directed at the whole and hitherto outlawed for that reason. Perhaps a valuable contribution from the generalists could win them yet the recognition and respectability so long withheld.

When once movement comes, if it is future-oriented, interdependent in scope and interdisciplinary in approach, then there will be uncontainable movement on all the other fronts too. Thinking ahead to the future, thinking with change rather than against it, working in conjunction with other sciences, broadening and shifting one's own limited standpoint towards total coherence and structural shifts — all these things make it impossible to maintain established positions. The shrinking, conservative science of sociology again becomes literally and figuratively progressive. The one-sided mask of conservative conformity can be discarded. The original function (role) of the expert social reformer will — once considerable resistance is overcome — ultimately acquire a new sparkle.

Connected with this is the removal of one of the heaviest and most damaging stumbling-blocks in the path of pure sociology. The defeatism of the "spectateur impassible" and the fatalistic attitude to future social developments will come to an end at last. It may be predicted, or at all events hoped, that the lack of a sense of responsibility inherent in the purism of "la science pour la science" will be a thing of the past. Applied sociology will be enabled to acquire new substance and significance through the involvement of the social researcher and prognostician with the developments which he experiences, follows, foresees and helps to shape.

The short-circuit between theory and practice on the one hand and between theory and policy on the other will, let it be hoped, come to a timely end in this new approach to the social sciences. Such a pragmatic reconciliation is now in full swing in America, and it is mainly due to the spectacular development of prognostics.

3. Revaluation

In previous pages I have perhaps been a little over-hasty and indulged in a measure of wishful thinking in anticipating a revolutionary movement which is actually still to come, in Europe at any rate. I am by no means sure that this optimistic prognosis will in fact be fulfilled in the foreseeable future, approximately along the lines I have stretched out. It is, after all, a masterly stroke of historical irony that social science would then have to be reshaped by precisely the same dynamic and disruptive forces that it has striven so earnestly and so long to exclude from its theory at all costs.

I think it is safe to say that the social sciences, with sociology at their head, have now fallen seriously behind the rapid social developments of the present time. If the arrears are ever to be made up, there is increasing danger in further procrastination: periculum in mora. The eleventh hour has already struck. What I have repeatedly referred to as an "absolute necessity" could become an unholy disaster if it is neglected any longer. The urgent need for a far-reaching accommodation between the science and the development of society presents the clear dilemma of a choice to be defined. Whether to achieve this accommodation *now, ourselves*: or whether to wait for others outside and without official social science, to seek practical solutions for the social problems that are piling up, and to find them, as they surely will.

If my hopeful expectations are fulfilled, albeit at the eleventh hour, and social science eventually chooses to renounce its escapist avoidance of confrontation with a rapidly expanding vacuum — to step into the branch itself where necessary — then it will be able, phoenix-like, to rise on soaring wings from the ashes of the fire which is consuming it.

As soon as it manages to shake off its self-imposed fetters and free itself of its own accord from the leaden weight of a rigid doctrinaire mentality unsuited to this age, a surprising and far-reaching restoration can begin. The pendulum may even swing back from one extreme to the other.

We have waited long, too long, for the rehabilitation of the humanities. This age, if any, should apportion very high priority to the human sciences and the development of socio-cultural future-research. Who in this ultradynamic and explosive period of human history could fail to be gladdened by another great leap forwards by the social sciences — sociology, if you like, since Comte places it foremost? By its taking the lead in a thorough investigation of the enormous social transformations and structural shifts of the future, which are now already in an advanced state of preparation, and by its giving a lead in the domination of them. Later historians will then enthuse over such a desirable initiative. If these conditions were fulfilled they could testify that sociologists were already doing their best to help write the history of the future in the right way. For this is, in essence, the dual function of modern social science or sociology:

(1) The study of the socio-cultural *dynamics*, the fundamental structural alterations, the revolutionary processes of acceleration and transformation and the kaleidoscopically shifting social patterns and relationships;

(2) The study of the ends and means of arriving, through the use of *human power* at a responsible and considered sense of purpose to guide, mould or reshape these social developments towards the best attainable society of the future.

CHAPTER 22

Normality as a norm for social science

So far, I have skated too lightly over one aspect, though it was of course implicitly under discussion throughout. Without an explicit statement of objectives, all prognostication remains a floating abstraction. The "futopological" problems of the "know what" and the "know where to" lie unavoidably across the path. Social science, with its new future-dimensions, is utterly disoriented without a future-*map* and a future-*plan*.

This too is one of the kernels of scientific resistance. The indoctrinated and hypostatized myth of the ideology of objectivity forbids — and brands as impossible — the scientific evaluation of objectives, norms and values insofar as they relate to the factual present, let alone the unknown future.

It is not without some diffidence that I approach this topic. For in so doing I am returning to a dissertation of some 20 years ago in which I sharply and extensively criticized this Weberian doctrine of scientific "freedom from values"[1]. At the time, almost every scientist found my novel views and unconventional standpoint extremely controversial. Too many still do. The fact of a clearly discernible swing in recent years — notably in America — is a source of some satisfaction to me. But to that I must add at once that it is definitely not justified to talk at present of a change of principle or the unmistakable effect of these new developments in the place where it would be most significant, that is in the social science, and sociology in particular. The most that can be said is that there is some cautious fence-sitting being done; the attitude is a reserved and predominantly hesitant one, waiting to see which way the cat will finally jump. On the other hand there can, I think, be very little doubt as to which way it *must* ultimately, inevitably jump; so that this period of watching and waiting for it gradually to set and embark upon a scientific course presumably cannot, or at least should not, last much longer.

I hope the reader will accept that I am not in the least concerned with making my point. Every student of the history of science will surely have learnt the rather odd lesson that it has often been possible to achieve the greatest progress only by carefully studying the faults and failures of precursors, and correcting them on the very point of derailment. But this has meant taking over the new approach, uncertain, groping and blundering but subsequently recognized as pioneering. Thus in some cases the enormous mistake has proved to be of far greater value than the smaller, but faultless, "added value". To have to admit later to being mistaken could therefore be a source of real joy. No, then as now, I was and am concerned solely with the question:

322

How can the social sciences best serve the general interest?
As was the case then and, unless I am much mistaken, is still predominantly or at any rate largely the established view[2], it must be assumed that almost the only way in which social science as such could further the general social interest was by providing decisive indications for working out what means, among those ready and to hand, might be considered the most suitable (most efficient, with maximum or optimum effect) to attain a goal *given* in advance.

Who was to give or indicate this *goal*; why this one especially; how the prior choice was to be made between divergent goals, or whether there was any choice at all because the given one could be simply deduced from almost wholly autonomous trends — mainly controlled by natural-scientific and technological development processes; these were questions of a quite different order. Questions, not of professional, but of personal and moreover largely political, judgment, and so not a subject for socio-scientific discussion; and definitely not permitted to enter into such discussion, it was thought, lest it fall prey to a chaotic confusion of entirely subjective and arbitrary opinions, of surging emotional tidal waves. For these are by their very nature tied to a rich diversity of particular views on society, life and the world, of party-political preferences and — almost worst of all, at least the crowning evil from the purely scientific standpoint — of fundamentally divergent, underlying or all-embracing socio-ethical and socio-philosophical points of view, standards and values. These last belonged to the elusive realms of meta-physics, ontology, axiology and ethics, with transcendental points of contact with religion, if not mysticism, and with humanistic but unreal Utopia. And so all this is inherently worse than the esthetic and accursed apple of discord that caused Paris so much trouble, being part of the feared and shunned controversy between a progressive-ethical attitude (which it again depicts as conservative-unethical) towards the pursuit of social reform on the one hand, as opposed to maintenance of the status quo on the other.

Social science was not prepared — and we must appreciate this reluctance — to get involved in that dispute and speak with an authority which, it declared in all honesty, it simply did not possess, never could possess and did not wish to possess.

But the consequences of this tenacious standpoint were calamitous, and possibly autodestructive. The revolutions in natural science and technology were allowed to proceed at will, as if they were possessed by an irresistible "innere Dämonie". Social dynamics advanced unhindered as it had done before under the classical economic system of "laissez faire, laissez aller", at an ever-faster pace, with an ever-wider radius of action, with ever-more drastic transformations, in short, with a complex of socio-cultural problems of constantly increasing magnitude whose scale is now planetary rather than national. The abstinence and escapism of the social sciences contributed to a growing pessimism and fatalism vis-à-vis the future, whose development as portrayed in

323

current counter-Utopias and science fiction could only go from bad to worse. Furthermore, concentration on the search for possible means towards given ends also entailed the growing risk that all-embracing social science would be degraded to an extremely limited form of social technology, which would become irrelevant and sterile into the bargain for want of donors. For new social goals were no longer given. To the extent that they had once *been* given, social science also became the conservative keeper of the existing order — sometimes unconsciously and perhaps involuntarily; it turned into the apparent defender of its proven version of the status quo. But that status quo slipped from under its gaze with pitiless speed. And so it was compelled to turn its back on the totality of a changing society whose future shape — the status ad quem — was neither known to nor, in its probable variability, likely to please it. Thus its fragmented activity was gradually reduced to forecasting the present, i.e. those little crumbs of reality which could still be dealt with as constant and abstract material in a comparatively short period of observation, by jumping as it were from one melting ice-floe to the next.

This study has already been told many times in a different context. The principle of "frappez, frappez toujours" that is needed may irritate, or even nauseate, some readers; yet its purport is different here. The point is not to establish, in a fit of pique, why and how social science might eventually bring about its own fatally tragic downfall in spite of all its good intentions. The main point at issue is that human society is now in a period of crisis that is rapidly approaching its culmination, because it is being swept along, almost wholly out of control, by a tremendous acceleration such as history has never seen before. Just when it most needs the assistance of a science once created for its especial benefit, it feels quite woefully abandoned, sold out and betrayed. It is my firm conviction that Sartre's *existentialist philosophy* which so vividly reflects this confusion in human society and the hopeless feeling of uncertainty about its prospects could *not* have evolved, let alone taken such an overwhelming hold, had not the social sciences made a very considerable contribution to this mood of despair, total abandonment and endless misery (a "Schrecken ohne Ende") by their complete absence and aloofness.

The complaint that is laid at the door of the social sciences here weighs all the more heavily because they now have a wealth of technical resources, indeed an astonishing abundance of them, at their disposal. Extensive and perfected means are now available, enabling human ability to be effectively applied to the study of our own future; they can be used to bring practically *any* objective within reach, within reasonable limits. But science has absolutely nothing sensible to say *about* that objective, about the selection of ideal goals. Thus, aside from the fate of social science itself, human society is faced in due course with the threat of chaos, confusion and degradation.

This criticism harks back to an earlier discussion in depth of the neglect by the social sciences of two new basic principles that are particularly important to them. One of them is the ousting of the concept of simple *changefulness* by the imposing idea of the deliberate *changeability* of social dynamics. The other, related fact is the supersession of the notion of fatal *forces beyond our control* by that of purposive *human power*, willing and able independently — and so with a fully developed sense of responsibility — to determine man's future destiny.[3] Both these fundamental changes of attitude have now reached their zenith, while the social sciences, by taking no notice of them whatever, have reached their *nadir*.

This then is both a *breaking-point* and a *turning-point*. It will be remembered that in Jantsch's extensive report on his findings as to developments in technological forecasting, two related conclusions are repeatedly brought forward. It may well be — as he rightly states — that the application of normative goals is still a bone of philosophical-scientific contention; the fact remains that in all methods of technological forecasting — quantitative and qualitative alike — the normative approach has begun to play an increasingly important part. And — his second premise — it must go on playing this part better and more convincingly. For the success or failure of the forecasting techniques developed clearly depends in every case on the presence in sufficient or insufficient measure (or the absence) of a future-oriented *normative component*.[4]

A convincing case appears to have been made out for the need to establish norms. Yet the question of *who* should indicate them and *how*, and *what* their nature and scope should be, remains unsolved. Moreover, it might still be thought that this normative component was intended solely for *qualitative* approaches to the future. But in my view, one of the merits of Jantsch is precisely his valuation of the great importance of the *necessity* of such "mission-oriented" objectives which are, after all, introduced time after time in the *quantitative* techniques employed. By repeatedly stressing this goal-setting activity, by analysing and — in its valuational character — again evaluating it himself, Jantsch has clearly demonstrated the leap-forward that has been achieved. It is amazing to discover how far the applied exact sciences have advanced in this particular respect, while the social sciences still go on imagining that they are pursuing a completely constant, exact cognitive ideal.

Just one example, but a characteristic one that is also closely related to prognostics, is the recent development of statistical applications of modern probability theory, based on a system of axioms elaborated and renovated by Bayes. Thus, for example, L. J. Savage in his "Foundations of Statistics" has evolved the concept of a subjective ("personalistic") probability, or rather probabilities, which are part of a normative theory indicating how an individual should behave in taking his decisions. This theory has met with criticism of course, but also with approval. But its rightness or wrongness — which I cannot judge — is not the important thing: the point is the existential possibility of the appearance and serious treatment inside the model-fortress of mathematical objectivity of a theory which by old-fashioned standards is wholly inexact, unsure and vague.

325

But this theory, which is no longer purely descriptive but normative, is concerned with application in the field of decision-making; it is itself a new form of "decision-theory".[5] But an unprejudiced examination of the facts reveals that this is far from being an isolated case. What terminology is used in particular circumstances is of little importance. Whether the subject is termed "decision-making" or "planning", "guided mobility" (e.g. from the country to the city), "monitoring", "social action", "social control", "social technology" or "social policy" (see also Chapter 23), it is always found at the "decisive" moment that in the scientific preparation of decisions (individual or collective) for the future, the normative indication of a *pre-established goal* is *indispensable*. Without clearly defined goals, all prognostication is *blind*: without prognostics, every goal is *empty*.

Prognostics and normativity form a *complementary duality*. Without normative justification, prognosis is irrelevant and meaningless.[6] A choice has always to be made not only between the ultimate goals to be attained but also of intermediate objectives, e.g. the choice of magnitudes, proportions and amplitudes of desired changes, the best rate for desired growth and expansion, the optimum phasing of the system selected or the course assigned.

Apart from this, normative goal-setting is certainly not one and the same task in all prognostics. The nature, scope and range of the goals to be set can vary within wide limits. Jantsch rightly emphasizes, at the very beginning of his report and in numerous places later, that the correct determination of social goals in particular is undoubtedly the source of the greatest difficulties. The problem exists independently, irrespective of the fact that the social sciences have caused this study to be totally neglected for so long. To be fair, it must be admitted that, on the contrary, these special difficulties, which can scarcely be overestimated, have helped to determine the negative standpoint of the social sciences. Feelings of impotence and inability have been veiled and overgrown by an unwillingness which is obvious on the outside. So it is certainly not true that this lost ground could be reconquered at one blow, even in a united effort. In order not to convey the false impression that this work would be simple to tackle and perform, I must not fail to show briefly, but clearly, the very considerable difficulties that would need to be overcome.

The essence of the problem always lies in the need to make (not to mention analyse, indicate or recommend) all kinds of choices that are of decisive influence on developments to come. These are:

(1) The choice between an autonomous development (dominated by natural scientific and technological determinants) of the socio-cultural scene, and the controlled (guided, corrected, monitored) development of social dynamics;

(2) The choice between possible alternative development potentials that are inherently probable ("futuribles");

(3) The choice between different humanistically — ethically desirable lines of development;

326

(4) The ("futopological") choice between social Utopias that are really achievable and realizable (approachable).

That is not all. Generally speaking, there are no simple arrangements of black/white or even either/or choices. Reality is not only filled with a multiplicity of values; even if all the "Western values" are collected together in one system, for instance, there remain possibilities aplenty of conflicting values or conflicting effects (by-effects) of particular choices. It is far from simple to establish a hierarchy of values, and yet one is compelled to determine priorities for the simple reason that it is impossible to realize everything *at once*, or even in a predetermined *order*.

Furthermore, it must be recognized that the preferences of the people — who have not been rendered very exactly choice-conscious — are well-nigh impossible to determine. What is, or what serves, progress, human happiness, well-being and harmony? How can the "summum bonum", the optimum human society be described? According to what criteria? *What values are the most valuable?*

In a both satirical and serious counter-Utopia the British sociologist Michael Young has shown how the value of everyone's acknowledged personal merits (the meritocracy) could in future collide head-on with the fundamental equality of human beings (democracy). Max Weber has proved himself an unequalled master of clear exposition of the almost insuperable difficulties in this territory of values, strewn with snags, snares, traps and pitfalls. Yet I have sometimes wondered whether some sociologists, who were by nature disinclined to change, have not fallen for his reasonable argument as if for an "artifice of reason".

However that may be, this conviction has now found its way from Europe to America and become entrenched in the sociological mind as an unshakable part of their doctrine, after a less disciplined phase of pioneers and idealistic social reformers. The inflexible dogma has since been passed on from generation to generation, from the classic textbook of Robert McIver[7], which has gone into countless editions, to the later sociological school of Chicago and the pace-setter in present-day American sociology, Harvard.[8] American sociology, serving in its turn as a model for its applied European counterpart, has unmasked everything and everybody in succession. But so far it has never woken up to the fact that one of Max Weber's greatest, and still acknowledged, sociological discoveries, that of charisma, still shines forth undiminished as the charisma of Max Weber himself.

Only two branches of social scientific practice have managed to break free from this negative vision. The first was economics, which initially ventured a few independent splinter-movements. Compelled by the Great Depression of the Thirties, the war effort, the expanding scale and influence of state economic policy, the Korean crisis, the almost universal spread of central economic planning from its experimental beginnings, and, last but not least, the growth of purposive research into economic forecasting, politics and programming, novel ideas and dynamic methods previously thought of as inconceivable forced their way into this static world of the imagination.[9] Economic aims such as adequate employment, structural growth, monetary stability, equitable income distribution, anticyclic economic policy and even — in face of some scraps or pockets of resistance — industrial reform, have gradually become self-evident notions, as have the establishment of priorities and the resolution of value-conflicts (e.g. between balance of payments deficits and certain allowable or impossible national expenditures, and the increase or otherwise of aid to developing countries). These and other value-problems are nowadays openly discussed by economists of every creed and color, with the result that interest in, and the importance of, this science (in which the original pioneers have long occupied a leading position) have grown enormously. Who really talks seriously these days about pure or positive economics?

The second branch referred to above, which has only broken away in recent years and has gone furthest in America, is technological forecasting, a development which has already been described at length and is gradually going in the direction of a separate, comprehensive and specialized area of prognostics, which of course has learnt its lessons from its economic predecessors. It is here above all that the problem of social goals has constituted an immediate obstacle.

It must be admitted that the difficulties were initially underestimated and also that the possibility of transplanting the highly successful renewal of quantitative economics mentioned above to sociology was thought a little too lightly of. Sociology just does not lend itself to organization as social physics or even (except for a small part) as sociometry. And there is no specific macrosociological statistics available to society as a whole either (again, except for certain elements, such as education). The social goals can definitely not be indicated so exactly and concretely as most of the economic objectives that have now crystallized out.

Because there was in fact nothing, everything had to be learned and built up from scratch. Painful experience showed that there was no simple choice like that of Buridan's ass, between two identical piles of hay, one on either side but exactly equal distances away. In reality the two piles of hay turned out not to be the same at all; there were far more than two; nor were the distances equal. But the strangest discovery of all was that the hay, the shape of the pile, the distance and position — in short, the number, quantity, value and attainability of the desired goals were all subject to continual change.

This complex of problems may not have been quite so elusive and insoluble as that in the famous historical legend of the papal election at the Council of Nicaea. On that occasion, every time the votes were being counted, each bishop changed into another bishop after he had voted, so that nobody could tell who had voted for what, and the heads had to be counted again and again, endlessly and fruitlessly. In dignified terminology, this is a mythological illustration of the really non-existent, or at least humanly ungraspable, objective reality and of the constantly changing, changeable and ethereal matter that dissolves before the eyes of the researcher.

In any event, it gradually became clear that this process of social change would have to be tackled mainly by stochastic techniques. The data of the basic situation, the effective means to be employed and, finally, the maximum goals to be desired and achieved, were highly variable in the nature of things. Consequently, all these possible, continuous and discontinuous changes had to be accommodated in an elastic prognostic framework by means of a particular type of specially designed probability calculation, in which prior account was taken of their built-in variation and acceleration and which were directly aimed at the passage of time into the future.

It was assumed in the light of experience that social goals must be equally subject to social change, and this enabled a great distinction, in degree and even in principle, to be drawn between these and economic goals, which could at least still be treated as comparatively constant in a given historical siutation in time and space, and made into "welfare economics". Nevertheless, as regarded the content of the social goals that were to be assumed or indicated, such economic material progress along these lines was by no means the same thing as social progress.

In the framework of social dynamics there is more often talk, and now more than ever before, of fundamental processes of transformation and reconstruction which can be set in motion by this same technical-economic progress. Understandably, however, this does not simplify one iota the complex of social problems that already exists. For a new attitude of mind has slowly taken root[10] (and is in itself heartening evidence of a more progressive, undogmatic and liberal mental approach) according to which the existing values of today need not, indeed must not, be the exclusive point of departure for these social goals. To an important extent, posterity (our future is their present) might decide for themselves to prefer quite different values and standards from those of the existing established order of our own day.

Naturally, this implied an entirely new type of normative thinking that again, as throughout the centuries, would draw its sustenance and inspiration from the vital sources of a socio-humanitarian, socio-ethical and idealistic-Utopist thinking that was fully removed and adapted to that *other, better* future. I have already baptized this as a modern form of dual-oriented futopological (*f-utopo-logical* as well as *fu-topological*) thinking within the comprehensive framework of prognostics.

Before a decision was taken and acted upon, the following postulate — which has my full agreement — was then made: we must not only acquaint ourselves with present social goals, we shall also have to learn how to work with *that type* of social goal that is *likely* to be adopted in the future.

Those who arrived at this conclusion were then bound to ask the *nagging question*: social ethics, social humanism, social Utopia, *where* and *what* art thou? Social science, why dost thou hide thy face from a human society that is rushing headlong, in a blind frenzy, toward the future? Where are the proper guidelines for the move towards humanistic self-determination? It is an endeavor that has been roughly propelled towards the future, mainly by technical-economic forces; but for that very reason it needs inspiring with fresh courage and new mental energy.

The response to this passionate appeal has so far been weak and sparse. Professor C. West Churchman of Berkeley has tried to show that ethical judgments too can be verified in the interests of a workable decision-theory.[11] Eleanor Sheldon and Wilbert Moore of the Russell Sage Foundation have carefully attempted to trace more exactly the outlines of social change in the sense of a social progress deliberately appreciated as such, with social action directed to that end.[12]

It is my personal opinion — and unless I am much mistaken, my friend and kindred spirit Ozbekhan thinks almost exactly the same — that the urgently needed elaboration of a new social ethic and a modernized social Utopism may receive enormous impetus and substantial support from a development the full scope of which is as yet almost entirely unrecognized and from a quarter which would appear least likely to provide it.

For I am convinced that the new techniques of computers, information, communication, games and simulation, which to date have scarcely been exploited at all in this direction, may prove to be extremely valuable in the normative field too by reason of their almost inconceivable range of possibilities for nearly complete collection, phenomenally rapid processing and purposeful calculation of results. Not only the most enormous quantities of arbitrarily varied sets or systems of data, but at the same time associated and likewise alternating *normative objectives* and *ethical value-systems* will be "run through", with a vast number of variables being handled. In this way their social implications and consequences, their feedback, interaction and interdependence can, as it were, be played out before one's very eyes. Thus one might *see* a copy and experience a foretaste, so to speak, of a selection of desirable, or desirable and somehow realizable, shapes of the future displayed in visual form. In other words, social experimentation (hitherto feasible only in strictly limited partial areas and within very small confines) would for the first time become possible on a large, even global, scale. Thanks to this totally new and original type of socio-scientific experiment, comparable in principle to the natural sciences, it will be possible to make alternative patterns of facts and values visible and surveyable over a wide spectrum, and amenable to scientific assessment and selected applications in their arbitrarily but quite logically consistent outcomes.

An amazing, indeed extremely paradoxical, conclusion! The *very same* second industrial-technical revolution of *automation*, which more than ever before threatens to reveal with unmistakable clarity the helplessness of the social sciences, with nothing but the emperor's clothes to hide their shame, now appearing at the eleventh hour as their only true friend in need! It — and it alone — if its helping hand is yet grasped firmly and in time, can contribute to the lightning and miraculous transformation of the *wedge* now driving deeper into their flesh into a sturdy *bridge* into the future.

Such a procedure might then prompt a number of sociologists who previously refused, as men of science, to be manoeuvred into one of two possible directions, to lean towards another point of view. The unacceptable directions were the religious-methaphysical, with transcendent values unamenable to any reasonable discussion; and a social-Utopian one with speculative values which no empirical test could verify. For neither of these two solutions did they feel equipped or qualified to make any scientific statement.

It is in no way my intention to give the impression that the solution tendered in outline here is a way to square the circle, or even something approaching a delightful "perpetuum mobile". In no single science, as has been established of old, is there a short-out, still less a panacea or simple recipe for the easy solution of all the constantly multiplying and more complicated problems. On the path to scientific progress the critical challenge is never removed; rather it is continually intensified, and the required response itself becomes increasingly problematic in a never-ending cycle.

But — and this is the full extent of my claim — it is now becoming possible, without possessing the philosopher's stone or calling the genie of the bottle to one's aid, to combat the process of petrifaction and to escape from the existing bottleneck which have hitherto prevented the social sciences from entering and exploring the realm of values.

Let no-one imagine that this territory can henceforth be trodden without risk or danger or, to use Berger's gloomy modern characterization of sociology, "as a pastime".[13] On the contrary, the point is not to pass the existing time of the present but to seek out that other time to come in the still unknown future, and so via new trails that have yet to be blazed. Even with the most recent and highly promising aids this is and remains a decidedly risky and precarious undertaking. But it offers fascinating prospects for the explorer in that country who again takes as his device the idea of progress, which is imperishable once it starts to be fulfilled. For he is the trail-blazer towards a social science that will be able both to *observe* and to *create* the future.

CHAPTER 23

Social technology and social politics

In 1965 Olaf Helmer of the Rand Corporation published a short but extremely interesting work entitled "Social Technology". Helmer is clearly no social scientist by calling, but he wants to do more than just add his voice to the chorus of disquieted thinkers who assert that the social sciences today are guilty of irresponsible shortcomings, that the traditional sociological methods have lagged hopelessly behind in our age of new techniques "ranging from molecular to planetary engineering" . . . "with eery implications" that must surely lead to "a dire view of the future".

He is intent on breaking free from this fatalistic resignation and apathy. He himself tries to apply new social methods to overcome the "potential disaster that may befall us" unless we succeed in suitably bridging the everwidening gulf, or in filling the now intolerable vacuum, between modern natural sciences and their antiquated social counterparts.[1]

Not surprisingly, Helmer would like this new "social technology" to be principally based on the prognostic methods of operations research, information theory, gaming, strategy, simulation techniques and decision-making developed in America over the last few years and, last but not least, on the Delphi technique with its novel electronic man-machine symbiosis, a specific long-range forecasting method elaborated by the Rand Corporation itself.

Helmer pleads not only for the application of these techniques in the sociocultural field; he himself goes a stage further by taking a number of concrete examples to illustrate how he envisages the practical application of this approach.[2] He deals briefly with the successive possibilities of urgent town planning and redevelopment, the likewise exceptional urgency of educational reform, the problem of juvenile delinquency which is crying out for effective treatment, and long-term economic forecasting which to date has been insufficiently attempted.

In addition, he mentions two other, more ambitious, undertakings of social technology that he sees as desirable and effectively possible, viz. political planning and programming on the one hand, and "the society of the future" on the other.[3] As for the political possibilities of social technology, Helmer cites the examples of operations research, gaming, etc., as employed by top diplomatic and military leaders to help solve or prevent international crises. He also mentions systematic exploration of the future, for the year 2000 for instance, by means of specially devised scenarios and "images of the future of a social-Utopist nature, that are also intended as "contingency planning", to draw attention to future socio-cultural trends that may present a threat, and thus expressly predestined to be self-defeating prophecies in this respect.

Finally, where "the society of the future is concerned", Helmer states emphatically that the social engineer's function here is a decidedly *normative* one. He describes its execution as "dynamic Utopian planning" coupled with "systems synthesis".[4] Helmer too, of course, stumbles on the inescapable problems of the definition of individual and collective preferences and the question of discovering these preferential values, to be expressed in the future-choices that will be based on them. However, as he concludes his argument somewhat abruptly and with an anti-climax, this takes the social technologist outside his terms of reference and into the realm of politics.[5]

Now Helmer's argument, which is finding acceptance and approval in America, leaves me terribly undecided. On the one hand, a great deal of his exposition, particularly the ardent appeal for application of the new prognostic techniques in the ultra-high-frequency, high-energy field of social dynamics, is an exact echo of my own feelings, needless to say. This is equally true of his forcible argument about the inexorable, decided and decisive urgency of the need to bridge the fearful, unimaginably dangerous gap between the application of natural scientific and social scientific methods as rapidly and as thoroughly as possible, in a balanced and efficient manner, using properly founded piers, girders and arches.

On the other hand, I feel extremely uneasy about his "social technology" and more particularly, his ideas on the "social engineer" who must represent it to the outside world. As an emergency solution, as a powerful stimulus — either held like a carrot in front of the stubborn social donkey or wielded like a stick behind it — or even as a sinister means of menacing pressure or blackmail, a forced countermove on the chessboard of society, there is hardly any firm defense against it. No social scientist could brush it aside as an insulting insinuation or even as an undeserved criticism. He might possibly view this development with misgivings, but an honest, discriminating assessment would surely make him acknowledge its great merits. In the pitiless, time-limited game of challenge and response he would have to take account of the reaction to it, if it came in time and gave proof of a competent pioneering spirit.

It is true that the social sciences themselves (again, with the possible exception of economics) are entirely out of place in these procedures that Helmer et al. eventually take as their solution. In the last analysis, only "politics", whatever that may be, functions alone as a sort of nebulous "deus ex machina" reserved for the final dénouement. In this final, rather naive casting, there is still no escaping the lack of social-scientific training of thinkers schooled in the natural sciences and technology, however brilliant, sound and flexible they may be. In my opinion, any American "social engineer" who ended up in this political jungle would stand a good chance of breaking his neck in it. A man

333

like the European politicologist De Jouvenel, with a very profound schooling and wide experience in social history, is of course much better equipped.

So it seems that we have almost literally landed "between the devil and the deep blue sea". Are we now left with nothing but an either-or choice between Olaf Helmer's view, which dismisses the future of the social sciences out of hand as being quite decrepit and fit only for the museum of antiquities, and De Jouvenel's view, which, though it does strongly recommend a renovation of political organization for the requisite control of the future, nevertheless denies with equal firmness any possibility of constructing a social-scientific study of the future?

I am sure there is a *third way* which synthesizes and combines the best of *both* these visions. I have endeavored to outline this solution clearly in the detailed expositions given earlier, so that no further repetition should be needed here.

A new initiative towards effectively future-oriented, specifically social *scientific* research using all the *technical* aids of modern prognostics, is today both necessary and possible.

At this present point in history we must accept this as totally indispensable in three respects, and so give it top priority in matters of manpower and finance.

In the *first* place — as was indicated at the close of the last chapter but one — it must accompany (futurography) and control (futopology) the social processes of change and transformation that are now developing, pressing forward from the present, or even rushing towards the future of human society with unprecedented force, speed, depth and scope.

The *second* requirement is communication and exchange of information with all the leading sectors of human society, in order that their future-consciousness shall be sharpened and their obligation of choice be clarified and matured. This latter factor must find definitive expression in a declared willingness and explicit capacity to determine our own destiny by the purposive application of human power, which in turn will be made feasible by clear insight into the possible-desirable "where to".

Thirdly, there must be scientific preparation and a responsible advisory function on behalf of the appropriate government bodies who take the policy decisions. These government bodies must of course also involve one or more ministries with *responsible cabinet ministers* specially charged with questions of technological renewal and prognostic control of the future. The latter, however, are wholly *dependent* as regards the policy they pursue on the *independent* scientific apparatus and organization operating on their behalf at high level. This will take the form of their own research divisions, special social-scientific advisory councils, future-research institutes, "look-out institutions", modern communications media for future affairs and so forth.

334

Though somewhat over-simplified, it is by and large true that the final goal of all prognostic work or preparation lies in its utilization in some form of decision-making. Prognostics is an auxiliary science which serves this ulterior purpose — provided it does not confine itself to the study and evaluation of means but also includes desirable-possible ends themselves in its normative research. In this way it quite definitely indicates a well-considered, purposeful and future-oriented direction for this decision-making and is able to influence the design of the end-product.

Naturally, this scientific contribution and reflection are of the greatest importance in the making of policy decisions. I therefore shudder to think that — as Helmer is forced to suggest — social technology, conscious of its own limitations, might leave this work entirely to politics, and pass the buck to the politicians. As a former senator I may take the liberty of observing that as a race, they are wholly incompetent to undertake it in any country under the sun and that the result of such a course of action would be worse than useless. I am unfortunately unable to recall who it was who said that politicians are a species of professional idiots produced by mammalian evolution, or the worst example of the "naked ape", or words to that effect; but who could put his faith in any kind of "big brother"? What Helmer's suggested solution really boils down to is the replacement of one yawning hiatus (between natural and social sciences) by a chasm at least as bottomless — between a well-equipped social technology oriented towards the natural sciences and simply *unqualified politics*. The link of the social sciences, though, sad to say, they now function only poorly if at all, simply *cannot* be removed without fatal consequences.

As I have already remarked, the economists have finally realized, albeit only through bitter experience, that close ties between economic analysis and economic policy in the framework of theoretical economics and economic research have become scientifically permissible, and indeed essential. No politician who completely ignored the results of economic forecasting, planning and programming could hold his place for long today.

Yet a close marital bond of this kind between the practice of social science, or a particular part of it, and the formulation of social-political programs is by contrast, practically everywhere, almost entirely absent. And the prospects of realizing this dream, to parallel the development of economic science, look relatively dim at present, despite the extra attention given to the special sociology of government. The tendency to shift this important step in accordance with the motto of "mutatis mutandis" still seems too strong.

There is something stirring, but closer examination reveals it as too limited and too conservative a movement. It is a sign of progress that the Dutch sociologist Van Doorn has recognized, for instance, that sociology can move within three different "relevance frameworks" — those of science, society and policy. The scientific circle is that of pure sociology, operating according to the age-old standards and conventions of strict scientific practice. It could be effectively complemented by a practical sociology to deal with the special social problems that arise. But this prompts two questions: 1. whether pure sociology is not in fact concerned with social problems, and 2. whether the methods of practical sociology are therefore unscientific. For our present purposes, however, it is much more important to define the third relevance framework of sociology: policy. Of this, Van Doorn says: "As a political sociology it ultimately *submits* to the criteria adopted for the policy in question" (my italics).

But this is almost exactly what Helmer proposes in respect of his social technology. It is also the main burden of my *insuperable* objection to it. Furthermore, it is evident in many instances, to my knowledge, in the methods of sociologists now working in a number of government departments. This type of sociologist is all too often — and quite understandably — so indoctrinated with pure sociology and so inseparably bound to the dogma of freedom from values that he does not dare, when requested, to give any opinion on this or any other approach. These administrative sociologists thus refrain *as a rule* from making any advisory contribution to decision-making; how much less likely are they to criticize the criteria set down for them, or to re-structure the existing structures? In a word, these so-called political sociologists are on the whole what their education and training obviously make of them, i.e. political conformists.

If I earnestly plead for the enlistment of social science (or sociology), rather than leave an open field or vacuum to be filled by an almost autonomous "social technology" that itself, as it recognizes, must perforce refer all important questions back to an equally autonomous and so wholly separate policy, my motives in so doing are in no way chauvinistic or professionally biased. It is essentially immaterial where and by whom a problem is dealt with, provided that it is handled in the best way. This technique, however, provides no guarantee whatever that this will happen; on the contrary, there is a serious danger that it will not. Although social science has failed on almost every score, I am still convinced that it can, and therefore must, yield something else, and something better — particularly as regards the development of socio-political policies.

Policies cannot simply be the result of the availability of a scientifically operating technique. They must be carried and shaped by a scientific élite: in the case of socio-cultural policies, by a socio-scientific group that in our own day must also be strongly future-oriented. The shaping and reshaping of the future has at all times been the task of a competent, creative minority, communicating its inspiration, conception and visions of the future to the great mass of the population.

Technology, and modern prognostic techniques in particular, are a very important aid to political management. But a close watch must always be kept so that the means does not become an end in itself. Technology can be used

336

and abused by politics. It offers infinite possibilities. Nearly always, there is an automatic tendency to preserve and protect that which exists. In the absence of critical supervision and normative goals established by the social sciences, there is a fair chance that every new social technique will be eagerly seized on and exploited in the service of conservative rather than progressive forces, for rigid absolutization instead of relativizing reorientation.

This is all the more true since in the areas in which social science has progressed, the structure, character and methods of the corresponding political organs and institutions, the party political systems and media, and the executive and bureaucratic bodies often date from the pre-industrial era. They are not just old-fashioned, they stand out as a dangerous and well-nigh fatal anachromism against the background of the second industrial, and socio-cultural revolution that is now under way and of the processes of transformation that are pushing it forward with ever-greater dynamism. In order to keep up to date and to control these socio-cultural processes in the future, by channeling them along the best possible lines, we desparately need parallel, corresponding transformations in the field of policy. But it is here that the innate lethargy is greatest and that the laws of inertia have their most retarding effect. Opportunistically and with an appeal to historical continuity, politicians would, if possible, give the present a permanent commission.

Here more than anywhere else then, there is need — considerable need — not only for modernized techniques but also, if not primarily indeed, for socio-scientific analysis and a systematically studied approach to purposeful renewal. Both are indispensable, both for the criteria to be applied to future policies and for the ways in which concrete social problems, as they arise now and as they will probably develop, should be approached and tackled.

Among these possible and desirable institutional innovations in the political field, it will surely be wise to make room for De Jouvenel's proposed "forum prévisionnel". This forum would enable a varied élite of experts to elaborate future-problems and future-alternatives in depth and formulate carefully considered advice (or minority opinions) before particular points directly or indirectly related to these problems are discussed at parliamentary level.

Like social technology itself, such a discussion forum for future affairs that are soon to affect the political scene strikes me as being extremely useful.

These should never be regarded, however simply, as political extensions and accessories, dissociated from their only real, substantial foundation, systematic scientific investigation of social dynamics and the all-embracing totality of the shapes of the future — probable, desirable-possible, and therefore attainable. It is still within our power *now* to decide whether what emerges from the social cocoon that is at present solidifying and will soon burst open is to be a monstrous, congenitally deformed technocratic and ultimately self-destructive freak of natural history, or a form of society that is humanly decent, evolutionally viable and qualitatively acceptable to the human community.

337

The answer lies in our own hands, provided that social science breaks its vow of silence and joins in the debate; provided it also applies the modern technique of decision-making to itself and exchanges hesitant abstention for purposeful resolution; provided, at long last, it once again realizes its social responsibility for the future of human society ... and proves that it was once the jewel of the humanities, destined indeed to be their crowning glory. For me though, it need not sit on any throne. Time, the inexorable arbiter, will judge it from his own seat of supreme authority, as he will judge the future fate of humanity which, willy-nilly, it will have helped to shape for good or ill.

PART FIVE

Prognostic problems, plans and prospects

"It's a poor sort of memory that only
works backwards"
(The White Queen in Lewis Carroll's
"Through the Looking-Glass".)

Looking back and looking forward

If earlier chapters have given the reader the impression that the author considers everything possible and achievable, accepting no problems as insoluble and no limits as absolute, he is right in principle but wrong in practice. In reality, the labels "optimism" and "pessimism" cannot be applied without qualification. Nor can those of "idealism" and "realism". Not everything is moonlight and roses. Even to cherish the hope would be to surrender to treacherous illusions and to invite a rude awakening. On the other hand, events repeatedly prove the unrealistic idealist to have been a long-term realist after all. My plea is for a proper balance of existentialist pessimism and volitional optimism. Prospects at present are decidedly not too bright. But things might turn out reasonable well, if only . . . The "if only" is a twofold condition; first of all, of course, it calls for the application of the required purposive thinking backed up by the appropriate effort. Secondly, and just as inescapably, it calls for the prompt bringing into play of sufficiently strong and fast-acting counterforces.

All this does not come about of its own accord. And still less all at once. On the contrary, the room for manoeuver between challenge and response is constantly shrinking. As time passes, time becomes ever shorter. As I have remarked before, *shortage of time is the greatest shortage of our time.*

But the ever-increasing shortage of time does not only mean that when the shortage is most acute, it is necessary to react much faster and take certain drastic steps almost at once. It can and often does mean also that the later these steps are put into effect, the less influence they can eventually have on the already very disturbed force field of social dynamics. Appropriate intervention at the right time has much greater potential influence. The man who first understands and masters the self-created dynamics of human society stands the best chance of progress through self-conquest. Activated *revolution* aimed at changing ossified habits of thought and dogmatic attitudes of mind, which lead only to a state of passivity, thought of as a sensible "wait and see" attitude, is now the best quarantee of a continued *evolution.*

I The pressure of the past

CHAPTER 24

Old bottlenecks and new problems

1. Casting off the myth

The spirit imprisoned in a bottle, held in by a narrow neck and a solid stopper, is a myth. So, alas, is the miracle-working genie, released by breaking the neck of the bottle or withdrawing the stopper. True, many spirits are still imprisoned, crowded together by the pressure of dogmatics, in tight, restrictive containers. But simply to release them all would only mean volatilization and loss of something to go by. The liberated spirits — and Mannheim's "free-floating intelligentsia" comes to mind — must be given guidance and new, tenable sheet-anchors if they are to reach a new order at a higher stage of evolution.

In this section I should like to restore to some of these long-incarcerated spirits their hard-earned freedom, and in the following chapters to show that, without demanding miracles, it will be possible through our own efforts, achievements and plans as yet unfulfilled, to open up really new perspectives and — it is no exaggeration — magnificent panoramas.

It is surprising to discover that in our own time — a time apparently so sober and, to many peoples' minds, increasingly dominated, or at least strongly influenced, by a hardboiled, matter-of-fact and realistic younger generation — nevertheless some of the most antiquated myths continue, like so many clichés or axioms, to reign almost supreme and essentially intact.

To try to catalogue them all here would be a herculean task.[1] I shall mention again, by way of a résumé, only those tyrannical, patriarchal or parochial myths which earlier discussion has revealed as the main snags (sometimes intentional obstacles, sometimes unconscious barriers) in the way of social-cultural advance.

To begin with, the myth still predominant in many spheres is one of age-old religious origin: the future is not mankind's, the future is God's. Thus the future as such is unknowable, let alone in principle controllable, still less amenable to purposive creation or transformation on the part of humanity. Since the beginning of human history, however, mankind has striven, with increasing success in many respects, to struggle free from the paralysing hold of this dictum, as from an inescapable knock-down argument. The epic story of these enormously varied, wide-ranging, heroic-tragic bids for freedom is also in essence the history of human civilization, though it has virtually never been written from that standpoint. It is at the same time the history of the evolution of the human species. And finally, also, the history of idealism and volitional optimism; it has often been forcibly repressed, and has constituted many bold experiments, often wholly or partly abortive, but nonetheless has never been suppressed completely or for good and has constantly reappeared in new areas and with new resources. I have defined the joint intellectual part played by idealism and volitional optimism in the history of culture as the evolution — with its ups and downs — of *human power*. This has found twofold expression in the field with which we are concerned — as an empirically reliable anticipation of the future and an inextinguishable volitional activism to decide one's own future fate, individually and/or collectively. Since the Renaissance this striving, at least in the first instance, has ceased to be regarded as a criminal and therefore severely punishable activity, wickedly daring to exceed the bounds of human behavior; on the contrary it is held to be the purest and finest expression of the idea if human dignity.

And yet, though a high value might be set on the determination of one's own historical lot for today and tomorrow, and if need be even for the day after tomorrow, from the religio-philosophical point of view the future as a total dimension remained God's preserve, and as such was labeled as inaccessible "terra incognita". On this ground, seers, prophets, and social reformers could not but wreak the most fearful havoc.[2]

It is unnecessary to invoke or subscribe to the modern "God is dead" theology in order to state that, even if it be true, the only future time which should be regarded as a divine preserve is that which coincides with eternity; or to use Spinoza's terms, with the "infinite expanse" and "eternal necessity" which would at the same time represent the essence of the highest, divine bliss. In other words, even if one holds this view of life on the basis of a religious outlook, expressing itself in some kind of metaphysical-ontological system of values or in a transcendental eschatological future-expectation of the "end of time", the historical future can still be interpreted as a purely earthly process. The Utopian "diesseitig" view of future human society need no longer be regarded as inherently opposed to any kind of religious "jenseitig" approach. On the contrary, the shape of future society could and should constitute an indispensable, though too long and too thoroughly neglected, complement to every kind of religious inspiration.

Besides this, of course, the myth of religious origin lives on in a secularized and indeed stronger form, in which the "the future is unknowable" doctrine is asserted with just as much confidence and pressed home by monotonous, gratuitous repetition. If it were said only that the future remains veiled, or that the future is not completely predictable, i.e. in every detail and for every point in time, then that in itself would be a reasonable statement. We have clearly established that at every juncture there is a variety of possible future developments, only one of which can ultimately stand out and reveal itself as the real future which will then replace the present. But the frequently held view that nothing of any value can be said even about these probable, albeit alternative future possibilities, stems from a thoroughly unscientific attitude of mind — a mentality which does not serve truth, but simply pays idolatrous homage to an indubitable though impossible certainty and so wishes to live on undisturbed in the self-contained cocoon of the observable present. It is on this point that the social sciences have led the way back to this extremely disquieting dogmatic starting-point, with the sole exception of economics itself, which has managed at length to struggle free from the anathema of being the "dismal science". For this reason they have largely become, or degenerated into, *asocial* sciences.[3] *Non-sciences*, in short.

It is now undeniable that we can know far more about these future possibilities of development and the potential shapes of the future — while the time dimension considered is continually being lengthened from an initially fairly short period to an ever-longer one — than has often been supposed and systematically elaborated hitherto. It is a long time since the future was a book sealed with seven seals. The future, as far as our foreseeable earthly fate is concerned, no longer depends on prophetic revelation of divine inspiration. We now have numerous, quite recently developed and reasonably reliable means which we have designed and tried and tested ourselves for seeing ever better and ever further ahead, and for exerting an independent influence on the shape of things to come. And not only on the future shape, but also quite definitely on the essence, of the things themselves.

This view of the eternal essence of things, of a divinely ordained unchangeability in nature, has readily accommodated another idea likewise derived from antiquity: that there are no leaps in nature ("natura non facit saltus"). The movements which man has elicited from nature, however, include leaps of phenomenal proportions. Again we are struck by the paradox that man, obedient to the law of inertia and to his own human nature, nevertheless tries as hard and as long as possible to hold fast to the myth of a state of affairs set up once and for all, in principle the same for ever, and subject to only insignificant change, if any. While we ourselves, in contrast with this myth, could with far greater justification borrow from Greek mythology another image already frequently employed, viz. that of a metamorphosis brought about as if by magic.

On the one hand we are compelled nowadays to work with vast concepts such as exponential acceleration, explosion, revolution, transformation, fundamental structural change, etc. On the other hand, all our energies are devoted to the establishment of timeless and wholly abstract social theories which submit to a "role distance" from reality carried to extremes. There is a desire to continue as always with the task of establishing constants in a "frame of reference" which is made to serve the purpose. Thus it is detached from the obstructive, kaleidoscopically shifting patterns which habitually occur in the forcefield of social dynamics. Attempts are made to escape from, or to soar

344

Olympicly above, the increasingly turbulent social scene — a kind of shunting yard with its continually changing points and switches (manual or automatic), different track and route arrangements, signals changing color like chameleons, variable driving orders, steering systems, motor power ratings, intermediate stations and terminals. In so far as there are leaps they are accurately planned in advance as if by a lion tamer in a circus, and made through narrow hoops at exactly regulated heights and distances, by wild animals first broken to a manageable tameness, showing obedience to the crack of a whip as the result of the Pavlovian reflexes cultivated in them.

The stubborn clinging to the social myth I have described — which I stress, and so exaggerate, as almost always "ideally typical" — the myth of a concrete and variable reality which can be divided up and filed in abstractly arranged pigeonholes, is itself closely related to another myth which still enjoys a similar popularity. It may be referred to as "la science pour la science". This is tied to the neutral scientific idea of "le spectateur inpassible", which happily has long been abandoned by modern economics but was still valid and indeed predominant in the scientific code of classical economics. "Impossible" would be a more appropriate adjective. This type of socially unmoved scientist is shocked by nothing — no emergency, disaster, crisis, explosion or derailment. In his research he is governed by the taboos of puritanism, asceticism and abstinence. As such he is uninvolved, frigid and stiff, and in no way whatever responsible for anything which may happen. Only certain facts are valid and useful to him (to the extent that they fit into a theoretical scheme or can be made to serve it), but as a man of science they do not concern him. They make no appeal to him, and nor does he to us. Facts which do not fit, do not exist for the time being, until a new theory is found which can absorb them; though meanwhile the subject of study has again undergone a transformation, so that, fortunately, there is always work for new researchers to do. In the meantime the cultural lag between constant research and variable society leaves an ever-wider hiatus. The direction in which this change is going is scientifically irrelevant; the final purpose is a matter of indifference.

The myth of "la science pour la science" is completely different in kind from, for instance, the tenable maxim of "l'art pour l'art". At any rate, its application to the social sciences makes everything topsy-turvy. Referring to a proposition concerning Feuerbach, Marx commented "Philosophers have explained the world, now we must change it". Conservative practitioners of social science may object to this, rightly or wrongly; but they cannot deny that the world is now, in our own, time, *being changed* evermore forcefully and rapidly; that it is *changeable*. Albeit willy-nilly, when once they have chosen society as an object of study, they should in no circumstances shirk the job of concentrating most particularly on a study of the nature and operations, the causes and consequences, the size and speed, the scope, the quality, the continued development and the probable significance of these characteristic processes of social change.

If we try to dig down to the grass roots of this abstinence and self-denial, which in itself is incomprehensible, we come up against a connection with yet another myth. In fact we uncover an inner trinity of myths. The first holds that the future lies in God's hands; only He has *knowledge* of it, in accordance with His preordained Plan for mankind. The myth of secularized science runs roughly thus: we *may* not wander from the paths laid out without sinning against absolute rules of true scientific practice — our task is coolly to observe the here-and-now, as far as the outermost limits of our day. Our task involves only reshaping what has obviously coagulated in the context of an abstract theoretical system, explaining why things have turned out in precisely that way and why therefore *no other* situation than that which obviously, existentially, exists today, is in practice conceivable.

If emphasis is laid on these words "no other", which are generally only by implication deducible from the theory, we at once touch on a third approach which may be the most important central idea. It is the idea — a delusion indeed as a myth — that, even had he wished to, man could not have achieved any essentially different result . . . nor can he now for the future. Setting aside the fact that this line of thought puts an eminently realistic science under no idealistic obligation to assist the course of human endeavor, the execution of such a task would be condemned to futility in advance, and so entirely superfluous. Man, even social man vis-à-vis his fellow-man, is unwilling to perform and incapable of performing any future good. Here we are digging round the very roots of an often unconscious but firmly established conviction about human *impotence*, from which other religious notions such as human presumption (hubris) and original sin have sprung. The *may not* of science goes hand in hand here with the *cannot* of mankind. The earlier view of the future as being in God's hands alone has a direct corollary, namely that the future is therefore not in mankind's hands, and this has continued to survive in its own right even after secularization, with much added weight. But most of this weight is due to the authority of science with which the idea has been linked. After all, it is the passive, agnostic attitude of social science to the future which intensifies existing feelings of pessimism and resignation and turns them into fatalism and negativism.

Here too ancient mythology or mythical tragedy itself provides the means of casting off the myth. Whom the gods wish to destroy, they first make blind, as the wise dictum has it. We have been made blind, especially to the future. To see clearly again, for the scales to fall from our eyes, we must first unmask the false gods. Even if they are scientific deities, and even if we must adapt Marx in regard to sociology and exclaim: the unmaskers unmasked!

The unmaskers unmasked: it is easier said than done. The social sciences are still intertwined with yet a whole arsenal of other myths. What, for instance, can man do in the face of the autonomous forces, incalculable and unpredictable in their effect, of inexorable technological advance? Strange to say, the roles are reversed in this continuous offensive. Statics are suddenly abandoned, and dynamics find themselves called upon to support the justice of the standpoint previously adopted. It is an illogical volte-face, hidden behind a logical argument. This myth will be recalled when expressed as follows: technological progress is indeed unpredictable, since to forecast it would imply inventing the things which will be invented in time but are wholly unforeseeable at present, and which will then prove to have at least as much influence as e.g. radioactivity, the atomic bomb, space travel, penicillin, transistors, lasers, etc., which at one time were just as unpredictable. This argument is formally quite watertight, though, as we have seen, its foundations are being increasingly undermined in a material way by the technological forecasting which precedes present-day technological advance and is gaining ground at least as quickly, with astonishing success. It remains valid to the extent that we certainly cannot foresee every future technological development, though we can foresee more and more. Furthermore, even the sketchiest and most approximate forecast, even here, after deducting a wide margin for error and making nominal provision for shots wide of the mark, always has a value considerably above nought point nought. A rough prognostic figure is always more, and better, than none at all. Strange that this particularly exact statement has been ignored, so completely and for so long, precisely in those inexact circles where figures are revered as divine.

Moreover, even if we could know nothing whatever of future inventions, the possibilities of technical development which already exist, or represent a trend, always need a period of diffusion. Calculations have been done on the rate of this diffusion. There is also much one can say about the probable direction and effect of the diffusion. When it is in our interest to control a technical development process, the process in question is more likely to be the one which is *now* on the point of expansion-automation, for example — than a technology which will surely be invented in due course but as yet does not exist.[4]

Other myths, it is true, do not appear quite so emphatically in the shape of logical contradictions, but they do take on the form of impossibilities or insolubilities. As the irreconcilable antithesis between natural sciences and social sciences, for example. Or as the irresolvable opposition of facts and nonfacts (read: present and future) or facts and values (read: scientific judgments and value-judgments). The allegedly unbridgeable gap between theory and practice (read: between objective science and political discretion) is of course important here too.

I must break off here. Not because I underestimate the problems which confront us, though they can be solved, but simply because this would call for a thorough and complex methodological analysis, save where points have already been raised and refuted in other places.

Just let me say this: to the extent that the social sciences — now in clear opposition both to the applied natural sciences and, for instance, to economics — hide behind problems of this kind and refuse to participate in studies on future social developments, their mythology takes on a rather fairytale character. Even if we render unto Caesar the things which are Caesar's, we must inevitably discover sooner or later that he is wearing little more than the emperor's clothes, whose beauty is only apparent. At most a few, small, isolated and shielded portions can boast a scant covering of mini-mini-fashion.

2. The connections between socio-cultural problems and socio-cultural sciences

Science is, almost by definition, conservative. It takes quite a long time for a given subject of study to be clearly defined and for particular links to be satisfactorily explained within a soundly reasoned corpus of systematic theory.

The tragedy of the social and cultural sciences is that their subjects are now changing so drastically and so dramatically that their work is beginning to seem like a labour of Sisyphus. The difference being that they do not have to keep rolling the stone uphill, but that their map is out of date and even their compass has ceased to point in the right direction. They have to cope with avalanches, or hurricanes and cyclones, or even volcanic eruptions, which block their path, completely wipe out existing landmarks, and give rise to a multiplicity of new phenomena and processes.

Faced with this convulsive, explosive form of social dynamics, social science is also confronted with the soaring problems of its own dynamics. I do not think it valid to say that no science would manage to adapt itself so radically in such a short space of time. If we consider the enormous revolution which has taken place in the last 50 years — and particularly in recent decades — in nearly all the natural sciences (physics, chemistry, biology, astronomy), in medical science, in mathematics and in technology, we are less readily inclined to apply the word "impossible". It must be admitted that manpower, financial resources, research effort and equipment have flowed in massive quantities into these fields, or been concentrated in them. To pin down the "prime mover" here, to disentangle cause and effect, has become a chicken-or-egg problem. Must we ascribe the flood of resources to the obviously achieved, or achievable, progress, or vice versa? Or is this a close-knit mesh of interrelated effects? Or, as I think, mainly a difference of mental approach?

However that may be, the social sciences have as a rule neither had this wealth of imported resources at their disposal, nor managed to achieve even remotely comparable or spectacular results. Perhaps, to be fair, we should concede that there is probably no single sphere where such great difficulties exist as in that of the social sciences; for their original field of study, human society, is whirled along in a maelstrom and cast increasingly adrift. But on

348

the other hand it is precisely now, if ever, that greater knowledge of this social evolution and its expected developments has become completely indispensable.

This is no mean task, indeed. The social order is already in need of reconstruction. But, at the same time, reconstruction is also needed in pure and applied social science.

We have unconsciously got into a position which virtually compels us to do what I jokingly suggested many years ago in the conclusion to my thesis: leap before you look! Olaf Helmer has reached a similar conclusion in his plea for the adoption of a "social technology", which has already been discussed. He argues that the need for radical control of social processes has now reached such a peak of urgency that we cannot possibly wait for the eventual advances in socio-scientific theory — perhaps a generation or more later — "until satisfactory, well-tested theories of human relations are available".[5] Begin, therefore, he advises, with a reorientation (i) of "operational model building" and (ii) of "systematic use of expertise".[6] For lack of a solid theory, this must be done on an ad hoc basis, tentatively, experimentally, but must in any case be "future-directed" and "policy-oriented".[7] Helmer's hope is that any aversion or compunction there may be will disappear from social science "when the pragmatic step is taken from the perfectionist demands of pure theory to the more modest reliability requirements of practical technology".[8]

My own agreement with, and objections to, this approach have already received attention.[9] But not only the gap between social science and social technology, directed mainly to social policy is problematic. More than Helmer, I continue to believe above all in a rapid, adequate capability for adaptation, in particular as regards sociology.

Only if social science fails entirely, or if its renewal takes place too slowly for the times, in other words only in a situation of extreme urgency, is there little left but Helmer's purely technical approach.

But it is also worth reflecting that a usable social technology would after all have to deal with a number of precisely those problems with which social science at present has to wrestle. I mean that to some extent it will turn out to be a mere shift in terminology.

This does not hold for prognostics, which will be indissolubly bound, as it were, to the development of a social technology. Nor does it hold — this is in fact Helmer's starting-point — for improved chances of bridging the gulf between the "hard" and "soft" sciences: such a bridge is in fact already constituted by social experimental and prognostic techniques. Finally, social technology will also have much less trouble in effecting a really comprehensive, structural and interdisciplinary approach.

On the other hand, however, the great problem of social science is a far greater problem still for social technology. If the social scientist cannot, may not and therefore will not make judgments on aims and values, how dare we leave such judgments to the social engineer?

The socio-cultural problems lie essentially in their future-directedness. Every approach — whether purely scientific or "only" technically appropriate — demands a thoroughly schooled, socio-historical and socio-ethical insight and a "normative-idealistic attitude of mind". This insight and this attitude of mind must be based on both socio-scientific knowledge and a sense of social responsibility. In addition they call for the application of thinking directed to future developments, together with a *sensory* perception of possible changes, a *moral* feeling for desirable changes and a *reasonable* ability to combine these two factors properly.

I can of course well imagine that many a reader will be inclined to think that, to put it mildly, my thesis has so far paid very little respect to the practitioners of social science. But I do not wish to be wrongly interpreted. Desperate cases require desperate remedies. Major surgery has become unavoidable; this I have certainly tried to express as clearly as possible.[10]

Let us make no mistake. The picture above is the roughly sketched outline of a sheep with five legs. We can no longer make do with less. But let me state quite unequivocally that my answer to the question where such strange animals may be found is this: look for them, not among the social technicians, but among the scholars of social science. That they are to be found there is, I think, more than wishful thinking, confirmed as it is by much important work performed largely before the withering and paralysing influence of the puristic encapsulation process began to assert its dominance. Besides conservatism, all scientific practice also is subject to oscillation.[11] The time is more than ripe for the reappearance of the latter phenomenon. The link between social problems and social sciences can still be realized if the latter manage to surmount their own internal and external difficulties.

3. Prognostics and democracy

After my ardent plea for the development of prognostics, it would be wrong for me not to show the other side of the coin and the problems connected with it. The Baconian dictum "knowledge is power" has already been changed by Comte into "prévoir pour pouvoir", so that the earlier maxim can surely be expanded today into "foreknowledge is power".

But who are the people who at present can claim a virtual monopoly of such foreknowledge? They can be counted on the fingers of one hand.[12] They are of course principally the military chiefs of staff, a few forward-looking industrial concerns, some central executive government offices, presumably the large intelligence and security services, and some scattered criminal investigation services, on a national or international scale (e.g. Interpol).

This exclusive concentration is decidedly not desirable from a democratic point of view. The new power afforded by automated information must not remain solely in the hands of the official executive bodies but should be at the service, not of parliament alone, but of the whole populace. Mass participation along these lines is possible through the installation of a central computer system to which everyone would be connected, for a moderate fee, just as with other public utilities.

But there is much more to the question than simply making available and distributing collected and processed information to all interested parties on request. True, it marks a communal advance, to the extent that such information, as complete as possible, is indispensable to all ultimate decision-making. But the process of decision-making involves more than that; and the "more" is just where the danger lurks — in cauda venenum, the sting is in the tail.

For we have had to point out emphatically and repeatedly that prognostics, as an instrument for decision-making, requires a distinctly *normative* attitude, a clear setting-out of the object in accordance with certain scales of values and priorities.

In the narrower sense, a military objective might be the attainment of superior combat strength; an economic objective, that of sufficient employment or continued growth; an industrial objective, increased profitability; a police objective, maximum efficiency in crime detection, etc., etc. The objective of an administration or of the political party or parties in power may consist simply of increasing, or at least maintaining, their existing power.

In other words, without democratic safeguards, though prognostics itself is progressive in orientation, it can be used (abused) to consolidate conservative positions of strength.

This signals once again the danger of not having clearly outlined social objectives, set out on a broad basis and longterm in character.

Whoever decides the aims decides the shape of the future. This cannot be left to big industry, the C.I.A., the Pentagon or the President of the United States, nor to similar concentrations of power elsewhere. This above all is a matter on which the views of the people as a whole should be heard.

The people, however, can only really be drawn into the deliberation and discussion of the question if information is available multilaterally and impartially. This involves first of all the cooperation of the social sciences and of independent socio-scientific institutes for future-research. These will have to be attached to universities; in addition, there would have to be an official Central Bureau for Research into the Future, (along the lines, for example, of the Dutch Central Bureau of Statistics and Central Planning Bureau) vested with scientific authority, to act as catalyst. In addition specific non-profitmaking communication media will have to make accessible to the public at large the possible and desirable future developments, in certain fields and in their interrelation.

As I have mentioned, Jantsch has shown in his excellent report that leading American enterprises do *also* try to integrate future social objectives into their normative technical forecasting.[13] This is both laudable and indicative of outstanding insight. Of course — it cannot be otherwise — the main emphasis must still be placed in the task entrusted to the social technicians: the future optimization of costs and returns in further research and technical development. In a private enterprise system — and this is no place for a discussion on the merits or demerits of a particular production system — this is entirely justified; a bounden duty, in fact.

But it is no less a bounden duty for a counterweight to be created, such that the collective aims of future social development are set out just as clearly and without the prejudice of certain vested interests. Not by guesswork on the part of particularly influential large concerns which bear no responsibility in this respect, nor of social engineers who may be attached to them, but in accordance with the "will of the people", effectively consulted and always apparent. To organize this efficiently is again no simple task, and I shall come back to this point.[14] We are concerned here only with the question of principle: who is the steward responsible, not only for managing the treasures harvested from the past but, more important, for the ultimately preferable, and so transformable, future?

If we agree with Lord Action's "power corrupts, absolute power corrupts absolutely", then clearly we are witnessing the tapping of a new source of power of the highest energy yet known, but also of a new form of abuse of power bearing a power factor which makes Orwell's terrorist dictatorship of 1984 seem like a child in the art of evil. For we are able not only to exercise complete power over the present: we can already control the future of generations still unborn.

If wrongly applied, the power of prognostics can also have the same malignant effect on distant posterity as can the radioactive radiation emitted by a freely released cloud of nuclear energy. As the evil is lessened somewhat by the attempt to make a "clean" bomb, so the aim should be to achieve "clean" prognostication, exercised by unsoiled scientific hands and democratically managed.

To have drawn attention to this aspect and the cardinal importance of the matter is among the greatest services rendered by that champion of the future Robert Jungk.[15] He is right to point out, besides the deliberately set tasks, the "hidden parameters", the concealed value-judgments. These can and will possibly exert an unconscious influence on prognostic researchers attached to private institutions or to semi-official bodies which have particular interests to serve. On the one hand, for instance, one can, like the author, have great admiration for the Rand Corporation's famous model of long-range forecasting. On the other hand, where for instance questions of war and peace or of new weapon techniques are involved, we must still remain critical and remember that this brilliant "think-tank" is the brain-child and purveyor of ideas to the American Air Force. The attentive, color-sensitive reader will have no difficulty in recognizing this mental attitude in the report in question. It by no means detracts from its exemplary value or technological usefulness, nor from the methodological pioneering work; but, somewhere, a warning light comes on.

If the reader is acquainted with my views on the value of *explicit* scientific value-judgments, he must willy-nilly agree with me in greatly preferring them to the *implicit* value-judgments contained in the prognoses of certain, mostly one-sided, interested parties. This valuable and inescapably normative set of instruments cannot be left solely in the hands of private interests or those which aim at one limited goal. We are concerned with a capital which in the future will become infinitely more important than the possession of economic-technical means of production. Neither monopolization nor reservation for an oligarchy can be permitted here.

Independent public bodies should take a hand in administering this overwhelming large spiritual capital on which the future of everyone of us depends. Nationalization is required, and in the future the major, or even only, need, will be for public internationalization. For the time being, besides application on the basis of private initiative or for a particular (e.g. predominantly military) purpose, I think it is enough thoroughly and quickly to realize how necessary it is for the comprehensive future aims of human society as such to be synthetically and universally pondered, crystallized out and balanced against each other in an independent and, as far as possible, unprejudiced manner.

If human society is to be democratic and just, if it is to change for the better, the future "to be or not to be" is now at stake on this sensitive point.

II The pressure of the future

CHAPTER 25

New notions and progressive plans

1. Study related to research into the future

Today we are left with only one magical formula which can be used as an "Open Sesame" for the breaking of new scientific ground: research and development. Our spiritual ancestors were able to found a science by writing one oracle book. Thus Quesnay and Adam Smith created the science of economics as an independent whole. Vico, at the beginning of the 18th century, did not exactly pluck his "nuova scienza" ready-grown out of the ground, but the many modern ideas it embraced had a strong influence on both the romantic idealism of Hegel and on the historical materialism of Marx and the later empirical history of culture. Auguste Comte, it is true, needed a number of volumes to construct his system of philosophy, but in doing so he established three quite new directions: positivism, the science of politics and sociology. One of the last figures who was able to stake out a new scientific field by means of one published book is Norbert Wiener; the field, cybernetics.

In fact, however, the science of cybernetics was the product of years of modern methodological research which preceded its foundation. As far as the present status of prognostic research is concerned, we have to thank the O.E.C.D. for a survey which at the time of its compilation could still be considered up-to-date.

It shows two things. Firstly, a still rather chaotic and for the most part isolated, uncoordinated complex of developments. In America these have stemmed mostly from the "think-tanks", which in turn owe their existence to official military and civil projects, but also to independently pursued initiatives inside certain military organizations and Federal government authorities. Partly — in a very important measure — pursued by individual business concerns either within their own organizations or by outside contracts. Partly by certain research institutes available to everyone, and also by large, private, business organization offices and consultants. And finally, through university and academic institutions which have eventually been set up, with or without business or government support, either with definite terms of reference or "without strings attached".

In contrast, the picture in Europe is a poor one indeed. To my knowledge, very little is being done in this field at present; and if there are a few people active here and there, they do not know what is happening elsewhere, nor where and how; they generally know each other hardly or not at all, and lack the possibility of establishing contacts of various kinds which their American counterparts would certainly require as an absolute necessity.

There is as yet a complete absence of any sort of international coordination in prognostic research which is now beginning to develop and flourish, and likewise of a comparative study of the methods employed and a sound assessment of the results achieved as against the objectives established.

One of the projects recently initiated by the organization "Mankind 2000 International", which comprises a large number of thinkers about the future, was a plan for the setting-up of an internationally based institute for research into the future along these lines. As soon as sufficient funds are available a research facility of this kind could be built and set into operation. More of these research units, however, should be established in other European centers.[1] In East European countries, too, a similar development has started.

There can be no doubt that a similar conclusion will be reached in America and that efforts will be made there to achieve coordination either nationally[2] or on a wider basis, so as to further a better institutionalized approach to prognostics. There cannot be the slightest objection to this; on the contrary, from the scientific point of view it is a matter for rejoicing.

The widening, technological gap between America and Europe is being watched with Argus eyes.[3] The observer viewing this and the related brain drain with some envy, if not anxiety, should, however, realize that if Europe continues to stand aside and shows no interest in accomplishing something itself in this new field, which may assume a decisive influence in the future, these phenomena will probably snowball. The right to self-pity will be reduced in inverse proportion.

It is quite certain that if Europe goes on importing technology from America and exporting intellect to America, it is condemning itself to a slow decline to the status of underdevelopment area. By the year 2000, Europe could be entirely dependent on America for all inventions and developments. It would tend to be simply a massive, modern continental colony.

A reasonable prognosis forecast yields the (to my mind) inevitable result that America's present lead in the field of prognostic research will itself very soon repeat the already familiar sequence of effects — acceleration, explosion and transformation.

According to the experts, there is already scarcely any chance of catching up on the American lead in certain technologies. I am convinced that this is not yet true of prognostics. But even here, delay is positively dangerous.

I am just as firmly convinced, though, that a European contribution to the development of large-scale prognostic research could undoubtedly display its own originality and inventiveness, and could furthermore be of great value in tackling both specifically European problems and future problems of an international kind. Ce n'est que le premier pas qui coûte.

Once it was in Europe that these first steps were actually taken. The 14th and 15th centuries saw the foundation, in different European countries in succession, of the first scientific institutions under the pertinent name of universities — pushing up northward from Italy, via southern Germany and France, as far as England and the far north of Scandinavia. The Low Countries too were affected almost at once, and to multiple effect, by this new, booming, intellectual movement.

I do not think it fanciful to draw a certain comparison between the modern establishment of universal institutes for research into the future, as championed here, with that earlier movement towards comprehensive organizational renewal and towards the raising, at least of the intellectual elite, to a generally higher academic level. Indeed, it is once again a question of adding a new dimension to scientific investigation, springing from that same urge to qualitative improvement, synthesis and an essentially "university" approach. It is truly nothing less than a second Renaissance.

Why should we leave its discovery to the historians of the future? Purposive future-thinking can and must deliberately create it now, and give it life.

2. Future education and education for the future

In the past too, man has been continually faced with the future. But this confrontation with the future has now assumed a quite novel character. The dividing-line runs right across our own age, and as a result, *our* today is *different* from any today before it. Different in that the future will no longer be a continuation, but will usher in an entirely new age with entirely new problems of much greater proportions, rooted in structures of a totally different kind.

The younger generation now growing up will live its adulthood in a wholly transformed situation. The most characteristic feature of this new situation will be the ever-faster tempo of ever-greater, more wide spread and more radical change. In the space of this one generation's few decades of mature adulthood, more and vaster changes will take place than have previously spanned a number of generations. More than have ever occurred in the course of a hundred or even several hundred years, in some respects possibly even more, comparatively speaking, than during the apparently uneventful millennia of history. How can this initially gradual, then more intense, reversal, mainly of quantity and quality, this substitution of a slow development process by a sweeping revolution, this compression of endlessly progressing time into fast fleeting moments — how can these colossal processes of tranformation, or even entire mutations, be tackled at the level of the psyche?

How will this generation of the near future manage to accustom itself to living a life of incessant, violent change and instability, to ever-changing family, social and community relationships, to a lack of continuity in human relations and structures, to continual, profound revolution in work, leisure activities and daily timetable, in patterns of behavior and styles of culture? Alvin Toffler is quite right to talk of "The Future as a Way of Life" in his interesting article under that title.[4]

We should really be a little ashamed that there seems already to be a clear realization in America that the golden age of the current "American Way of Life" is gone for good, and that the new way of life will from now on, and for the first time, be determined wholly by the future. In America and everywhere else. Toffler has also fully studied the consequences of this, and concludes that our great problem today is: how can we prevent the generations who will succeed us from succumbing to the traumatic experience of everfaster changing change — what he calls "Future-shock"?

I have already drawn attention in previous chapters to a couple of important consequences. To meet the challenge of continuing acceleration and explosion in social dynamics, the prime requirement is a revolution in the social sciences, and especially in sociology. The second requirement, which may or may not be a part of this revolution, is a scientific foundation for, and responsible elaboration of, prognostics. There is, however, a correlative or complement to these two developments, just as indispensable a copingstone, which I have kept, last but not least, to complete this edifice. It is the simultaneous revolution, equally reorientated toward the future, in our whole system of education, schooling and training: in short, an *all-embracing educational revolution*.

The use of this revolutionary, or at least radical, terminology is no longer so shocking nowadays. At any rate there is much more level-headed discussion of the need for renewal in education, or didactics, pedagogy and methodics, or in educational research, since the need has been at length recognized. Often the emphasis is laid on the future use of modern teaching methods, such as audio-visual aids, teaching machines, programmed instruction, educational media such as radio and television, computer teaching, etc.[5] All this is of very great importance, but it is mainly restricted to *means*. What I am concerned with here aims much higher — at the *ends*, the scope, the vision and general direction of all education and training. Of every kind of education, at every level; for all ages and sexes, for all existing and new trades and professions, for industrial training as much as for education for leisure, for elementary, primary education and for all subsequent stages of higher education, up to and including the post-graduate level. Education leading to specialized research, adult education of a more general kind, artistic and cultural training, sport and recreation. It includes education for clerics, civil servants, labor union members, diplomats and managers. In short, this vision of mine extends to everything which is, or is called, education, whether or not it leads to diplomas, titles or qualifications. The only thing for which everyone must be qualified, competent and prepared, is to be able to live a fully human, meaningful existence in the new type of human (or man-machine symbiotic) society which looms up in front of us.

As with so many other matters, I can only point to the need for this *total educational revolution*; I can do little more here than allude to it, albeit with some emphasis. Let others, more qualified than I in educational matters, develop this idea in their own writings; bearing in mind as they do so that our own latest organizationally comprehensive Dutch creation in this domain, the Education Act of 1963, must be regarded as being out of date even before it was passed, at least in the particular respect which I have mentioned. I fully realize that all educational legislation is a codification of what already exists or prevails; perhaps its function, by definition, is to seize, date and fix historical continuity at a given point in time.

This does not alter the fact for our own future, that is, the future of those for whom this plan is intended, it is *dis*continuity which will come to be the most significant factor. Those who receive this education will have to be specially well prepared, in particular for the disparity of events. Present-day education, in all its forms and at all its levels, is still based principally on assumptions of an unchanging world, of an essentially uniform substance and consistency. Education, as it will have to be in and for the future, will only serve a purpose if it makes sense of, makes informative acquaintance with and provides flexible preparation for, unchangeable changeableness, abrupt mutations and astonishing metamorphoses, confused and confusing scenes and structures, variable settings, and shifting social relationships, processes and groupings. It has no meaning except as a mental preparation for changes in jobs and changes (which are already with us) in home town, district, country and language. It must prepare men in advance for the future dissolution, or at any rate evaporation, of existing values, traditions, conventions, customs and standards, whether they like it or not. It must give itself and its recipients the means to face a continual, breathtaking reshuffle of what is "in" and what is "out", a constant kaleidoscopic and chameleon-like confrontation with new attitudes, institutions, authorities and regulations, with the resultant modified attitudes to social codes and taboos, to what may not — or must — be done, to what may presumably be considered proper or improper in situations other than our own. It will probably be necessary to consider the future possibility of different views on celibacy and virginity, even on increased variation in sexual partners, marriage partners, free or steady relationships, changes in family ties and connections, even in one's very identity. Account will have to be taken too of new technical developments in labour-saving, travel, transport, information and communication, of entirely new conceptions of time and space, perhaps of creation and God or religion, of the position of earthbound mankind in a cosmos which is expanding and fleeing from his grasp. Needless to say, account must be taken of all the increasingly numerous, almost inexhaustible, and perhaps bewildering changes with their widening radius of impact, which will inevitably arise from the even-closer links between theoretical science, research, discovery, invention and practical application.

There *may* be totally divergent opinions about the nature of what I have suggested may happen in the future, and what may seem fitting to later generations. Indeed, one *might* think about this, decide on a justified socio-ethical attitude in this respect. The actual shape of the future is by no means clearly established: there is a variety of possible futures. But whatever form and substance the future may eventually take, there is one phenomenon which, in its content, can be established in advance: the future will undoubtedly bear the stamp of far-reaching change and revolution. Failure to make adequate advance preparation for this will mean running the enormous risk of becoming completely disoriented at some stage, and the chance of severe symptoms of neurotic mental illness. It is this essential preparation for profound future change which must also determine the basic framework of the *revolution in education*. Here, indeed, is both the reason and the justification for my using the word revolution, which is all too often misused. The revolutionary nature of the sweeping educational reform which is now needed will be the subject of a few further explanatory remarks. Remarks, not firm instructions for the instruction of the future; after all, this must still be completely rethought.

3. Between the poles of history and future-sociology

The nucleus of a revolutionary thought process generally consists of an axiomatic reversal, expansion or transformation. The structure of most education has, in broad outline, been twofold: how did the present situation come about (*history*) and how far have we progressed today (*vocational training*). What we now know, however — or think we know — has gradually expanded, in ever more minutely differentiated specialist fields, to such an extent that it presents a growing threat to the first part, history (which includes other antiquities such as classical languages, philosophy and so on). This is a great pity, for two reasons. Firstly because a good grounding in history is the best frame of reference into which the when and the where of all human life and endeavor can befitted, and because it indicates the need for great caution in taking anything to be absolutely true or finally or generally valid, as we are continually tempted to do. And also because it teaches excellent psychological lessons about earlier human stupidity and folly, to which, alas, even the leaders of society are never immune.

In the second place, this markedly growing tendency towards a constantly swelling knowledge of the present seems hardly even to be accompanied by the realization that, however much the study period is lengthened or the study requirements extended, no headway is being made. Once again, mainly as the result of the same, ever-faster, stirring-up of social dynamics and the technological revolution, even the best-trained specialist finds that an increasing proportion of the knowledge of the present thus pumped into him is obsolete within a relatively short time. It is estimated that acquired specialist knowledge ceases to be adequate after some 5 to 15 years, no more. The average specialist trained in this way thus finds that he is in fact completely, or at least largely, unsuited to his job after his 35th to 40th year. In other words, *our knowledge of the present is not conditioned by history only*, but just as much by *future developments, if indeed they do not reduce it to an even greater extent*. We must even take account of the fact that changes in acquired knowledge *in* the future will themselves be subject to all the factors *of* that future — acceleration, explosion and transformation. This implies that the rate of obsolescence is likewise accelerated, so that the obsolescence takes effect even earlier and at the same time affects an even larger part of the accumulated store of knowledge. In principle, of course, this does not — disregarding mutual shades and differences of phase — apply only to the case of specialists in the various fields, who are taken as the most striking illustration here, but also to all trained craftsmen (who may in any case disappear entirely as a result of automation), indeed to every kind of knowledge and wisdom taught, and every kind of experience and skill imparted. And it also applies, not least, to all the teachers themselves.

In these circumstances, what form then can an all-embracing educational revolution take? To my mind, the study of history should never be omitted from any system of education — whether vocational, academic or scientific — though clearly it must be thoroughly purged of unconnected facts and dates, and modernized to reflect intellectual or socio-cultural movements and relationships.[6]

But even more important, it seems to me, is that the *greatest possible* effective and affective attention be paid everywhere to *a new subject of study*, "*future*", as an accompaniment and complement to the modernized study of "history".

It is of course not my intention here to give an outline syllabus for the subject "future". In any case, there would have to be differences of scope and emphasis, according to the specific type and level of instruction. I should like simply to indicate a few general elements which to my mind would always have a part to play.

As I see it, "future", as a subject of study should surely comprise an explanation of its reason for existing, its right to exist and even its duty to exist. This explanation is implicit throughout the present work, and mentioned again more explicitly above. Briefly stated, it is this: *the future will be quite different*. Furthermore, it will continually *become different*, at an ever-increasing pace.

Secondly, "future" should cover the *future-thinking* of socalled primitive and civilized peoples, from earlier times, right up to the present day. To a considerable extent, therefore, the subject "future" also belongs to the subject "history", simply because, throughout history, thought about the future has had an extremely important bearing on the rise and fall of human civilization, and of our Western culture in particular.[7] I refer both to prophetic-religious (eschatological) visions of the future and to inspiring social-humanitarian projects as seen in various ethic-humanistic types and models of Utopia (from Plato through Francis Bacon to Campanella, Thomas More, Fourier, Marx, Lessing, Morris, Herzl and Bellamy). A handful, so far, of the essentials of the history of culture and the sociology of culture.

But it is already possible to trace the outline of what, for the sake of convenience, I shall refer to as *future-sociology*. It would, for instance, include earlier writers such as Wells, Stapledon, Haldane, Russell and H. J. Muller. Not forgetting the celebrated counter-Utopias of Huxley, Orwell and Virgil Gheorghiu. In addition, I find personally that some of the best products of science fiction and science fantasy (Asimov, Campbell, Heinlein, Bradbury, Bester, Arthur Clarke, C. S. Lewis, Boucher, Bretnor, van Vogt, E. E. Smith, Fletcher Pratt and others) definitely offer important food for thought. Finally, the programme should include some modern future-thinkers such as Gabor, Bertaux, Baade, Fourastié, Robert Jungk, De Jouvenel, Gordon, Harrison Brown, Helmer, Daniel Bell, Donald Michael, Michael Young, Tinbergen etc. No, I am wrong: the very last chapter might be added by the up-to-date Utopia clad in its Hollywood trappings — Herman Kahn's "scenario".[8] This could be appended to the results, not yet fully analysed, of some of the other, more spectacular long-range forecasting techniques, e.g. those of the modern "think-tanks" such as the American Rand Corporation.

The last element, however, would not be included as a curious, somewhat sensational development, but as the entirely regular, though most recent, manifestation in an almost endless series of studied and continuously perfected visions of the future. Running through the subject "future" like a thread there is always the idea of human dignity, as it was clearly reformulated in the Renaissance by Pico della Mirandola. This was at the time, as essentially it still is, an illuminating ("enlightened") exposition of the faith which has ebbed and flowed throughout the history of civilization, always receding for a while and then returning afresh, which has believed man to be capable of achieving social progress by virtue of his ability to determine his own destiny. To determine one's destiny by the conscious application of human power calls for purposive future-thinking. The chosen form of inventive, expressive, idealistic vision of the future is a very important means to this end, but not the only one. For real social progress to be achieved, these idealistic visions of the future must always be crystallized and given concrete shape in the realistic, pragmatic channels of social politics and the corresponding social technology. "Future" as a subject of study will also have to aim at the formation of personal char-

362

acter as a social volitional activism oriented towards the future, a schooling directed at volitional optimism which will be purposive and responsible and have faith in its own knowledge, ability and discrimination. It must be clearly stated that social dynamics does not only demonstrate an increasing, though mainly capricious and fortuitous, historical mutability, but that increasing importance must be attached in future to the element of considered and so *normative* social *changeableness*.

The function of the subject "future" must surely not be to foster in its pupils the illusion that the future can be known in full, accurate detail. It would, however, be advisable to stress that the possibilities of reconnoitring the future generally tend to be underestimated rather than overestimated. And, furthermore, that a rough, overall approximation which does cover the ground in many respects is always infinitely preferable as a tentative forecast to total ignorance of what is to come.

An orderly arrangement of the selection given above is in itself really a minimum syllabus to cover present requirements. At a somewhat higher level — certainly during the second half of the period of secondary education — the subject will undoubtedly have to be extended to include a clear exposé of a number of modern methods and techniques by which, in general, a reasonably reliable knowledge of the future can now be obtained with an accepted, satisfactory degree of probability. Some insight into the material referred to in this book as "prognostics" must be demanded of every highschool leaver as being indispensable to his future everyday existence. To be wholly ignorant of the methods of modern prognostic experimentation would have to be counted, after a while, as the illiteracy of the age. In this respect I should prefer to see a kind of prognostic snobbery or future-mania arise than that dogmatic agnosticism, which, I fervently hope, will soon be classed as cultural barbarism, should continue to exist much longer.

The educational revolution which I have mainly incorporated in the subject "future" has an equally revolutionary aspect which is closely related to it. A facet which I consider so important that I have even chosen to use it as the motto for the whole of this last part. The introduction of the subject "future" into the curriculum also involves an entirely new approach to learning-memory and the exercise of the memory. This same conclusion plays a significant part too in Toffler's work which I have quoted. Until now, memory, as used in education, has always served two main purposes which have already been mentioned, either to remember how things came to be as they are, or to impress upon oneself what subject-matter of theory is valid and authoritative at the present moment. In other words, it has been above all a *historical* memory and a *present*-memory, and in view of the ever shorter-lived pleasures of the present-memory, it is the historical memory, surprisingly, which is often able to render the greater services, where the teaching is good.

But the system is wrong in principle, or at least very incomplete. Current

363

education teaches us to memorize established facts, figures, events, propositions and explanations. Indeed, as Toffler says, we have only an inheritance from the past at our disposal, nothing of the future. I would add to that, however, that we have received a tremendous legacy, a commission of vast proportions, from the future. We must also develop a memory for non-facts and apply it to the non-existent. We must begin to transport ourselves more and more into conceivable, possible and desirable futures and stretch our "memory" out to encompass them. To this extent I willingly endorse the opinions of Roger Revelle[9] when he says: "It is far more important for young people to obtain some understanding of what is not known and what may be discovered than to memorize (and soon forget) logical outlines of existing knowledge."

But the concept of a "memory for the future" essentially embodies more than a few mental voyages of discovery to reconnoitre the terrain of a future which it will be possible to penetrate ever further and, thus, becomes ever-more fascinating. Thus the revolution in education, if consistently carried through, will be more fundamental than may appear at first sight, despite the somewhat ironical Alice-in-Wonderland touch. I have already written at length especially about this, (especially, though not exclusively in the context of Higher Education) and will therefore content myself here with a few brief remarks in reference to it. If education really does give effect to the implications of a future-memory, then two more essential renewal processes will be required.

In the first place, education will increasingly come to mean the imparting of abilities such that the pupil is *subsequently* capable of tackling and solving new and different future problems, independently. In the second place, the special aim of all education must henceforth be to make *final* education only a *beginning*. In view of the accelerated obsolescence of all knowledge about the present, good education must teach its pupils that they must go on learning continually after their studies are finished, and must show them how this can be done, so that they may remain up to date, partly by self-tuition, partly by extra tuition and post-tuition, as much and as long as possible. Purposive future-teaching along these lines is the sine qua non of "permanent education", which will become more and more necessary. It does not stop at teaching why and how learning should be a continuous activity. It also means that people will be able to train themselves in advance for fairly sudden changes of profession or trade, if necessary or desirable, without too great an effort; they will, as it were, be able to renew their own schooling or undertake their own retraining. The right educational preparation for the future will purposely transform all study into both elementary and auto-generative pre-study. Such apparent *relegation* is the only way to truly possible *promotion* in the future.

And therefore to the question of what a revolution in education basically means, the answer, as the above remarks indicate, is that it means more than can be suggested by concepts such as the establishing of the "future" as a subject of study and the fostering of a "memory for the future". In fact it really boils down to a conscious *shifting forward* of the whole range of education, carefully projecting it, so to speak, from the outset towards an unknown, or at least only partially known, future. Present-day education is losing more and more of its value and its hold because of the expected impact of the future. Only education directed to the future will be able to maintain and prove its value in the future; only then will it attain full development and application.

This reorientation can also be expressed in another way. The education which will be of value in the future will in fact exist in a completely different world and so, as regards the values at which it will aim and the characteristic and intellectual skills which it will seek to impart, will indeed be worlds away from education of the traditional kind. Revelle (q.v.) has taken the trouble to draw up a balance sheet of modern and traditional educational values (13 in all). As a non-expert, I shall not venture so far, nor try to draw a complete picture (or contrast). But I want to finish by highlighting once again those educational aims and mental prerequisites which embody the arguments repeatedly set out in this book in favour of the future-mobility which I see as an undoubted necessity.

This mobility is closely related to the exploring of various different, or even opposed, development possibilities, elaborated in the form of Utopia, counter-Utopia, science fiction and scenario. This whets the appetite for change and renewal and teaches one how to transpose oneself into new situations, real or fictitious. These can quite wel be *crisis* situations. The social game of "crisis role playing" is already being used in America as a means of advance acclimatization to them. And indeed, the new system as a whole is more in the nature of play — and as such fits in with both Jean Piaget's child studies and Huizinga's homo ludens. It is play, but not just for transitory relaxation. Consequently, this transposition to completely strange situations must not be left to the romanticized dream factories of Hollywood with their automatic happy endings which they still never fail to engineer. The important thing is to be able to cope with painful and unexpected emergencies by dint of good practice in counter-attack and resilience. One must know how to deal with emergencies as painful as they are unexpected by practised counter-attack or resilience. One will have to learn to adopt an extrovert attitude to the extent that one is not upset when the bottom drops out of things. In all circumstances one will have to possess deliberately built-in shock absorbers.

Among prognostic techniques, therefore, "gaming" and simulation are very important teaching methods. Helmer and Gordon, who elaborated the Delphi technique for the Rand Corporation, also devised the game of "Future" with the aid of Kaiser Aluminum. The aim here is to estimate the probability factors of certain future development that are considered possible (based on the results of their "long-range forecasting study").

All forms of play, and the action of playfully thinking oneself into, and experimenting with, a different future set-up, demand — and sharpen — one's powers of imagination, fantasy and inventiveness. These qualities can then be brought into play again to solve new, unforeseen problems of one's own. And the possession of an adequate ability to absorb shocks, and sufficient reserves of resilience to start again whatever happens, even though a good cry may first be necessary, can be positively learnt and acquired with the help of shining examples and systematic exercises. Nevertheless, this capacity to overcome difficulties and obstacles also calls for other qualities which must be nurtured as much as possible by future-oriented education. Independent perseverance, indestructible volitional optimism and inexhaustible creativity, for instance, are an indispensable trio.

These qualities are essential to the subsequent steady building of one's own individual future, even though it may be built on quicksands; together with a consciously applied sense of social responsibility they must form a contribution, according to individual ability, to an optimum collective future in accordance with a built-in, optimistic outlook on the future.[10]

Without a firm basis of independence and self-confidence, hardened by systematic schooling, even self-study continued almost perpetually could not be expected to achieve much. A combination of all the characteristics I have mentioned does more than remove most of the fear of the unknown and the changeable, by familiarizing one with them from one's earliest days through play, simulation and fantasy. The instilled ability to play one's own part in shaping the future also leads us to the most pressing future requirement: the capacity for making decisions. Education had already made the students acquainted with the prognostic process of decision-making. In practice, when finding themselves in constantly different situations, people will be able time and time again to make difficult decisions at the right time without too much hesitation, thanks to the "Aha experience" or recognition in the manner of J. B. Priestley's "I have been here before"; for they will have already seen and heard and even felt them before to an almost excessive degree: that is what life will be like in future!

We should now be early through, were it not for the eternal platonic problem of teaching the teachers, on which every innovation in education threatens to run aground. Precisely because — mutatis mutandis — it always comes to the surface, there is no sense in doing more here than touching on a few specific points.

(1) There is no doubt that, as has already happened in some places in America and is now in full swing (Europe limping behind with too great a cultural lag) it will be necessary to create a number of *university chairs* in the teaching of prognostics or the science of the future.

(2) Attached to these will be institutes for *research into the future*, where theoretical and practical courses can be followed and experimental research carried out. I have already discussed the need for international coordination,

and also on both the requirements and the task of the government as regards future-policy and future-information.

(3) An *international association* of future-scientists and future-research workers must be established to organize, inter alia, regular congresses and personal contacts.

(4) There must be an *international journal* (and later several), giving information on the nature and progress of future-research, prognostic publications, applications of long-term thinking and long-term decision-making, etc. etc.

(5) Thought must certainly be given also to the drafting of a special future-encyclopedia, somewhat popular, and as far as possible international in character.

(6) In all higher education, an important place must be given to the mutual relationship between a changeable society and changing future-values, sufficient attention being paid to the parallel changes in religious, philosophical, ethical, natural-scientific and social-humanistic future-thinking. The didactics and methodics of the subject "future", or "future-sociology", would have to be elaborated in greater depth to this end.

4. Creation of a new elite: generalists and Utopians

Revolution can also accommodate rehabilitation. Both generalists and Utopians were once held in high esteem. Generalists stood at the summit of the human intellect as philosophers and encyclopedists. They represented the incarnate ideal of the "uomo universale". Among these many-sided, versatile spirits, who were often men of genius, must be counted Socrates, Plato, Aristotle and Da Vinci; Pico della Mirandola, Descartes, Pascal and Leibnitz; Kant and Goethe, I assume; Bayle, Rousseau and, for a number of admirers, Voltaire too; for many, probably Comte and Marx; no doubt for countless disciples, Schweitzer and Buber; and finally Einstein, quite certainly, and possibly Robert Oppenheimer.

The unrealistic Utopians, stretching in a long line from Plato to More, from Bacon and Campanella to Bellamy and Wells, were regarded, until about the turn of our own century, as visionaries and social idealists with exalted intentions who, though we are not always aware of the fact, contributed much to the actual creation of our most treasured institutions.

The undoing of the generalists was the diligence of the work-distributing specialists. It came to be considered impossible for one person to take in even the bare essentials of so many branches of knowledge when they had grown so large, except in an abysmally superficial way.

The Utopians were brought down by the counter-Utopians. It came to be considered impossible for one person, under the threat of so many and such menacing dangers, to go on believing in the advent of another, better society, unless he were the victim of infinite naivety.

367

Thus, synthetic and visionary thinkers have long been overwhelmed with scorn and mockery, been disregarded and despised. They once served as the great creators of the future. Their absence today has torn great holes in the future of our future.

That this vacuum must be filled as soon and as well as possible can hardly be disputed. But the question is, how? Generalists and Utopians do not grow on trees. They do not reappear as if by magic as soon as the concertina of society, tight shut for so long, is once again jerked open, pulling out all the stops and sending up a loud chorus of appealing voices. They belong to a race which is finally almost extinct. In this sense it is certainly not fair to talk of "le trahison des clercs". These "clercs", at least, have been themselves betrayed, sold and enslaved in all respects and everywhere.

It is not just a question of status and respect. It is not even a question of remuneration, though nobody stops to consider how a generalist or Utopian can be expected to live in our specialized and professionalized society, in which Maecenases have ceased to be. It is above all else a matter of education and investigation.

It must be admitted that fortunately (or unfortunately, from our limited point of view) the tide is already beginning to turn quite noticeably in America, in these two respects.

As for educating generalists, it is a remarkable fact that in American universities there is a move towards courses and programmes, and even whole departments, which combine different disciplines; inter-disciplinary faculties and special institutes are being created. Apparently with increasing success — that is to say there is a ready market for the resulting intellectual product.

There is likewise a clear revival of interest in, and a reappraisal of, Utopian ideas at the present time. Once again there is a growing recognition of the dynamic drive of inspired and inspiring visions of the future, in the force field of progress. There is a new awareness of, and respect for, the outstanding pioneering work done in this direction, particularly by the idea of Utopia. Counter-Utopia has also achieved its own quite definite counter-effect, however. Like a barb left behind by the past, there is a certain ambivalence of attitude: on the one hand, Utopia is seen as a nostalgic yearning for paradise, and on the other, as the mainspring of social reform.[11] But the burgeoning of prognostics and the positive appreciation in this connection of scenario[12] and science fiction are also restoring Utopia to its seat of honor, its rightful place in history which has meanwhile remained unfulfilled.

There is, however, one respect in which America too, or perhaps America alone, is showing great weakness which could have insidious consequences. There are indeed unmistakable signs of the rehabilitation of the visionary, sometimes rather eccentric minds, the non-conformist, heretical and rebellious seers or social reformers, the creative and critical future-thinkers, the Utopian idealists and inspired innovators of the future. Homage is being paid to them. They are no longer immediately brushed aside as idiotic, or at least "crazy", or branded as ridiculous crackpots, muddleheads or phoneys, or simply as obscure eggheads.

But vision, idealism and optimism are necessary prerequisites of progress, though insufficient in themselves. For progress to come about, there must first be criteria, standards, values and objectives. These, however, can only be determined philosophically, socio-ethically and humanistically, with eye and heart, knowledge and conscience, voluntarism and a sense of responsibility consciously directed toward the future of human society.

America, with its understandable preference, pragmatic aptitude and instinctive liking for ingenious experiment and applied technique, has not been notably successful in establishing these socio-philosophical foundations and objectives. What the gifted "Founding Fathers" set out along these lines in the Declaration of Independence and the Constitution was almost entirely a further development of a theme composed from the revolutionary body of thought of European enlightened philosophy, which in its turn had borrowed heavily from the progressive Utopia and social-reforming intelligentsia of the West.

European thought displayed its strongest side here. And the testators of European civilization left no heirs behind them. Although Europe rightly allows itself to be overawed by American technology and now by its most recent manifestation, prognostics, the fact remains that in an America of European origin and in a subsequently largely Americanized Europe, a great and palpable void has arisen. Where but in Europe should we hope to find the best, most valuable contribution to the modernization of social philosophy and social ethics?[13] European thinkers need only reach back into the unsurpassed, though now neglected, intellectual achievements of the original masters of humanism, the generalists and the Utopians, who matured in their own cultural circle and radiated their ideas in all directions. It matters not in the slightest whether they are then labeled "futurologists", "futurographers", or "futu-pologists", or anything else. All that matters is that they make their own contribution to the new values and major aims of future humanity.

5. Future-consciousness and future-choice

All increase in our knowledge of the future avails us little or not at all unless we know with sufficient certainty what we must do with it. Know-how remains a floating abstraction without a clear indication of the know-what and know-where-to. This is essentially another way of expressing the conclusion reached in the preceding section.

Even if a new elite of synthetically and Utopistically oriented thinkers about the future were to resume their former supreme function as a creative minority,

369

then, however gratifying this might be, it would in itself mean nothing more than the resurgence of an intellectual elite as such.

And although this aristocratic, intellectual elite may be functionally quite indispensable, and even capable of giving satisfaction all round, even in a platonic ideal state, the fact is that we have clearly made up our minds, partly under the influence of social philosophy and the socio-ethical Utopia, that our social system is to be a democracy.[14]

This implies that future social evolution should be determined by the will of the people, and so eventually by the world community of peoples.

Generally speaking, the executive has at present not the remotest notion of the extremely weighty matters with which we are concerned; nor has the parliamentary majority which is elected by the people and takes the ultimate decisions — it may even comprehend them far less. In all government administration the future — long-term, that is — plays a relatively small and subordinate role. Opportunist motives, day-to-day opinions, and short-sighted interests are usually the deciding factors, although what is done, as well as what fails to get done, has a great influence on future developments.

As is known, De Jouvenel has urged that this gap be plugged by the creation of a "forum prévisionnel" or "look-out agency" where all kinds of problems and aspects of the future could be thoroughly debated, at a high level of expertise and trained insight into future development potential, by generalists, socio-scientific future-thinkers and professional prognosticians before the decisions are taken by governments and parliaments.

This strikes me as a highly commendable proposition which could certainly exert a favorable influence. As such, however, it is still only a politico-organizational intermediate solution. As a former member of the Dutch Social and Economic Council I can say that it seems hardly possible to me to contend, for instance, that the Council's resolutions and suggestions reach or affect the great mass of the people. The traffic is mostly one-way, towards the Government, Government departments and the two Chambers. From one section of the elite to another, so to speak, or if you prefer, from one group of managers to another.

The great unsolved problem remains the liaison between the top of the social pyramid and the broad underlying layers toward its base. A problem which can only be fully dissected and broken down in modern terms of communication, information, participation and identification.

Expressions such as "national consciousness", "sense of justice", and the like give rise to much dispute. While I am quite well aware of the pros and cons, I still know of no better description of what I mean here than "future-consciousness". Future-consciousness of a religious kind has existed for centuries, predominantly focussed on a "hereafter", equipped with the attributes of heaven, hell and purgatory, or on a kingdom of God soon to descend on earth. A parallel development has been that of a strong socio-humanitarian

370

future-consciousness, aiming at a different and better society, no matter whether Utopian in color, classical-liberal or social-Darwinian in flavor, or marxist, and later socialist, in inclination.

In our own day, future-consciousness has been continually undermined and very greatly weakened. Where it has survived, it has been characterized by a growing ambivalence and fragmented into two contrasting elements: on the one hand it has indeed gratefully acclaimed the recent blessings of technical miracles; on the other it has been just as voluble in voicing, in a mood of depression or panic, the potential dangers which they also bring with them (counter-Utopia, ultramodern weapons technology, perfected dictatorship, nuclear destruction, automation, psychedelics, biogenetics, etc., etc.). Our future-consciousness itself has been completely and extremely technicalized, in a one-sided way which the Utopian and spiritual ancestor of technical evolution, Francis Bacon, could not have foreseen.

Now modern prognostics in itself is no more than a particular scientific branch on the tree of modern technical knowledge. But with one reservation, which is in fact decisive and points the direction. Prognostics can advance no further — as has been repeatedly explained, to drive the point home — without normative aims, and without a clear and justified indication of the *route to be followed.*

It is precisely this preoccupation with direction which must be injected with new life, positive and volitionally active, in the general future-consciousness.

All available modern technical media — or media that have to be especially created for the purpose — must be brought into play, where possible in concrete and preferably visual form, to bring home to the maximum number of people what possible futures may be open to them.

Nevertheless, it must also be shown, and proved, in the most impressive way possible, that these are no more than inherently probable possibilities. That there is also room to give expression to certain wishes which can be fulfilled to a certain extent, i.e., within given limits, in a carefully considered way.

I would stress that it is not simply a question of instilling a *future*-consciousness: that is only the broad and firm foundation. Ultimately, in the most profound sense and in the last resort, it is a matter of instilling a *choice*-consciousness. The people will eventually have to decide for themselves, via their elected representatives, the direction in which they want to go, and the targets which they will choose and approve. It does of course entail making a declared, though never easy, choice between good and evil. But this choice, when further refined and seen in the light of the future, becomes a choice between the more or less good, what one hopes may be better, and what in the circumstances may reasonably and morally, properly and justifiably, be supposed to be the very best.

We should only be deluding ourselves and others if it were not frankly acknowledged that this dual job of inculcating in a majority of people a con-

371

sciousness both of the future and of their own power of choice would mean a *single* and *simple* task.

True, this ultimately means a conscious return to the highest of Renaissance ideals, the idea then formulated in humanistic-Utopian terms and later equalled only by Lessing and Kant, of what would constitute the quintessence of human dignity: determination of one's own destiny, the purposeful, rational exercise of well-intentioned human power, under the inspiring and enthusiastically followed leadership of an intellectually creative elite. On the other hand, though, there is no shadow of doubt that in our modern society, increasingly complex and subject to evermore profound structural changes as it is, the gap in understanding between the elite and the masses had widened immeasurably. This is already true of existing positions and situations; how much truer, then, of future developments and phenomena which as yet have hardly seen the light of day. The elite now tends to be identified with "the Establishment", with administrators of an established order and so protagonists of the status quo; certainly not as the progressive avant-garde of a new future.

I can only outline here the decisive significance and ominous proportions of this problem. There is in fact much room for doubt whether and in what measure we really do have a democracy today, or whether on the contrary the managerial revolution has not simply carried to the top a different intellectual class, ruling traditionally, authoritarian and dogmatic in approach, and thus conservative in character.[15] There seems, however, to be an almost complete loss of contact between this new ruling class and the mass of the people, and between it and future developments. I cannot prescribe a simple remedy for this situation. The best hope of a cure for it lies undoubtedly with the younger generation, if ever it manages in time to free itself from the stranglehold of future-dogmatics, and remains sufficiently critical and alert to burst once again the barriers to a fundamental reconstruction of the future.[16] This book attempts to indicate in broad outline how such a change of front might be achieved. Its detailed execution will call for an extensive and concerted effort on the part of many people, and as rapidly as possible. I must just add that the organization "Mankind 2000 International", which is spreading fast throughout the world and attracting widespread support, views this process of inspiring mankind with a general future-consciousness and choice-consciousness of what will and must come, as one of its major tasks.[17] It hopes to be in a position before long to propose a number of new plans and instruments for the attainment of this goal. Part of its intention is effectively to encourage others, where possible, to follow its lead.

III The future of the future

CHAPTER 26

Positive visions and meaningful prospects

1. Present and future applications of prognostics

I have reported in detail, relying heavily on Jantsch, on present-day applications of "technological prognosis" in America. A provisional assessment shows that, on the whole, industry and commerce are succeeding in making more money thanks to this new development and to management with a keener eye to the future; the military authorities consider that these techniques, effectively handled, can ensure greater national security in the future; a number of public services can be more efficiently administered as a result of them; and they can therefore, in principle, lead to a system of management which is both more effective and better qualified to make decisions.

It is of course also apparent that much of this development is still at an experimental stage, so that, naturally enough, many mistakes are made and the techniques are sometimes wrongly applied. But nothing ventured, nothing gained, and we learn from our mistakes. The saying "knowledge is power, foreknowledge is wisdom" is generally regarded nowadays as a sound guiding principle. Above all, more and more areas of fundamental and applied research are increasingly following the lines suggested by preliminary prognostic studies.

The new phenomena and trends in America, as pointed out by Fortune and also by Toffler in his article which I have already quoted, are of especial interest. In America, of all places, where the greatest emphasis always used to be placed on conservatism and feet-on-the-ground realism, free speculation, combined with a knowledge of scientific forecasting methods and prognostic techniques, is now not just tolerated as a passing phase, but actively encouraged. Large American concerns have begun appointing "staff prophets", people who are prepared, and presumably able, to see far ahead; such people — and the concerns employing them — would have been considered crazy only a short while ago. But bitter experience has taught the lesson that such unreliable speculators or half-baked dreamers have hit the nail on the head all too often in respect of future developments, while it has been the so-called "sound thinkers" who have made fools of themselves as soon as they made any assertions about the future. All values are turned inside-out when acknowledged experts become idiots and crackpots are spiritual advisers. What had hitherto been regarded as a purely academic, and so largely unrealistic, question, is found to have the greatest possible reality and significance for the future. One

374

giant corporation has already offered a post to a science fiction writer, to draw up a report on the future situation of that concern in fifty years' time.

In any event, the idea of employing "prophets", "wild birds" or "blue skiers" is beginning to catch on. Toffler advocates following the example set by big business and setting such people to work in "all the major institutions at local, regional and federal level, in all cultural organizations and educational establishments and, last but not least, in Congress and all legislative bodies too.

When I published my article "Prognosis of Prognosis" exactly twenty years ago, I confidently predicted a further upsurge in prognostic techniques and applications. But I certainly did not foresee the last-mentioned possibility at that time, and indeed I am still waiting to see it. Generally speaking, however, I still cherish the same idealistic optimism as I did then, though much re-inforced of course by actual developments, especially in recent years.

I am convinced that we face a historical watershed of major significance. Our present age has reached the point of no return. A quite different future is already "in statu nascendi" — on the point of being born. A midwife's services are urgently needed. Before long it will simply be incomprehensible that prognostic techniques were not used much sooner, on a much wider scale and in a much more intensive way. I believe that the number, size and speed of such applications will increase within the foreseeable future to such a degree that this alone will mark a clear dividing line with our present civilization. *The future is a prognosis of the future.*

Future exploration will come to be the most commonplace thing in the world — much more so, and much sooner, than the continued exploration of space. This will mean a sharp break with the past, and a new era, if only because the *short* term will be extended with increasing confidence to the *long* term, and *short-sighted* measures will continue to be ousted by *farsighted* leadership.

2. Futuro-cracy and futuro-creativity

The primary aim of the development of prognostics is to provide the exact opposite of the laissez-faire and fatalism which have pervaded so many areas for so long.

Social legislation — itself the successor to the extremely infirm and "indigent" poor laws — was the first step forward, the necessary outcome of the (first) Industrial Revolution.

After the Great Depression it was the turn of economics to break free from the paralysing spell of human impotence, with purposeful anti-cyclical and structural policies.

Maybe the dictatorial terror and the Second World War, together with the atomic bomb and the advent of automation, inter alia, were needed to free the human spirit from the vice-like grip of drifting socio-cultural forces.

375

Perhaps then we, at last, have reached the point where we have learnt to realize that the future development of human society *must not* proceed unattended: that, if we exert ourselves, it *can* be controlled to an important degree.

This job of social control requires analysis, diagnosis and prognosis. The combined socio-scientific application of all three might be referred to as futuro-cracy.

The main import of such a concept is however largely negative. Control of future developments would in the main, after all, mean simply that wherever great danger threatened, an "early warning system" would enable man to intervene in time, either to prevent the danger from arising at all or to avert its unpleasant consequences as far as possible — or at least to alleviate them, smoothing the sharp edges and redressing the imbalances produced.

But the reader who has borne with me in the preceding chapters and not just glanced through these final pages is well aware that the idea of prognostics as canvassed in this book is in principle, if not something different, at least far more than that.

As I see it, once prognostics has been developed and refined, it will not be limited to the preventive control of future events. It is not just a tool of futuro-cracy, but also a means of aiming higher, of attaining futuro-creativity. Futuro-creativity is the ultimate, purposive substitute for the "blind play of forces". The substitution has begun in two spheres, economic policy and social legislation. But is only a first, and still rather lame, beginning, supplemented in recent years by a "Dritter im Bunde" in the form of the budding programming of development aid. There is still no systematic, comprehensive grip on the future as such. Even the continuing efforts at peace remain a rather vague ideal as long as they are not part of a concerted attempt to master and mold the *future* as a *totality*.

In the last resort, what is needed is the perfecting of operational equipment by means of which the future, as a complex whole, can be shaped. One day, by the purposive application of human power and intellect, mankind will be able to create and recreate the future to conform to a future ideal. This is where futopology, with its feedback research into desirable-possible futures, comes in. This is why futuro-creative planning must be instituted to support long-term socio-political management. And finally, this is why social science is now earnestly entreated to cooperate fully and positively, as future-science or applied future-sociology, or under whatever title it may choose, in the constructive realization of this objective under its auspices and on its responsibility, aiming at a new and better society.

3. Prevision and revision

Throughout this book such great emphasis has been laid on the need to evolve a science of prognostics, and on the urgency of projecting ideal visions of the future as norms for a futuro-creative course of action, that confusion and misunderstanding might arise on one point as the result of exaggeration.

It must of course be understood that *this work is endless*. To have achieved a revaluation or reform, some sort of renewal or transformation, can never be enough. The horizon never gets any nearer. Rather, because of the ever-increasing tempo of change in the future, and the social revolution which may have more and more drastic consequences, to stand still is to fall behind, more than it ever was before. We can never come within a mile of the ultimate ideal in its perfect form. At all times, in all its variations, or precisely because of them, the future remains the future. Every true future-minded approach calls for a new, elastic and dynamic reorientation and reconstruction.

As long as the threesome of acceleration — explosion — transformation[1] are in supreme control and continue to exercise a determining influence on the social pattern, the fact must never be lost sight of that they also influence, quite radically, the means and the ends of prognostics itself.

Neither Plato's ideal Republic, nor Thomas More's Utopia, nor Bacon's New Atlantis, nor Campanella's Città del Sole, nor yet Bellamy's ideal socialist state or any of Wells' fanciful visions of society, are inspiring or electrifying as far as their contents go. They are no more than important milestones of the spirit on the road to social progress and improvement. Fanciful, stimulating, alternative forms and ways of determining and improving one's own social lot. Instructive models of thought, but somewhat primitive for our own day, and in any case outmoded and fictitious. Models of visionary power, still possessing functional qualities of play and simulation, and in that respect still exemplary and expressive.

Precisely *these* future visions teach us that future visions themselves must remain up to date. They too are caught up in the acceleration processes of social dynamics and, as if reflected in distorting mirrors, made into whimsical or even nonsensical images. Madame Tussaud's Waxworks always remain horribly real, despite the passage of time. Those visions of the future which were quite unreal and seemed completely unattainable (and were therefore so fascinating) have subsequently become reality in part; but to the extent that this is not the case, or never can be, it is the passage of time that makes them truly, wholly, unreal.

Classical future-visions from the past are only an illustration. All prognostics, and this kind especially, is subject to the ravages of time. Too many forecasts fail to observe the golden rule that at repeated, periodic and comparatively frequent intervals, assumptions and objectives must be very critically examined to decide whether they can be retained unmodified.

The aversion to dogmatics and the progressive urge are equally applicable to prognostics. Failure to adapt in time to the passage of time inevitably leads to wrong prognoses, which devalue prognostics itself. Leaving aside chance successes, prognostics is practically always *incorrect* in some measure. By definition, it contains its own coefficient of uncertainty. For this reason we must constantly strive to reduce the inevitable margin of error as much as possible, and never to let it grow wider. *To predict the future, you must keep up to date.* Behind our present-day future-problems we shall discover heaps of new ones, probably still more complex and comprehensive. There is no break, let alone an end, in scientific work on the future. There can never be an "end of time" for this work. The building of cathedrals in the future and castles in the air is in principle like an unfinished and unfinishable symphony of unchangeably changeable future-music.

Where there is no vision, the people perish (Proverbs, 29:18). I have often reiterated this — itself a vision of great truth. But besides *vision* and *prevision* there continues to exist a pressing need, too often neglected, for *revision*. The principle of *changeability* discovered here applies not only to the incipient history of the future, but equally well to the future history which will be written and made and contained in forecasts and prognoses. Chronicles and visions of the future are also changeable; rewriting and revision are constantly required. Continual reconstruction of the past is extremely informative; but continual reconstruction of the future is a sacred commandment. Historical visions of the future form a series of consecutively short "stills". They have affected history, sometimes very powerfully. But these visions of the future must themselves acquire the aspect of a motion picture; they must on all occasions give evidence of their social involvement. Periodically revised vision of the future must remain as topical and up-to-date as a live telecast. More than this, they must continually polish and re-touch their antedated view of future time so that the original, speculative exploration remains, when seen from a later viewpoint, as reliable as possible a forecast. In philosophical terms, Bergson's endless duration (durée) must be pregnantly imprinted and depicted as "creative evolution" of the everlasting future. Not time which is inherently characterless and arbitrary, but a future-crystal repeatedly shaped in advance and subsequently polished, is what we must try to create. Constant reorientation to the foreseeable part of the future-dimension continuum is an absolute essential.

This incessant process of future-creation likewise demands, unconditionally and unceasingly, an act of re-creation applied without parti pris to one's own creation. This "creatio continua" is the only way of achieving our supreme objective, which is to ensure that *the future will be on our side.* The processes of social transformation constantly involve death and degeneration, which again and again require further-seeing regeneration, just as disorganization requires reorganization; demolition, reconstruction; displacement, transformation; and creation, re-creation.

Our life of permanent revolution is by definition incompatible with the unchangeableness of a final solution. The futuro-creative planning required is of a dynamic, possibly dialectic, kind, systematically keeping pace with the progress of time, or better still, overtaking and keeping ahead of it. Let us not forget that we can already reach any point on earth where there is an airfield in 45 minutes at most. Within less than 2 seconds, any occurrence anywhere on this planet can be seen in every living room, thanks to artificial television satellites. Cosmic events scores of millions of light years away, and travelling at unimaginable speed at similar distances in time away from the earth, can be closely followed by means of radio-telescopes.

Partly because of this universal process of acceleration, all prognostics, from the smallest beginnings to the grandest and most visionary pictures of the future, must respect this inexorable criterion of timely, adequate revision. Knowledge of the future is never absolute or definitive, but always relative and fragmentary. Anticipation makes sense only as a self-correcting process development, permanently revisionist in orientation.

Only in this way can the formerly cherished ideal of "the American Dream", for instance, materialize into something which will now serve as a model for "the Great Society". And so it might continue in other forms and shapes, during a never-ending pilgrimage, on or outside this earth in search of that other and better human society, of the ideal state which itself is subject to permanent revolution and will forever continue to bear the stamp of "future". The future of the future is both specific and unending. Man remains what he always was, albeit with immensely greater capacity and power: homo prospectans. But now, for the first time, he can grow, making full use of the power that lies dormant in him, into something else: Homo Creator.

The principal types of modern prognosis techniques[1)]

Jantsch states in his report that he has examined a hundred or so methods of technological prognosis which, with their variants, cover about twenty different main directions.[2] In his survey[3] there are somewhat fewer, and in the explanatory text rather more. I shall not follow that table here because it adheres rigidly to the division between exploratory and normative techniques, while a considerable number of these techniques are used in both cases. My intention here is simply to give the interested reader an impression of the way in which various important techniques are applied to the making of prognoses. I have therefore chosen the arrangement considered the most appropriate for that purpose, the development of which also appears to me to follow a decidedly logical line. However, didactic considerations have required the making of a number of corrections to the technical explanations given by Jantsch.

Before going on to give this stylized arrangement, I have a few observations to make. Firstly, I fully share Jantsch's opinion that it is not just a question of the value and capacity of each new technique considered individually, but above all of the new prospectivist approach which it brings to the fore, and the arsenal of techniques thus built up to equip this new armory.[4] Thus I am absolved here from the duty of giving a full and exact description of each one, such as Jantsch has attempted; moreover, their mathematical elaboration lies outside my sphere of competence.[5] I shall therefore confine myself to the summary outline and substructure of some essentials[6], reducing the techniques to a number of selected main types.

Secondly, in discussing these main types I shall not necessarily respect the time sequence in which these techniques and methods were first introduced. It is often difficult to draw an accurate line between older and newer techniques because of the continuous processes of growth, development and interaction. After all, we had been using some techniques for a fairly long time, including methods of extrapolation and analogy, input-output analysis, linear programming, regression analysis, graphical future projections and curves of various kinds, simultaneous comparison systems with or without constant coefficient, simple or complex economic planning models, containing prognoses for expected economic expansion and for the development of for instance the productivity of labor, national product, consumption, investment, savings, balance of payments and other macro-economic quantities. All these forecasts were usually lumped together as belonging to quantitative economics, which began to evolve as a separate and distinct branch in the Thirties. It is usually called econometrics nowadays. After the war this was further subdivided with a particular type of "operations research", also known as business econometrics, though it is not a clearly delineated specialist branch, and also by the new and rather broader name of "decision-making theory". The latter is directed especially at specific problems of business economics, business organization and management science or management decision-making, which it handles by predominantly modern mathematical and statistical methods.[7] On the other hand, in company with Jantsch, I shall certainly no longer need to abstain entirely from "appraisal". Such abstention could in his opinion lead only to "amorphous and meaningless statements on essential issues".[8] In addition there were, inter alia, the micro-economic calculations of business enterprises on investment and future yields, the result of forecasts about cost curves and consumer behavior, and of stock-market expectations, the latter again based principally on quantified Dow-Jones trends, cash flow, price-earnings ratios and the like. In this old field of business economics too, a powerful development is now afoot, with mathematics and statistics as its main spearheads. Initially, the new feature was mainly that existing, older techniques and concepts from other branches of science were transposed into new fields, notably that of business. There they were refined, for instance as regards linear programming and the approach to problems and prognostics specifically related to business economics. My point here is that "new" is certainly not always or in every respect equivalent to "brand-new" and that often — at the quantitative level especially — existing mathematical, statistical and probabilistic foundations are used to build upon albeit using details elaborated with this very goal in mind, together with (as has been said and will be said again) qualitative and normative viewpoints and, last but not least, with a characteristic future-orientation more deliberate than before, and often strikingly determined.

Thirdly, let me say this. A number of named types of prognosis techniques are distinguished, as I have said, in the following pages. A complete division is, however, not possible. For one thing, they frequently have elements in common. There are numerous hybrid forms and all manner of combinations. The distinctions made therefore rest mainly on a slightly different emphasis or a particular new or variant feature.

One fourth and last remark to introduce, or rather stake out, the infrastructure for this survey of a number of modern prognosis techniques. Such an introduction can perhaps best take the form of the question: what requirements should be made of a prognosis? People do talk in this connection of scientific and non-scientific prognoses, both of which, however, may be equally important and indeed cannot always be so sharply distinguished. The conditions that a scientific prognosis ought to fulfil have been discussed in depth by various authors over the years, and the currently prevailing views of these writers lend themselves very well to the present objective. The following stringent requirements are generally set for a prognosis to merit the epithet "scientific".

(1) The prognosis must be capable of verification. This means that it must be entirely clear in what circumstances a prognosis has proved true and in what circumstances it has not. In other words, it must be possible after a lapse of time to establish unequivocally whether a prognosis is correct or not, it being frequently stipulated that *both* possibilities should be present. The first condition implies that there may be no ambiguity regarding the concepts that are introduced and that above all, the point or period of time to which the prognosis relates must be clearly established.

(2) It must be possible for persons other than the forecaster to follow step by step, fully and identically, the way in which the prognosis is arrived at, i.e. the forecasting mechanism. This does not of course imply that there must be agreement with the forecaster about the method of forecasting. Briefly stated: the prognosis must be based on a theory or theoretical scheme, however simple or open to doubt this may perhaps be. This means that such a prognosis technique starts with the construction of a theoretical model.

A model can be taken as the abstract representation of processes which take place over a shorter or longer period of reality. The art of constructing a model consists in finding, for each case, a manageable simplification of the process while preserving in tact its essential features. Only then will the model be able to provide a usable imitation of reality and acquire prognostic value. Of course, the greater the reality value that can be ascribed to the underlying theory, the greater the prognostic value. Obviously, experience acquired with particular models is an incentive to the construction of other — often more useful — models. Success achieved with this technique in one science may also influence developments and methods in other disciplines. For instance, the recent attempts to apply information theory to economics are of interest in this context. It is perhaps important to point out that there is not just one model, even inside one branch of science such as science or economics, but that every problem calls for a model of its own.

(3) The prognosis must be based on information, that is to say on observations, however rough and uncertain these may be.

(4) The reliability of the prognosis must be specified. That is to say, the probability that the prognosis will turn out right must be indicated in advance as precisely as possible. This last requirement has a particularly important implication: it means in fact that the theory on which a prognosis is founded must be *stochastic* in character. A stochastic theory is a theory in which, besides ordinary (mathematical) variables, stochastic variables also appear. A stochastic variable is one the ultimate value of which cannot be stated in advance; such variables (random variables) can assume a series of values, but every value is assumed in advance with a certain degree of probability.

Many prognoses which are made and used in practice are, however, unable to satisfy this last, exact condition. Thus, if the four above conditions are imposed, a considerable number of prognoses are not strictly scientific in this sense. The fourth requirement has been expressly emphasized by a variety of authors. It is a requirement more easily met in the context of the natural sciences. In the social sciences, though, it is frequently impossible to satisfy it; and yet it is precisely here that the application of modern prognostic techniques is so urgently needed and should not be handicapped at the outset by excessively severe or over-stringent conditions — particularly as the differences between theoretical model and reality tend to be larger here than elsewhere.

The above will in any case have shown that in all forecasting techniques the calculation of probability or chance, to whatever degree it is applied, is of great importance in arriving at reasonably useful and acceptable prognoses. We shall therefore begin by examining in greater detail this sphere of scientific activity,[9] which is passing through a period of great progress and exerting a powerful influence on the development of modern prognosis techniques.

1. The calculation of probability

The calculation of probability is, according to Theil, nothing but surveying in the field of uncertainty. It is concerned with uncertain phenomena, the outcome or which cannot be positively foreseen. These phenomena, also called *chance* phenomena (or random phenomena), constantly produce different results even when they occur in circumstances which are as identical as they can be; they have what is known as intrinsic variability. Examples of such phenomena are: the result of tossing a coin, the life of an electric light bulb, and the length of inter-city telephone calls.

Now these phenomena all share one significant characteristic. While each separate experiment may involve unpredictability, as soon as long series of similar experiments are taken into consideration, an important phenomenon is discovered: the average results of long series show a marked regularity. This can be referred to as the phenomenon of "stable relative frequencies". The regularity has been confirmed by research studies involving, inter alia, long series of coin tosses. The statistician K. Pearson, for instance, tossed a coin 24,000 times and obtained heads 12,012 times. The relative frequency of the number of times heads came up was thus 0.5005 in this case.

A new coin was tossed 20,000 times at the Rotterdam Econometric Institute, with the following results:

No. of tosses	Heads	Tails	Relative frequency of number of heads tossed
5,000	2,529	2,471	0.5058
10,000	5,067	4,933	0.5064
15,000	7,604	7,396	0.5069
20,000	10,086	9,914	0.5043

The remarkable thing about these experiments is that, although the individual experiments reveal nothing about the result, the relative frequency is found to be fairly stable, namely about 0.5, when the number of tosses is large. This means that, although we cannot say *when* the coin will fall heads or tails, we are able to predict fairly accurately *how many* times heads or tails will turn up provided that the number of tosses is large. In other words, *unpredictability in an experiment does not mean unpredictability in long series of the same experiment.* This is the fundamental fact on which statistics is based. We might say that statistics is the science of "how often" when the question "when" cannot be answered. This "how often" is therefore based on the empirical law of large numbers. A similar regularity to that seen in games of chance is also found elsewhere. For example, the annual frequency of births, marriages, deaths and similar demographic phenomena per 1,000 inhabitants is found to be *approximately* stable, at least unless there are major changes in social conditions.[10] One result of this regularity is the coupling of the notion of probability with the phenomenon of stable relative frequencies. In this connection, a further distinction can be made between a priori and a posteriori probabilities. In the first case (a priori), probabilities are attributed on the basis of an assumed symmetry or equivalence of outcomes. The phenomenon of chance has not yet taken place. In the second case (a posteriori) the behavior of the relative frequencies concerned is first studied, and the probability determined from the findings. Thus we frequently decide to consider that the chance of tossing heads is equal to $1/2$, or the chance of drawing an ace from a deck of 52 cards is equal to 4/52. It is of course self-evident that these a priori probabilities must subsequently agree with the a posteriori probabilities. Naturally, it is possible for errors to be made and for deviations to occur; and, in principle, preference must be given to the a posteriori probabilities when the highest degree of certainty is sought.

Nonetheless, a priori probabilities are important because they enable us to predict the probability of events in circumstances where it is difficult or virtually impossible to repeat an experiment on an extensive scale. This, therefore, is the plane of contact with various prognostic techniques, notably in the social sciences.

The examples given above are of course extremely simple ones. But the application of prognostics in social fields calls for a command of highly complicated statistical and mathematical methods.

It must be realized that the uncertainty which is by definition inherent in many future-problems cannot be entirely resolved by probability calculations. Nevertheless, it can safely be said that insofar as the uncertainty is enclosed by particular mass functions or densities, the degree of uncertainty is reduced somewhat, which is a distinct step forward from the state of complete ignorance previously endured.

The highly interesting ideas on statistics of the English clergyman Thomas Bayes, originally published in 1764 by the Royal Society, have only recently been reintroduced and elaborated. Bayes was the first person to talk about the probability of causes. His theory is also known nowadays as that of inverted probabilities. The modern development of Bayesian ideas is frequently referred to as a new interpretation of "subjective probabilities". Briefly, the essentials are as follows.

In certain cases, notably in the social sciences, the notion of probability is taken as a measure of the confidence which an investigator has in a specific assertion. If the notion of probability is used in this way, we speak of personalistic probability. Since this depends on a given person, it can happen that two people, because of different insight or information, may a priori attitude two totally different subjective probabilities to the same event. This contrasts sharply with the objective probability of an event which is the same for everyone.

The conception of personalistic probability originates from Savage, who developed the theory of it in his "Foundations of Statistics".[11] He bases this concept on a number of premises about coherent behavior which most people would in fact be willing to accept as guidelines for their intrinsically consistent actions. He demonstrates the existence of a measure of subjective probability for an individual acting in accordance with these premises. That is to say, a person whose behavior in an uncertain situation is coherent in the sense of Savage's axioms behaves as if he attributes numbers to those events which are relevant to himself. These numbers satisfy the axioms of probability calculation.

The remarkable thing about Savage's theory is that he does not need to presuppose the existence of subjective probabilities; their existence follows logically from his axioms. According to logic, therefore, on the basis of the premises postulated, this theory is also normative. Its practical usefulness lies in the fact that a person accepting Savage's axioms as guidelines for his actions can be helped by the explicit rather than implicit attribution of probabilities when taking decisions in situations of uncertainty.

Incidentally, it is extremely interesting to note that this application to the exact sciences is now expressly admitted by a number of leading lights, while as a rule it is still strictly forbidden in the inexact sciences — not without some criticism, of course — with reference to the earlier dominance of the exact scientific model!

This means in fact that the dogmatic criterion of pure and complete objectivity as a sine qua non of scientific practice has ceased to be imposed here. Years and years ago I pleaded earnestly for this to happen in the social science, on grounds of epistemology. The odd thing is not only that this view — a dissentient one as regards the pursuit of irrefutable exactness — is now significantly confined from the source of scientific advance and possibly approaching that exactness more closely. Further, it is precisely in the social sciences and the prognostic techniques[12] which they employ that the application of these new ideas is of greatest importance.

Jantsch also reports the development of the new Monte Carlo technique. When so many chance "random" factors are present that there no longer seems to be much sense in a strictly scientific treatment, the computer can be called upon. The computer can be used to process a very large number of runs with different and combined random probability values, until a sufficient quantity of statistical material has been collected to decide what outcome can be assumed to be the most probable.

The probabilistic technique may partly coincide with the curve technique discussed below. In simple terms, a probable curve can for example be plotted between computed maximum and minimum curves.

In addition, of course, there are much more complex techniques. Jantsch singles out two of them, both still in an experimental stage, for special mention.[13]

The first of these is "parametric sensitivity analysis". Here, the probable combined effects of internal and external factors are linked with whole "families" of mutually influential curves and with the resultant parameters which are consequently, in their turn, variable. By means of this procedure, the latter yield a graphical probability picture reminiscent of a forecast showing meteorological expectations in the form of a weather map.

Another interesting technique under development departs from the classical Newtonian mechanics and statistics which served as a starting-point for Gauss. It is a technique founded on the principles of quantum physics, and in particular on particle processes and their distribution by path and place, resulting in the more recent statistical theories of Boltzmann and Gibbs. Wiener too had earlier set cybernetics moving along the same path. The technique enables individual behavioral forms and non-deterministic elements to be introduced.[14] As with almost novel, specific probability technique, this new one is inevitably faced at present with considerable problems.

2. Matrix algebra

A commonly used mathematical method, especially in modern statistics, is matrix algebra, also called linear algebra. It is employed in a variety of prognostic techniques.

The technique can be applied at different levels. The extension of mathematics repeatedly pointed out in the text has led, among other things, to group theory and symbolic algebra. Matrix and vector mathematics are concerned with hypercomplex systems. Matrix algebra serves primarily as an elegant script or compact notation for complicated forms or relations, and is used as such in input-output analysis, for example (cf. point 4, Linear Models).

It may also be employed in an abstract manner, by attaching a spatial connotation to a vector or matrix. The spatial interpretation of matrices can sometimes lead to a surprisingly simple proof of very complex propositions. In this way, linear algebra is used in linear programming (cf. point 7).

Matrix algebra is not itself a prognosis technique, though it can constitute a valuable element in a number of such techniques.[15]

According to Jantsch, matrix algebra proves most valuable in normative prognosis techniques[16], which are employed, whether or not in combination with other techniques, in France and other countries (besides America) for planning of the future and prognosis.

The U.S. National Academy of Sciences uses a periodically modified "missions/materials" matrix. Whereas most matrices are two-dimensional, NASA employs for its space programmes a very ambitious three-dimensional matrix originally developed in the research division of Noravi (North American Aviation), "that reaches to the highest end-use levels of society".[17] Which illustrates a comment I made earlier on the gradual merger of purely industrial objectives, in a wider framework, with national or even international and social objectives.[18]

Thus Jantsch already sees appearing on the horizon a long-range, mission-oriented matrix-management in both industry and government and in combination of the two.[19] Exact mathematics and inexact normativity are thereby fused together.[20]

3. Curves

As I have said, a prognosis should ideally rest on an underlying theory. If a particular curve is used for prognostic purposes, therefore, it should in principle also be founded on a theory, although this will probably be a relatively simple one in many cases.[21]

The "Gaussian" curve is now famous. It is a curve shaped as shown in Figure 1.

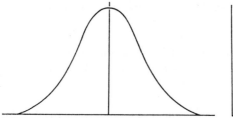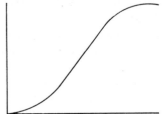

The familiar S-shaped curve in Figure 2, which satisfies the requirements of a prognostic theory, is a logistic growth curve which has the following mathematical form:

$$y = \frac{K}{1 + ce^{a + bt}},$$

where t denotes the time, K the maximum value of the y variable (also called the saturation level of y), e the base of the Napierian logarithm (so called after the Scottish mathematician John Napier, who lived in the second half of the 16th century) and a, b and c arbitrary constants. This curve is applicable if the phenomenon under investigation satisfies the following two conditions:

(a) the absolute increase of a phenomenon is inversely proportional to the magnitude of the phenomenon in the period of time in question. This means that the increase falls in proportion to the increase in the phenomenon itself;

(b) the absolute increase is proportional to the difference between the phenomenon in the period in question and the saturation level. This is also expressed by saying that the increase is proportional to the tention.

The following illustrates the form of this growth curve. If a phenomenon is subject to a logistic growth process it begins by showing very fast, powerful growth. This period of almost exponential increase is followed by a gradual leveling-off in growth until the saturation level is reached. The saturation level K must not be taken as being too absolute. The formula given above can be generalized simply by making the saturation level dependent on a newly introduced variable. For economic applications it would seem realistic to regard this level as a function of for instance national income. The utilization potential of the logistic curve is significantly entranced by a generalization of this type. Other examples of S-shaped curves which are also amenable to some measure of theoretical foundation are normal and lognormal distribution functions. The shape and regularity of these S-curves give them an aesthetic and satisfying appearance. How far this mathematical beauty also foretells future truth depends in part on the reality content of the underlying theory. Prognoses made by means of these curves are generally regarded as scientific, which cannot be said without qualification of some of the curves discussed below.

Where we are concerned with the continuing explosive or revolutionary development of technology, it is highly debatable whether S-curves are not the product of wishful thinking, whereas we should perhaps be thinking in terms of an uninterrupted exponential growth, or at least a growth moving upwards in a spiral.

A new subject of study in this connection, I believe, concerns the so-called "envelope curves" or "envelope cycles" described by Jantsch[22], which may serve the above purpose better. These are in essence another rather more refined, or at least modified, form of trend extrapolation. We are beginning to think in terms of a succession of cycles of technical innovation, with a constant or constantly variable rate of change. The curves of innovation systems developed in this way are now seen to lie over and across each other, at an ever-higher level, on account of kinks and crossovers, in a sort of escalation process. We have a simple example in the continually increasing maximum speeds of respectively horse, train, automobile, airplane, jet, rocket, etc., or of particle acceleration in high-energy physics, from the very first to the most modern types and those future types already on the drawing board. It is clear that, once again, the phenomenal pace of technical advances and the drastic reduction in the time taken for their implementation and diffusion have themselves tremendously heightened the need for new prognostic techniques, which indeed they ultimately create. But an essential element of technical evolution is precisely the making of discontinuous, sudden breakthroughs; these would then have to be expressed in a "disaggregative" curve form in which they would as far as possible be foreseen, calculated or accounted for in advance. This preconceived idea can and must be perfected to form another specific and distinct technique.

Of great interest and importance in this connection are the so-called "learning curves".[23] The establishment of such development curves may in fact follow one of two courses. They may be purely an extrapolation of existing trends, in which case they mostly lag behind completely novel or renewed developments by excessively neglecting the time factor. Or they may attempt to include the unforeseeable, or at least still unknowable, to the best of their ability, using a prognostically accountable method from the outset. This is done by means of "evaluation" and the power of creative imagination[24], it being accepted a priori that the effects of future events, including possible breakthroughs, may be either overestimated or underestimated. Learning curves try to eliminate as far as possible the overly personal element in projections, mainly by the comparative study of historical prognostic errors and by the application of specific counterbalancing corrections. An important element is the discovery of agreements with or similarities to earlier forecasts which have since been shown up as too pessimistic or too optimistic. Thus by closer analysis of the causes of over-pessimistic or over-optimistic future predictions, the lessons of the past are used to provide guidance for the future, while at the same time the development curves originally plotted on the basis of particular opinions are modified accordingly. It is, of course, very much open to question whether and to what extent "l'histoire se répète", whether or not the surprising and renovating "breakthroughs" will gradually become dominant as our age of continual acceleration strides or races onward. Maybe the earlier, over-optimistic forecasts about technical developments will prove over-pessimistic from now on. Exactly the same holds true in reverse, of course. It is not inherently inconceivable that the experience of the past might be excessively "set" by this procedure, vis-à-vis the ultradynamic and extremely radical transformations of the future. The question then arises whether the operational usefulness of these past-adapted projections might in fact ultimately not be increased, or at any rate not in all respects, but maybe even reduced on occasions. This risk can of course be lessened only by the correct interpretation and evaluation of these historical pointers.[25] So the wheel has come full circle and in manipulating prognosis techniques we are, as always, thrown back on personal, intuitive insight and the visionary, imaginative and creative powers of those who devise and use them.[26]

4. Linear Models

The linear model is much used for prognostic purposes, particularly in econometrics.

Unlike the curves discussed above, whose character tends rather towards trend-fitting, the linear model is generally built upon a considerably more refined and advanced theory.

A linear model may be defined as an equation containing random variables, parameters and mathematical variables, which is linear as far as the random variables and parameters are concerned. Its mathematical formulation will in many cases rely on matrix algebra. By the introduction of chance as a disturbance factor, the theory is presented with a stochastic component.

Although the mathematical notation is difficult, the model itself can be relatively simple. Let us take the case of a model illustrating the textile consumption of a country. Economic theory teaches us that the consumption is principally determined by a deflated price index and by the income per head of the population. Of course it is also influenced by a great number of other factors, though it is assumed that these are not of critical importance. In the model, all these latter factors are accounted for by an assumptive method, using a so-called disturbance term (assumed deviation). The object is to estimate unknown parameters affecting the future, mainly by means of observations from the past. Such a model provides a classical illustration of the combination of theory, observation and stochastics.

Prognoses arrived at by means of this linear model satisfy all the prognostic requirements and are considered worthy of the adjective "scientific". By dropping the linearity restriction, however, the model can be generalized, and this frequently happens in practice.

Stochastics, mathematically allied to the Markov processes or specific Markov chains, is also important in connection with the prognostic technique which employs linear models. In a Markov chain, the question is no longer how a particular phase of a process came about at some time in the past. Once a given situation is seen to have been reached, however it arose, it is regarded as leading, according to probabilistic (not deterministic) principles and time-series, to the possible phases and processes that may follow.

Irrespective of specialization and different sets of assumptions, all linear models employed in prognostics do of course aim at giving a usable cross-sectional picture of processes taking place over a shorter or longer time in the context of the dynamically unfolding reality of the future.[27] (See also point 5 below).

5. Simultaneous equation systems

Curves and linear models are still concerned with only one equation, whatever its mathematical form.

The transition to a whole set of equations constitutes a logical generalization. Such a description becomes necessary, of course, as soon as one has a large number of interrelated or interdependent variables. The theory underlying systems of this kind must likewise be further elaborated. The models based on it are applied particularly in macro-economic prognostics.

Besides the economic and econometric models based on such system of simultaneous equations, there are many other models also employing this technique which can be distinguished by form and content. They include social, political and psychological models; industrial and management models; cybernetic and computer models; strategic and tactical models; game and simulations models; input-output models; information models, optimum models, system models, feedback models and lastly, of special interest to extended time dimension prognostics, long-range and transformation models.[28]

In this sense, such a model might in some degree be likened to the externally observable phenotype which ultimately appears as the end product of various gradually developed genotypes. This analogy with genetics is not wholly correct, however, in that the construction of new, refined prognosis models does not simply constitute the termination of divergent theories and experimental techniques, it is at the same time quite definitely a new, independent starting-point for renewal and improvement.

There is no point in going into greater detail here on this variety of models based on simultaneous systems. But I should like to add three observations.

In the first place, experience has shown that in many cases the simpler models are no longer adequate for an increasingly complex reality. The system of simultaneous equations offers the most advanced technique for scientific forecasting yet devised.

391

In the second place it is essential to consider that stochastics, which we have encountered several times already, will occupy an increasingly important place in this system of models based on simultaneous equations.

In the third place, this refinement represents a provisional scientific rounding-off. True, many other kinds of prognostic techniques are employed, likewise calling on the assistance of mathematical and statistical processes and tools; but their scientific and theoretical foundations are usually regarded as less secure. This does not mean that they are therefore necessarily inferior, only that for the time being they are of a slightly different rank from the methods considered so far. A number of them — to be touched on next — have on the contrary been found, for want of better ones, to be usable and effective in practice.

6. Networks

Prognoses cast in the special form of networks place particular emphasis on the complex interdependences (also called "communalities"), the widely branched interrelations, and the pluriform mutual connections between all the subsystems of one ultimate total system which are still considered separately. The main object is to split up the different activities of an overall process into the most efficient sequence of time phases.[29]

Several such network complexes have been rearranged or refined in a separate way. Three methods for such analyses have received special attention in America[30], and are termed respectively PERT (Program Evaluation and Review Technique), CPM (Critical Path Method) and DEMON (Decision Evaluation Market Optimal Network). CPM is, I believe, the oldest of these techniques, and PERT is probably the first to have found its way to Europe, where it has also been adopted by some large industrial and governmental consultants — more so than the other two.

As is so often the case, some of these modern network techniques have their origin in the military sector — as do the fundamental "operations research" and "systems analysis" methods. For example, PERT originated in the special planning and programming of the American navy's Polaris missile. It is an instrument of management, not only for design and execution but also for the periodic adaptation or review and control of complex functions extending over long periods and using detailed calculations; having been processed and discussed in a European context, it may be assumed to be familiar, or recognized, there too.

CPM is based on flow charts which, by analysis of all multifariously interrelated partial tasks, make it possible to select the best path in a network of paths, an optimum which has repeatedly to be determined afresh in the presence of critical circumstances, to lead to the realization of given comprehensive projects or objectives. From the first time-phase up to and including

392

the last, the optimum is critically reassessed from time to time, finding expression in lowest cost, shortest time, etc. Both methods involve evaluation of alternative ways and means, and more particularly the pointing-out of critical points, factor and bottlenecks which arise during the realization of the fixed objective, which may be attained in a better, faster and cheaper way by virtue of certain switches made along the way.

DEMON follows somewhat analogous procedures, but primarily on behalf of industry, it involves market analyses capable of adaptation where necessary, in the interests of manufacturing and advertising new products marketable in a society developing and changing according to expectations and thus likely to be attractive to a future consumer public.

The Battelle Memorial Institute, which occupies a leading position in America and has European affiliations, has conceived a "Design Method"[31] with a "strategy for concept-oriented forecasting" based on CPM. Here too the target is the most probable, and at the same time optimal, implementation of a pre-established design (i.e. a normative idea as fixed objective) amid a variable course of events.

General Electric is experimenting with special network techniques, aimed among other things at the further development of nuclear energy applications and the building of improved, faster nuclear reactors.[32] And so on.

These specific methods are very closely akin to the dual prevision-and-revision system which I have described as a generally indispensable principle in *all* effective prognostics.[33]

7. Programming

The word "programming" itself is a blanket term indicating what programs (plans, projects, objectives) it has been decided to establish on the basis of the appropriate forecasts and prognostic techniques. In fact, any scientific-technical preparation for a long-term policy can be referred to as programming. The term "development programming" has already become current in this sense. Besides development programming, mention must also be made of long-term programming in education, science and research, for which the need is growing. Employed in this sense, prognosis and programming form a duality because the programs will, after all, be supported by a theory and the associated prognoses. In other words, prognosis serves as a rule for the establishment of programs.

On the other hand, while this does not conflict with the above, to many people programming still means *mathematical* programming — that is, linear, quadratic and dynamic programming. The best-known technique is linear programming, which looks for the optimum in a linear relation (also called target function) under a number of linear restrictions.

Quadratic programming differs from linear programming only as regards the function to be optimized: here it is quadratic in the model variables, the restrictions normally remaining linear. Dynamic programming is especially suited to the optimization of dynamic problems, i.e. problems involving variables which relate to different periods of time. In such problems, variables from different periods occur both in the restrictions and in the target function to be optimized.

With dynamic problems it is often important to employ strategics which make it possible to use the information that becomes available in the course of time. A strategy can be defined as a decision-making rule which indicates what action must be taken in any conceivable situation that may arise within the existing problem. The art, of course, consists in finding optimum strategics. Dynamic programming as a technique can often be used to determine an optimum strategy in a given problem. It may be asked what these techniques have to do with the forecasting of particular quantities. In fact they were not evolved with prognostic problems in mind. But it is possible to use these techniques as part of a more comprehensive prognosis techniques (see also point 8).

Jantsch's report does not mention a comparatively new method applied, I believe, in Euratom and elsewhere, and known as indicative programming. If I am right, the procedure here is to take divergent detailed prognoses based on different assumptions and alternative choices but elaborated in accordance with one and the same overall calculation method, and use them to derive a whole series of possible lines of development. By means of these indicative prognoses it is possible to analyze which development trend is best suited to particular targets and corresponding investment decisions or research projects — in this case, with regard to the energy policy to be followed.

Quite possibly, however, Jantsch does not list this form separately because he presumably sees scarcely any difference in principle between it and the modern techniques of economic analysis and planning in particular, or the recent evolution of all up-to-date R & D (research and development) in general, or the recent combination of the two in the form of "development planning" and technical-economic "research into research".

There is as yet no standard nomenclature, uniform terminology or organization in these new fields of technological forecasting. Everything is still in a state of flux, moving, shifting and developing.[34] The accent is on the development of development.

8. Games, Strategy and Simulation

Considering the growing importance of this trio of prognosis techniques it is, I think, best for them to be dealt with as a separate group, though they are of course, intrinsically, special modern development methods for the calculation of probability.

The original "Theory of Games" of John von Neumann, later elaborated, with Oskar Morgenstern as a theory of economic behavior[35], is also known in Europe. The prognostic theory of games depends on simulation, whereby the component parts of a simulated model are manipulated by means of a computer, by the players, or by both together.

In the "game technique", also known as "gaming", the model is so designed that multiple, simultaneous interactions of the various players (with or without computer) can be made to imitate reality.[36] It is then possible subsequently to assess who had the correct future expectations in the chosen case, and thus who made the best moves or choices as regards the management of affairs and the making of decisions.

The applications are numerous. Firstly, the prognostic game and simulation technique has assumed great importance in military planning and strategy selection. In addition, it is used to forecast new or future developments in the field of technology and the impact they may be expected to have (and which may be amenable to control) on the pattern of society. Business games, management and management decision games were first devised in America in the Fifties as being especially instructive for junior executives, and have also been exported to Europe. The "minimax" strategy, which gave greatest protection at least cost against the most unfavorable set of circumstances, won a certain popularity as a policy for cautious management. Against this, the subjective and intuitive probability model now provides a potentially important instrument, offering the overly cautious and possibly insufficiently dynamic decision-maker (who accepts too limited a risk) the opportunity of breaking through the conservative minimax attitude.

It may not be superfluous to point out that in these cases, too, particular models are utilized. These models will have the shape of a number of algebraic relations representing the decisions and the variables which measure the results of the decisions, normally related to a fixed (discrete) division into successive periods of time. As a rule the disturbance terms of these relations will again be included in a particular way, because the relations cannot entirely agree with reality, on account of factors not incorporated in the model. These disturbance terms, which reflect the uncertainty of the situation, are not the only source of uncertainty for the participitants in the game, however. Participants in simulated management games are deliberately not informed as to how the simulated model is constructed. They have to learn, as it were, how to discover this, and their strategy, for themselves.[37] Afterwards it is possible to establish which assumptions, reactions and decisions turn out to be wrong, so that future errors can be avoided, or at least the chances of their being committed can be lessened.

The authors of the Rand report, Gordon and Helmer, are now devising a "Game of the Future" at the instigation of Kaiser Aluminum. It will enable leading American industrialists and intellectuals to choose from various combinations of for instance possible developments in the next 20 years to come. The winner will be the player who gains the greatest following for "his" world of the future.[38] Mankind 2000 International is working on similar projects, in which the man in the street could also participate to increase his awareness of the future.

9. Family trees

The branchings of family trees, such as we know them from genealogy, have served as models for new prognostic techniques.[39] Jantsch usually refers to them as "relevance tree techniques". Most branches are vertical and so multi-level from top to bottom, though some grow horizontally sideways. The notion of "relevance" was originally "reliance" — discretion has caused the claim of reliability to be reduced to one of applicability. Taken together, the branches form an integrated whole.

A number of these family trees, in which the top corresponds to the highest aim to be achieved, are qualitative and normative. They indicate the separate events that must take place on each of the lower levels (which also extend sideways, right down to the base, for the chosen end-objective to be attached in an optimal way. (They may also give exact time divisions, estimated effects, costs, etc.).

This prognosis technique becomes more complicated when numerical values are assigned to each part according to weight, relevance, probability, activity to be performed, etc., in accordance with determined systems and criteria which are in part arbitrary and for which matrices are also employed.

The great industrial pioneer and perfectionist of these "integrated relevance tree schemes" in America is the Honeywell concern, which has in particular made them available for decision-making in defense and space matters. This integral prognostic model, now applied in other areas too, is called PATTERN (Planning Assistance Through Technical Evaluation of Relevance Numbers).

In spite of the great difficulties involved in the arrangement and evaluation of the relevant criteria and components, Jantsch regards this prognosis technique as one of the three most promising of all the new possibilities he has to date investigated, the other two being the morphological technique discussed in point 10 and the Delphi technique in point 14.[40]

10. The morphological method

The morphological prognosis method was evolved nearly a quarter of a century ago in America by a Swiss physicist considered at that time as eccentric; he was Fritz Zwicky, who was engaged primarily in pioneering research work on rockets and the new types of propellants to be used in them.

The technique was not rediscovered until very recently. Jantsch rates it very highly.[41] Its essentials are summed up in the following three questions.[42] What resources are needed to obtain all the information on a given complex of phenomena? What is the series of all the effects of a particular cause? Lastly, what are all the aids, methods and solutions applicable to a given problem?

The emphasis is on the word *all*. Its addition means that case by case, using the correctly evaluated parameters and matrices, it is really possible to find all the solutions in all-embracing systems and subsystems, and to indicate all future developments systematically and exhaustively. Until *all* the solutions are made available in this way none must be prematurely evaluated against the other, for this prejudices a correct choice later. Not until afterwards should all the (in the literal sense) possible constellations and configurations be screened and the best possible one selected from among them.

In Zwicky's own words, "the greatest successes of the morphological method may be expected in the field of human relations, where the prejudices have been most rampant and the activities in many cases tragically disastrous ... its application there is most urgent, because of the often appalling incapability or unwillingness of scientists and engineers to deal systematically, constructively and uncompromisingly with these human problems".[43]

Jantsch is of the opinion that a broad range of applications is both possible and desirable. At the present time the TEMPO think-tank, brainchild and brain trust of General Electric, is experimenting with this approach, as are the Battelle Memorial Institute and others.

Zwicky himself is a pacemaker among the space age prognosticians. He believes the method described above, which has indeed already proved successful in space studies and astrophysics, can also be used to deduce the future possibilities of, for instance, making the moon inhabitable (by producing water and oxygen on the spot) and to find ways of enabling planetary engineering to penetrate deeper into the universe; in particular, of achieving the objective of changing the heavenly bodies and planetary spheres in such a way as to make them suitable for human colonization and communication. Such projects would, needless to say, demand that his technique be applied on a far larger scale. He also reckons it capable of solving many of the problems of human society on earth. I am not competent to judge whether Zwicky's almost unlimited confidence and Jantsch's likewise boundless enthusiasm might not fall under the category unbridled overoptimism, and whether Jantsch's enthusiasm might not possibly stand in need of some disciplinary moderation by means of learning curves. Though it may be, on the contrary, that this optimistic-idealistic future-vision is in fact the "wave of the future"; who can tell?

11. Systems, structures, vectors, mosaics

There is an abundance of newer prognostic techniques, all striving along different paths, and in themselves quite rightly, towards a common goal — a synthesis of totality.

Two distinctions can be made. One approach is to try to put all sorts of pieces of the jigsaw puzzle together. This results in a mosaic or synopsis in which the term "iteration" is used for the fitting-together process. In this way one may arrive at a composite whole containing fragments from every conceivable sector, which Jantsch describes as "forecasting on the aggregate level".[44] In essence, however, this is really nothing but a kind of artistic pasting together of "disaggregated approaches".[45]

Attempts have also been made to reach the aggregate level in one jump. Initially, for example, Leontief's general input/output model aroused great expectations. Others too have expended much effort in the attempt to arrive at a projection of comprehensive patterns or structures, with the help of modern matrix and vector mathematics and of computers. Jantsch is rather sceptical about the results achieved so far with prognoses of this type.[46] Of course it is not inconceivable that advanced computers may soon be capable of accomplishing an integrated prognosis which extends over several spheres at once; by whatever means, all purposive prognostics *must* after all strive towards a total vision.[47]

Jantsch cherishes much greater hopes, on the other hand, that "systems analysis" may yield a total vision of this kind.[48]

Systems analysis is a highly personal art requiring great mathematical skill. It combines qualitative and quantitative elements at a high level. Its deployment in America, where it is also known as "total systems analysis", is still mainly the monopoly of the think-tanks such as the Rand Corporation, Tempo, System Development Corp. and the like. Rand, as usual, began studying it for military purposes. The System Development Corp. is doing pioneering work with it in the social field and also for cultural and educational purposes, among others.

Its application appears at bottom to be dependent once more on correct "evaluations". To set up a comprehensive system model, a particular preconception or vision is needed to break through, somehow or other, the multiplicity, complexity, intricacy and elusiveness of all the factors and relations. To this end, mathematical short-cuts and tricks are used to reduce the mass of possible combinations, eliminate those variables that are considered unimportant, or incorporate a number of them in composite elements. At the same time, in order to comply with the sine qua non of totality approximation, the way in which certain preferred parameters are used has to be evaluated, optimum criteria must be created, and more attention has to be paid to normative structure-ideas or the targets to be set, as well as to the interdisciplinary connections between science, technology and society. I suppose the secret of this method, which is evidently successful in certain cases, lies largely with the brillant individuals working at these institudes. Even Jantsch can find no more to say about it in the abstract. However, it is significant that a highly personal, sometimes almost ideological, appraisal once again appears, expressis verbis, to be inherent in all sound and successful prognosis techniques as an elementary and essential constituent. Without vision, there is no prevision of any value! But in all cases it remains a condition that the underlying vision, and surely all prejudices too, must be made as explicit as possible.

12. Contextual mapping

"Contextual mapping" is another broad conception containing qualitative and quantitative elements or versions.[49] It is a new and peculiar form of trend extrapolation which, while it does of course look ahead to future developments, is essentially independent of the factually precise chronology of events. The trend development is reproduced as a possible process or evolution in the pre-determined potential context of a longer term which itself is still under-determined. Thus the causal relations, and probable chances of development in the presence of certain conditions, of a number of new technological pos-sibilities, are established in the framework of ultimately expected social growth processes and structures of the future. According to Jantsch, it is a prognostic tool of use both for defense and for industrial ends. It has been, or is being, applied for new weapon systems, integrated circuits, fuel cells, VTOL (vertical take-off and landing) airplanes, etc., and is especially used in the interests of long-range forecasting not tied down to an exact date, i.e. with an open-ended future dimension.

13. Cost-effectiveness evaluation

This is essentially a greatly modernized offshoot of the cost-yield ratio of classical economics, normally known in America as PPBS (Planning Pro-gramming Budgeting System)[50]. Cost-effectiveness procedures introduce eco-nomic aspects into the task of achieving given objectives (arms techniques, civil administration projects), and make forecasts in which the achievement of these objectives can be measured fairly accurately by comparing the values thereby obtained with the investments, energy, time and resources to be expended. In other words, this too is a prognostic tool for all-cost-con-scious-top management, military, industrial and departmental, particularly where the most effective continued technological development is concerned.

From a technical point of view, the top of a "relevance tree" shows much similarity with the structure of this comparative evaluation system, notably whenever viable decisions have to be taken on the highest level regarding the results obtained. In defense matters and in civil administration, the highest national long-term goals are inserted at the top for the programming, which, by the way, is of a sliding character and so is subjected to periodic review. The programs, the planning and the prognosis results are continuously evaluated in accordance with the passage of time and on the basis of changes which occur in the overall situation.[51]

Jantsch regards this as a significant prognostic development, which is also gradually finding favor in Europe (Britain and Sweden, for instance), especially for long-term decision-making. The making of such long-term decisions is, however, as yet rather the exception than the rule. The development of prognostics serves precisely to activate it.

14. Delphi (in California)

In Jantsch's opinion, the technique introduced some years ago by the Rand Corporation in Santa Monica, which has resuscitated the ancient Delphic oracle in modern form, is one of the most important instruments for the future of prognostics as regards innovation and potential results.[52] It operates by means of questionnaires concerning expected future developments, which are discussed and analyzed in four stages by a select and sizeable panel of highly qualified experts from a wide range of fields, a staff of exceptionally competent collaborators and the collected data from computers programmed for the purpose. The extremely interesting Rand Corporation report on this long-range forecasting technique in stages (1985-2000-2050-2100 and after) has already been mentioned more than once in the pages of this book[53], and can be thoroughly recommended to the reader.

Although this Delphi technique originally derives from the rather wild and crude, sometimes confused and chaotic "brainstorming" approach, it has in fact succeeded in channeling it into orderly paths (via the four stages) and furthermore in relieving it of the overly subjective, and so obtrusive, psychological-emotional factors (by means of objective computer data, which literally form a feedback continually resubmitting statistically predominant or less favored opinion for further consideration in the following rounds). On the other hand, an equal effort is made to eliminate as far as possible the disturbing factor of the undesirable "bandwagon effect", a product of the swelling majority opinions. In short, the system is very well thought out, and its first published results were a source of astonishment to many people.[54]

Jantsch judges this Delphi technique to be extremely valuable not only for exploratory prognosis but equally well for normative prognosis, in which selected leading figures in various fields are consulted on "the selection of social goals, national objectives and broad missions".[55] Thus it is a technique which can be exceedingly useful in all "future-creative" thinking[56] and might also be of much service to a "look-out institution" organized with precisely that prognostic aim in mind.

15. Scenario (not from Hollywood)

While the Rand Corporation has taken the ancient Greek oracle as an example and kept the original name, Thomas More's conception of Utopia was apparently too highly charged for this. Modern utopistic techniques — which actually go back much further in time, to Plato's ideal Republic — have to make do with no better title than the devising of scenarios, of an intentionally unreal character. In their modern form they also resemble the best products of science fiction, though heightened in the sense — already applied in the ideal types of the sociologist Max Weber — that no matter how unreal and even extreme the future-fantasy may be, the strictest criteria of logical consistency and scientific method are nevertheless imposed. One of the leading methodological "authors" is Herman Kahn[57], an expert specializing in new weapon techniques, who was originally attached to the Rand Corporation and is now one of the foremost figures of the Hudson Institute. This Hudson Institute is likewise regarded as one of the leading American think-tanks; originally, it was mainly engaged on problems of defense, but is now extending its activities (partly on behalf of the American Academy's Commission on the Year 2000) to technological forecasting over a very broad front of interrelated socio-economic, socio-political and socio-technolgical future developments.[58]

The latter activity is well suited to the scenario approach which, by definition, is comprehensive, synoptic and simultaneous. It is a method whereby different possible futures are dealt with as a totality. A scenario suddenly skips across with a grandiose, even consciously dramatic dynamic movement to another such future, the starting-point being the phenomenal acceleration of fundamental changes and the end a supposed partial or almost complete transformation of the existing pattern of society.[59]

It is clear that the rather scarce *qualitative* properties of intuition, imagination, inventiveness and creativity, and also that of versatility, are required to compose operationally serviceable scenarios as "work of art". The artistic ability thought by De Jouvenel to be characteristic of *all* prognostic work comes very clearly to the forefront here — in the very type of prognostic technique he does *not* discuss. Furthermore, these future-depicting scenarios can be both exploratory and normative in character. It is in this latter ("mission-oriented") function that they most closely resemble the classical utopia.

Exploratory scenarios, by contrast, are much more likely to have the outward appearance of *counter*-utopias resulting from particular points of departure, such as Huxley's "Brave New World", Orwell's "1984" or a more recent vision, Michael Young's "The Rise of the Meritocracy, 1870-2033". However, they still bear as it were a figurative and implicitly utopistic stamp, as a kind of early warning system showing the form inherently possible developments might take and the risks they might entail, at least if the "laissez faire, laissez aller" attitude persists unchecked, and so unless . . .[60] The *pessimistic* exploratory scenario can thus act as a transition and means of approach to a more *optimistically* directed, normative scenario clearly indicating the conditions and requirements for the attainment of other and better future possibilities.

Jantsch has great expectations for the further successful application of projected, synthetic scenario-pictures of the future[61], though this technique too is of course highly person-tied. But the subjective element can be significantly diminished, if not altogether eliminated, by combination with other techniques such as the Delphi technique especially, which itself is broadened by the incorporation of the latest cybernetic information methods and computer techniques. This helds, pari passu, also for combinations with systems analysis techniques, game and simulation techniques, treetop techniques and cost effectiveness evaluations. In the famous PATTERN models of Honeywell, the scenario technique is combined with the treetop technique, which clearly indicates the highest achievable goals and the processual method of approaching them. In the technological forecasting of a consultancy bureau as authoritative as Abt Associates, this scenario technique also forms part of a greater and varied whole.[62] In the Swedish prognostic techniques described by Jantsch, especially those for defense purposes, the scenario method likewise plays a not unimportant role.[63]

In his general survey of creative thought and prognostics, Jantsch states[64]: "A central "idea", acting at a given moment and determining the set of desirable goals for that moment, also — spread out over time — guides the historical development towards that set of goals". An important line of thought or, as Jantsch says, hypothesis[65], for which he can find no rational basis but which nevertheless gives the notion of "long-range normative forecasting" its meaning. Now I myself, in my book "The Image of the Future" (TIF), to which reference has already been made, have tried to demonstrate extensively by means of a broad historical analysis that this hypothetical theory of cultural dynamics is indeed *absolutely right*; in other words, that inspiring and idealistic *visions of the future* in the past have to a very significant extent *de*-termined, or at least greatly *influence*d, later developments towards what was then the future.

The marriage of exploratory possibilities and normative visions of the future — scenarios if you like — can thus begin to fulfil in a much more purposeful way the prognostic, but also in a sense predictive or at least self-justifying tasks, as functions of the self-destroying and self-fulfilling prophecies respectively! It is for this reason that the refinement of this prognostic technique and its effective conjunction with all the other appropriate techniques appears to the author to be of considerable importance. I join Jantsch in assigning a high priority to this association of realism and visionary progressiveness for the development of prognostics.

16. Feedback and guided mobility

The systematic distinction which Jantsch rightly makes between exploratory and normative prognosis techniques reflects an extremely significant tendency now observable in America. Anticipation of possible futures (futuribles) is in itself a good thing — an absolute necessity in fact. But it remains a mere airy abstraction unless we pose the complementary problem: *what* future do we actually want? How does the desired "ought" stand in relation to the existing "is"? What influence — in what direction, within what limits — can and must we exert towards the determination of our own destiny? Thus the thought is beginning to take root that normativity and the scientific approach to social goals are wholly indispensable.[66] In addition, once again, there is a growing consciousness that these goals too are not fixed a priori and forever. It is equally valid here that in the purposive evaluation and choice of particular goals, not only is the best possible prevision required, but repeated reorientation and systematic revision are just as essential.

These views are at the core of truly future creative thinking[67] which provides the great stimulus to the effective application of normative prognosis techniques. But these are only properly formulated by the careful introduction of *socio-ethical* objectives and their effective feedback coupling with the exploratory techniques. Here, however, there is a transition to a social technology the problematics of which were discussed separately in Chapter 23. It was seen there that this socio-ethical examination in depth is far from being the strongest part in America today, at least in terms of scientific work, and has unfortunately been sadly neglected in Europe during the last fifty years.

As regards the purely prognostic aspect more especially, this is determined by the design of specific kinds of feedback techniques[68], on which the System Development Corp. — and notably one of its leading brains, Ozbekhan — are systematically working, by means of comprehensive cybernetic systems, transformation models and feedback loops. Interactions can be arranged, between, for instance, future-models (or scenarios) and present-models in general or, in particular, between future technical-social development processes and their outcomes in a number of widely separated or contiguous time phases, starting with the present. In effect, the point throughout all this is a purposive breakthrough from the present to the future. The greatest merits, to my mind, lie in the systematic linking of possible and desirable futures to form a future that in principle is effectively realizable and so can be achieved, or at least meaningfully approximated.

This technique has been applied (experimentally) by General Electric

(Atomic Energy Division), Battelle Memorial Institute, Zwicky (morphological research), and others. The methodological difficulties, however, are still enormous.

Ozbekhan bases his argument on my ideas in "The Image of the Future" about the dangers of the continuing, as it were timeless, prolongation of the present.[69] It means a clinging to the established order, a continual perpetuation of the status quo. Besides, in the normative ethical feedback techniques as propagated by him it is not possible simply to project present-day norms and values: we must take as our point of departure other future norms and future-values appropriate to other futures, future societies and future people. He sees this as a characteristic and essential feature of all true, and consequently very difficult, "futures-creative planning". In principle, Jantsch is fully in agreement with this view. He is consequently convinced that not only will the elaboration of such feedback techniques expand into an all-pervading problem in the years to come, but also that feedback control techniques (in which the feedback control will effectively transform the entire prognosis function by adaptation)[70] will be assigned, or have to accept, an important and expanding role.

I mention feedback and feedback control techniques as being the most promising so far advanced for the purpose at hand. They can and surely will combine with other suitable methods, either existing already or yet to appear. For instance there are already "by-pass" techniques on the way, aiming at the direct definition of higher level normative objectives (for future research and technological development too) without making detours or by shortcuts.[71] There are "guided mobility" techniques in statu nascendi, and analogous under various labels.

Computers are helping more and more in all the technical applications of information transfer, operations research and decision-making which have come under review here. But I agree with Jantsch[72] wholeheartedly that within the foreseeable future (within 10 years according to the Diebold Group, but I think probably much sooner) new "heuristic" electronic equipment, also capable of purposeful future prognoses, will appear on the scene. They may equally well be called upon to perform the normative tasks which are inseparable from such prognoses, to make the evaluations and decisions hitherto subject to the mental gropings and technical inadequacies of clumsy man — and then only of his ablest, most progressive and visionary, but consequently lonely, representatives. Though I must add in conclusion that, to be fair, we must admit to being further advanced now than ever — compared to the situation scarcely a few years back — in the realm of prognoses. If all the signs are not deceptive, this will continue in a rapidly increasing measure, as applications still controversial or uncritical are successfully raised on to a higher level.

The future of the combined exploratory-normative future prognoses seems to me to lie with the complex "man-machine-symbiosis" (also predicted by the Rand Corp. and the Hudson Corp.), which will prove capable of analyzing and synthesizing total systems and their coupling, or feedback, with optimum developments from the social standpoint.

Whenever there is talk of a new technical breakthrough, this must also be understood as technical *prognostics* itself breaking through its present limitations. Conversely, it will be able to apply itself more intensely and in a better way to ever-exacter anticipation of such breakthrough processes, bringing innovations, also in other respects. *Its perfection also contains the built-in propellers for optimal social structural reform.*

FOOTNOTES

Chapter 1

[1] Epoch and epochal were likewise later to acquire a completely different meaning and content, viz. as a certain memorable period of time, precisely with a concomitant temporal judgment.

[2] In the famous Anglo-Saxon genre of mysteries or murder stories the mastermind in his detection operates solely on alternative "conjectures", whose purpose is evidently to tempt the reader to guess wrongly, until he conjures up the true solution because only he holds the psychological criminal key.

[3] Cf. for this my The Image of the Future, quoted hereafter as TIF, and my Hoopvolle Toekomst Perspectieven, designated below as HTP.

[4] See for more about this Chapter 17.

[5] The man who thinks up the slogan "put a tiger in your tank" makes the car leap forward visually, but simultaneously and forthwith is also assured of his own leap forward to a better future on a higher rung of the social ladder.

[6] If I may mix a metaphor, most of the large European shipping lines missed the bus when back in the 1930's purposive research into the future already pointed to jet travel as the future form of long-distance travel. Now all that is possible is to get quickly into the world-conquering intercontinental door-to-door container transport.

[7] I am therefore expressly detaching myself here from the view of Jacques Ellul (The Technological Society, N.Y., 1964), who utterly condemns and rejects all technology, without any distinction as pernicious, and so going always from bad to worse. In identical fashion Toynbee is completely opposed to a technical use of the "time machine", i.e. the use of human power against the conflicting power of the future dimension, to save our Western civilization. I shall of course be returning to these differing views in more detail.

Chapter 2

[1] In return his name was given officially to Colombia in South America in 1863.

Chapter 3

[1] Cf. for a modern attempt at reconciliation H. R. Rapp, Mensch, Gott und Zahl, Kybernetik im Horizont der Theologie, Hamburg, 1967.

Chapter 4

[1] For the relationships referred to here between the models of the future of Leibnitz, Hegel and Marx, cf. also in particular Professor O. K. Flechtheim, History and Futurology, Meisenheim, 1966, sub I, History and Theodicy.

[2] Cf. also his pronouncement "Wenn der Mensch von den Umständen gebildet wird so muss man die Umstände menschlich bilden".

[3] Cf. my TIF and HTP.

Chapter 5

[1] It did so also, with a complete reversal to its spiritual opposite, when it was grossly misused in the National Socialist myth of the "Third Reich".

[2] In a certain sense one might regard Vico as the Tycho Brahe of history: inaugurating something that is entirely new while at the same time himself adhering to the old dogma. The only difference is that it took somewhat longer for him to find his Kepler. Vico himself was quite aware of the fact that his time was still to come. Who will some day write the revealing work on the highly mysterious "luctor et emergo" of the great historical renovators? Usually the truly great take considerably longer to get to the top than those who, revered as great by the spirit of the time, soon topple into well-deserved oblivion. Perhaps the answer to the question why the contemporary value-judgment is often so bewilderingly poor and cruel can be given in one word: dogmatism!

[3] This natural law instituted by divine Providence forms the foundation of historical prognostics. For this purpose Vico goes back to ancient, pagan divination. This also emerges from the pregnant words of Virgil which he chose as motto for the first edition: "A Jove principium musae" (Science begins with Jupiter). What is meant is that the divinatory interpretation of the awe-inspiring attributes (thunder and lightning) of the highest divinity formed the very beginning of all scientific prediction and explanation. Cf. for this Karl Löwith, Weltgeschichte als Heilsgeschehen, Urbar Bücher, Stuttgart, 1953, p. 121 e.v.

[4] Löwith, op. cit., p. 63 et seq.

[5] Cf. his "Philosophie du Progrès".

[6] Nietzsche himself propagates vigorously and with inspired enthusiasm new, aristocratic values, without apparently being aware of this self-destructive contradiction.

[7] We have encountered the same view in Voltaire.

Chapter 6

[1] See my TIF for a detailed discussion of this.

[2] The possible additional insertion of a millennium formed a variation on this main theme which, if realized, extended the division into three kingdoms to one into four kingdoms (the four beasts and the four kingdoms in Daniel's prophetic visions). A depiction which also led a life of its own, but without the powerful and lasting attraction of the tripartition, based on a number sacred from of old.

[3] I can give no more than some notes here on the tremendous scope of the concept three. Apart from its great role in the symbolism and mysticism of numbers, we encounter it everywhere, both in religious and in secular contexts. Before his imprisonment the next morning Jesus prayed three times in the night after having prophesied that Peter would deny him three times. The Pythia pronounced her oracles seated upon a tripod. Poseidon, the most dynamic Greek god of sea, water and land, had the trident as his attribute. According to the ancient Hellenistic world view the universe was tripartite (triplex) and had three forms: sky, sea and earth (including the underworld). Operating in that universe were three agreeable Graces (or Charites), three Fates (the Morai or Parcae) and three avenging goddesses (the Erinyes or Furies): aesthetic beauty, fatal destiny in life and death and ethically punishing damnation were entrusted to the rule of a supreme female triumvirate! The papal crown is a threefold tiara. The Roman triumvirate is a lasting creation of authority. The Roman people were divided into three parts (tribus), placed under

popular tribunes, seated on a tribune, pronouncing law through a tribunal, collecting taxes as tribute. In music the third, in tragedy the trimeter, in painting the triptych, in literature the trilogy are of elementary importance. The triangle forms a basis of scientific thought through astronomy, geometry and trigonometry. The third way repeatedly wrests itself free from the too narrow choice of the dogmatic either-or. The third child determines population growth. The French and Dutch flags display the tricolor. Third time is lucky. One, two, three is the usual starting signals. The trias politica (the threefold division of legislative, judicial and executive power) of Montesquieu still forms the basis of modern parliamentary democracy, etc., etc.

[4] For the ancient Oriental idea of this final victory that would come some day, for instance according to the religion of Zoroaster in Iran, see TIF.

[5] Translated into figurative language, the parabola can therefore be halved here.

[6] His main works – in this context – are, in chronological order of publication: Le Phénomène Humain, Paris, 1955; l'Avenir de l'Homme, 1959; l'Energie Humaine, 1962.

[7] See TIF and HTP.

[8] There is a still growing flood of (often contradictory) commentaries which not infrequently project their own point of view in part onto Teilhard (a fault of which I am perhaps also guilty). For instance, it is incomprehensible to me how the highly anti-Christian oriented Julian Huxley, who rationalizes in an exclusively causal manner in conformity with natural law, has completely appropriated to his own use Teilhard's finalism and has incorporated it in his own fiercely anti-teleological doctrine.

[9] Biologically speaking, Teilhard tends towards the rectilinear "orthogenesis" of macro-evolution, i.e. towards a steady succession of series of development without "mutations by leaps and bounds". However, it seems to me open to doubt whether, as he intends, one is permitted to use an equally linear and simple upward line for the schematic representation of the history of human progress.

[10] Since Joachim this idea of a new, third man has also found acceptance. It can be found among others in thinkers such as Berdyaev and Schubart. In America R. Seidenberg (followed by Kenneth Boulding, for instance) has introduced the term "Post-historical man", a rather unclear idea which, viewed historically, contains inner contradictions.

[11] Op. cit., p. 54.

[12] According to Collingwood nothing changed in what every Greek knew about the incessant historical change on account of Zeus' thunderbolts, Poseidon's earthquakes, the pestilence sent by Apollo or Aphrodite's urge for destruction. He consequently gives the Greek historian Herodotus an approving pat on the back: "The only thing that a shrewd and critical Greek like Herodotus would say about the divine power that ordains the course of history is: . . . that it rejoices in upsetting and disturbing things". Op. cit., p. 22. But hasn't Collingwood forgotten here the greatest Greek historian, Thucydides? The historical thinker who, two centuries before Polybius, described the incessant rotation and revolution of the historical cycle through action and reaction, thus quite definitely attempting to foresee the future from the past. Cf. Edith Hamilton, op. cit.

[13] Op. cit., p. 334.

[14] See for this my TIF.

Chapter 7

[1] Drawing broad lines naturally creates the danger of too great generalization. An important and courageous counter-figure from the first half of the 14th century was, for instance, William of Ockham (sometimes written Occam). As the chief representative of the aggressive nominalism mentioned in Chapter 4 (general concepts are not realities but names), he regarded current metaphysics not as a rational science but as a belief. He is a predecessor of empirical natural science and also of the Kantian, idealistic philosophy, as an opponent of the artificial synthesis between reason and faith, and also of the synthesis between philosophical-scientific thought and scholastic theology. His progressive supporters are called the "moderni" as opposed to the protagonists of the "via antiqua", the dogmatic old way. A case was brought against Ockham, who was an Oxford professor, before the Pope. He was able to escape conviction by fleeing to Germany. Neither modern philosophy nor modern theology can really conceive why this attitude of mind was regarded at the time as highly revolutionary heresy and condemned accordingly, the less so as the oldest Father of the Church, Tertullian (2nd century), had in fact already posited the same principle with his "credo quia absurdum". However, in the 14th century, together with mysticism, it was one of the great acts of resistance to the prevailing *dogmatism* (bound to realisms).

Chapter 8

[1] With, as sole exception, checking the effectiveness of possible means, susceptible to research, in the service of its objectives stated by others as valid.

[2] Cf. his The Open Society and its Enemies, 1952 and further The Poverty of Historicism, London, 1957.

[3] Cf. Inventing the Future, London, 1963, Ch. 1.

Chapter 9

[1] I do not mean only technical: for instance, the connection between railways and telephones, aviation and radar, space travel and computer miniaturization. But above all theoretical too. No modern astronomy and biology without physics, geology, mathematics. No nuclear physics without chemistry. No biogenetics and biomedical science without cybernetics. No psychology without information theory, etc., etc.

[2] This also shows from his famous lecture "Religion und Naturwissenschaft", Leipzig, 1938, in which he concludes that religion and natural science should take joint action misbelief *and* superstition, and may never stop fighting against both skepticism and dogma.

[3] Of course, there were other, equally progressive, scientific thinkers and Nobel prizewinners, as for instance, J. J. Thomson, Wilson, I. I. Rabi, Pauli, Langmuir, Urey, Otto Hahn. Besides, there are some important upsetters of basic principles missing, as, for instance, Lise Meitner and Max Born, who did not share in this highest honor.

[4] On this last point see the recent fascinating report concerning CERN by Dr Robert Jungk, "Die grosse Maschine", Bern, 1967.

[5] It goes without saying that I will have to bring up, in my own way, many things which may be common knowledge by now. I think it should not be necessary to

apologize for that. Those for whom this is "old hat" can, of course, skip the following. They need only ask themselves whether they have acted according to this wisdom.

6 As we know now, earth is only a rather small planet among the approximately 100 billion stars of its galaxy which, itself, is only one of the 100 billion galaxies calculated to be the total number existing in the universe. Our own galaxy has a diameter of about 100,000 light years. One light year (converted from time into distance) would be the equivalent of almost 6^{12} miles.

7 The meaning of the concept paradox itself has changed almost imperceptibly too. At first, it related primarily to an apparent absurdity or contradiction, which in reality does not exist so that, on closer study, the accuracy of the statement doubted could nevertheless be established. Gradually, however, a shift has been taking place to real contradictions which definitely exclude unlimited application of formal logic. This proved undeniable in the – of course initially disputed – mathematical theory of infinite aggregates built up especially by Cantor and Fraenkel in which A and -A can be true at the same time.

8 E. C. Berkeley, Symbolic Logic and Intelligent Machines, 1959.

9 In natural philosophy there have been, since ancient times, many different ideas about the first beginning (archè). According to Thales primordial matter consisted of water; according to Anaximedes of air; according to Diogenes of breath; according to Heraclitus of fire; and finally, according to Empedocles, of fire, air, earth and water. For Pythagoras numbers formed the basis; for Anaxagoras the mind; and for Parmenides thought. With Leucippus and Democritus, there comes a new materialistic change into an infinity of atoms. Since Kant and Laplace, clouds of gas have appeared for the first time as primordial matter. The place of ether, at present, has been taken by plasma which definitely is not the last word. The cosmos, in spite of all our greater knowledge, is, at present no more than it ever was: a mystery – Mysterium tremendum.

10 It is most remarkable to realize that not only Kant, as he said himself, "was awakened from his dogmatic slumber" by reading Hume on the problem of the inevitable insufficiency of facts for the devising of a theory. Later on, Einstein was emphatically to state, in exactly the same way, that reading the brilliant views of Berkeley and Hume had awakened him for the first time to the deeper realization that the physics of Newton could not possibly (as Newton himself argued) be deduced exclusively from the facts. Precisely these new ideas brought Einstein to the conviction that Newtonian physics could not be exclusively and universally valid either. This gave him the courage to create new, further-reaching and more comprehensive theoretical, though still speculative, hypotheses and theses.

11 See the special issue of Science Journal, "The human brain", May 1967. In addition, see especially, "Information and Prediction in Science", ed. Dockx and Bernays, N.Y., 1965.

12 The linguistic history of the word speculation really also testifies to this typical bivalence. For the stem means to look about, consider and investigate. It is the same stem as that of species, specimen, special and speculum (mirror). Initially there is, at most, only a shade of difference between the spectator and the speculator. The speculator, besides being a spectator, is a scout and surveyor. With a far-seeing mind, he already takes a step forward. His task is not only contemplation, reproduction of what he sees reflected in the mirror, but, in addition to this, gradual prereflection. From viewing the present the concept widens imperceptibly into viewing the future at the same time. The most famous encyclopedia of the Middle Ages (ca. 1200-1250) was entitled "Biblioteca Mundi" or "Speculum Majus". The old cyclopedia (as it was originally called) was not only one-eyed, comprising the whole cycle, but also developed a *third* eye: a future-eye. In other words, at first speculation was pre-

eminently observing, considering, investigating verification. These concepts were far from antithetical, but, on the contrary, complementary. Without such sound speculative consideration and reconnaissance, no real verification was even imaginable. Speculation was the main instrument of verification. The gradually developed linguistic contrast is an artificial, anti-natural, i.e. unhistoric and also unscientific one. Scientifically founded speculation is still a *sine qua non* of renewing scientific work. Every new hypothesis is, by definition, speculative. A science without hypotheses is a dead science.

[13] A. D. de Groot, Methodologie, Grondslagen van onderzoek en denken in de gedragswetenschappen, Den Haag, 1961.

[14] Likewise, Alexander von Humboldt could give his famous book "Kosmos" (1845) the subtitle of "Entwurf einer physischen Weltbeschreibung".

[15] Paradoxically, this rapid obsolescence is due, according to De Groot (op. cit., p. 101 note 1) less to the accelerated pace of events than to the researcher himself, since his plunge into the "deep end" is an attempt to escape verification. A remarkable sample of depth-psychology!

[16] Op. cit., p. 120.

[17] Op. cit., p. 69/70.

[18] Op. cit., p. 101.

[19] Cf. especially Chapter 21.

[20] Allgemeine Erkenntnislehre, 1925.

[21] See especially his contributions to the International Encyclopedia of Unified Science, Chicago, 1947.

[22] Cf. for example H. Reichenbach's Experience and Prediction, Chicago, 1938. Also his contribution to the Policy Sciences, ed. Lerner & Lasswell, Stanford, 1951 and The Structure of Scientific Thought, ed. E. H. Madden, Cambridge, Mass., 1960.

[23] Op. cit., p. 360 et seq. It surprises me rather that De Groot mentions Von Mises (Kleines Lehrbuch des Positivismus, The Hague, 1939) in this context, but, except in a rather stray footnote, not the genius who founded and completed this philosophy, or at least not the "later" Wittgenstein, Philosophical Investigation, 1953 (in which his own earlier work, the "Tractatus Logico-Philosophicus" of 1922 was fairly thoroughly demolished). Or is this self-repudiation possibly the reason for De Groot's neglect? After all, it was for the same reason that that great logical neo-positivist Bertrand Russell kept his protective hands off Wittgenstein.

[24] I have dealt in detail with the historical and philosophical significance of this fundamental distinction in my TIF.

[25] In principle, such a concept of "differentness" is also valid in relation to the supposed eventual discovery of an anti-cosmos, or of anti-universes.

[26] Cf. especially Chapters 21 and 23.

[27] Cf. in detail Chapters 15 to 18.

Chapter 10

[1] Ossip K. Flechtheim, History and Futurology, Verlag Anton Hain, Meisenheim am Glan, 1966.

[2] The first edition of TIF (1955) bore the daunting subtitle of "culture-futuristic reconnaissance", which I chose partly as a counterpart to Huizinga's "culture-historical reconnaissance" – at the time, certainly, no great success as a scientific proclamation. Compare this, however, with the sympathetic and well documented essay "The Futurists, looking toward A.D. 2000" in Time Magazine (Atlantic ed.) of 25 February 1966. See also Chapter 1, 1, sub B.

[3] L'Art de la Conjecture, Editions du Rocher, Monaco, 1964.

[4] G. Berger, Phénoménologie du Temps et Prospective, Paris, 1964.

[5] Réflexions sur 1985. La Documentation Française, Paris, 1964.

[6] Cf. also P. Massé, Le Plan ou l'Anti-Hasard, Paris, 1965.

[7] Plaidoyer pour l'Avenir, Paris, 1961.

[8] Recent publication: Les 40.000 Heures, Inventaire de l'Avenir, Paris, 1965.

[9] The recent German edition "Mutation der Menschheit", Berne, 1967, contains an important addition in its "Nachwort".

[10] Les Hommes du Future, Utopies ou Réalités de Demain, Casterman, Tournai, 1965. The same publisher also gave us Henri van Lier's Le Nouvel Age, 1962.

[11] Since published as a Pelican paperback in 2 parts, The World in 1984, ed. Nigel Calder, Penguin Books, 1965. A forerunner was Ronald Brech's Britain 1984, An experiment in the economic history of the future, London, 1963.

[12] Man and his Future, ed. Wolstenholme, Churchill, London, 1963.

[13] His theme "Die Zukunft hat schon begonnen" inspired a number of variations including Günther Wollny's "Die Zukunft ist anders", Boppard am Rhein, 1962.

[14] Between 1964 and 1966; publishers Verlag Kurt Desch, Munich.

[15] Die Menschenmacher, Die Zukunft des Menschen in einer gesteuerten Welt, Fischer Verlag, Hamburg, 1964.

[16] Die Atombombe und die Zukunft des Menschen, Munich, 1958.

[17] Wer beherrscht die zweite Hälfte des 20. Jahrhunderts? DTV, Munich, 1963.

[18] E. M. Vassiliev and S. Gouschev, Live in the Twenty-First Century, London, 1961. The final conclusion is less interesting than the background information.

[19] See W. Sukiennicki, The Visions of Communism, in Problems of Communism, No. 6, 1960.

[20] The Hungarian Kremlinologist George Paloczi-Horvath foresees an enormous and sudden advance in Russia, brought about mainly by the automation revolution and purposive research into the future.

[21] Cf. also his "Between Dystopia and Utopia", Hartford, Conn., 1966.

[22] Understanding Media: The extensions of man, New York, 1964.

[23] For a more detailed account see Chapter 11, 3.

[24] The Challenge of Man's Future, Viking Press, N.Y., 1954, followed by The Next Hundred Years (with Burner and Weir), from the same publisher, 1963.

[25] Cyborg: Evolution of the Superman, New York, 1965.

[26] The Future as History, New York, 1959/60.

[27] Science since Babylon, New Haven, 1961, and Little Science, Big Science, New York, 1963.

[28] The Next Generation, New York, 1965.

[29] The Future, New York, 1965.

[30] Of its many publications I shall mention only: J. Tinbergen, Shaping the World Economy, New York, 1962.

[31] Landsberg, Fischman and Fisher, Resources in America's Future (1960-2000), Johns Hopkins, Baltimore, 1963.

[32] Four parts have been published to date: World Resources Inventory, Carbondale, Ill., 1963-66.

[33] A survey appeared in the journal Daedalus, Summer 1967.

[34] Of the many books he has written, the reader is referred especially to The Design of Development, Baltimore, 6th impression 1966, and Lessons from the Past, Amsterdam, 1963.

[35] Voorspellen en Beslissen, Utrecht, 1964.

[36] Bouwmeesters van Morgen, Pantoskoop, 1964.

[37] Published by Paul Brand (Hilversum, 1966) who also published a number of

Prospect Books produced by "Working Party 2000".

[38] See, inter alia, the reports on Public Health and Town and Country Planning. (The second report, of 1966, is still not sufficiently advanced as far as overall outlook is concerned.)

[39] E.g. the method of the British "The World in 1984", the German "Modelle für eine neue Welt", the Russian "Life in the 21st Century", and the Studium Generale 1966 futurology courses at Leyden.

[40] Cf. Chapter 25, 4.

[41] Cf. Chapter 25, 2.

[43] Cf. in particular Chapter 15.

[43] Cf. Chapter 22, 3, and Chapter 25, 5.

[44] Cf. Chapter 25, 4.

[45] Cf. particularly Chapter 21.

[46] Cf. Chapters 14 and 21 to 26, and Appendix.

[47] See especially Chapters 11, 12 to 14, 15 to 18.

Chapter 11

[1] A few exceptions to the rule in the Netherlands' favor were mentioned earlier, in Chapter 10. As a rule however, the Netherlands contrasts unfavorably not only with America but also, of late, with other Western European nations.

[2] I have deliberately mentioned in the text only those men of genius who directly activated progress in their own fields, especially as regards existing ideas or notions of time. Other Jewish scholars, inventors or artists from the German-Austrian language area have also touched on this time dimension, albeit somewhat less directly. I am thinking of Hermann Weyl (topology), Heinrich and Gustav Hertz (electricity and electronics), of doctors like Semmelweiss (prophylaxis), Paul Ehrlich (chemotherapy), Eugen Steinach (rejuvenation) and Karl Landsteiner (blood grouping), of Elise Meitner (nuclear fission) and the atomic physicists J. J. Rabi and Max Born, of the philosophers Cassirer, Husserl, Scheler and Buber, the individual-psychologist Alfred Adler, the inaugurator of the plastics era Sigmund Politzer, the semanticist Sapir, and, last but not least, one of the greatest inventors of all time, Emile Berliner (pioneer of the aero-engine, the helicopter, the telephone microphone, developments in radio, gramophone and recording acoustics, pasteurized milk, etc.). I must not omit the Utopist and founder of the Zionist movement, Theodor Herzl. And artists of another time dimension like Kafka, Marc Chagall and Kokoschka. I have not of course considered the children of Jewish immigrants in America such as Norbert Wiener and J. Robert Oppenheimer.

[3] Major works are "Geist der Utopie" and "Das Prinzip Hoffnung".

[4] Quite dissimilar but still more or less mystic movements have also found favor there – witness the following for the "Institut de la Vice" and the more popularly styled "Planète", and not least, the meteoric (though posthumousè) surge of interest in the work of Teilhard de Chardin. Cf. also Chapter 6, 2.

[5] Cf. Chapter 1, 2, sub B.

[6] It is curious that De Jouvenel, in a characteristically cautious address given at the invitation of the American Rand Corporation, was almost knocked off his own feet, as the report reveals, by the surprising force of the "wave of the future".

[7] This, and the reason why I later came to a different conclusion, is made clear in Chapter 13, 2, Chapter 14 and Appendix.

[8] Reorientation, because America has always from the oldest times been strongly future-oriented. The kernel of the "American Creed" was the belief that Americans

could determine their own destiny. One of the most influential of their philosophers, A. N. Whitehead (see "Adventures of Ideas", Mentor Books, N.Y., 1955) describes foresight as one of the basic human principles.

[9] For example, a gigantic electronics firm also buys up a large publishing house, a very important radio and television station, a very influential news-paper business or a firm distributing widely read weeklies, magazines, popular phonograph records, film companies, etc. etc.

[10] Research and Development: but the accent of research is being placed more and more on *development*!

[11] The long-term project Seabed (Sea-based deterrence) is the best known of the Navy's projects. The Army's include FID (Forecasts in Depth) and the Air Force has the Forecast project, among others.

[12] American business is in turn heavily subsidized by the government for this purpose.

[31] This institute has organized several conferences in recent years on the theme: "The next fifty years: 1967-2017".

[14] The following have, to my knowledge, already been designated: Professor Christopher Wright (Columbia Univ.), Professor Werner Hirsch (Univ. of California, L.A.), and Professor Lerner (MIT).

[15] The work of comparable European foundations is little known. The German ones of Volkswagen and Thyssen appear to support predominantly German projects. The relatively new and much smaller Werner Reimersstiftung in Germany is both international and future-oriented; it supports "Mankind 2000 International," among other projects. The same holds for the small Ciba Foundation, which is established in London. The Foundation Européenne de la Culture, established in the Netherlands, is also future-looking. We must hope for collaboration and coordination between all foundations anxious to promote studies on the future.

[16] We know only that future-institutes have been or are being established there on a broad front.

[17] In 1964 the Swedish National Bank allocated to Parliament the sum of 500 million kronor (about 100 million dollars), so that a special institute could be financed from the annual interest accruing, to conduct and publicize forward-looking research on "man in a changing society".

[18] Hamburg and Berlin, however, are two places where much hard work is being done.

[19] The American weekly Time (Atlantic edition, 25th February 1966) gave a brief survey of some "futuristic" developments in America and France in its role of a sensitive mirror of fashion. The French monthly Réalités followed suit in June 1966. Elseviers Weekly (26th November 1966) in an article entitled "De wereld van overmorgen" confined itself mainly to reproducing the best known long-term-future report of the Rand Corporation and again aroused, or strongly confirmed, a slightly unscientific science-fiction impression, thus falling largerly in line with the prevailing tenor of public opineon in the Netherlands. So I do not suppose it jolted many people out of their slumber, although the editors rightly described it as one of the most important pieces of reporting ever published in their paper.

[20] An exception is Ronald Brech's "Britain 1984", a forecast prepared for Unilever Ltd. (London 1963).

Chapter 12

[1] Cf. also J. A. Schumpeter, "Capitalism, Socialism and Democracy", N.Y., 1942.

[2] The conquest of the Chinese continent by Mao Tse Tung was possible only by

reason of a completely mistaken American orientation or, to put it another way, by the lack (following) of a well-informed prognosis.

3 We are not yet in a position to know whether, and if so to what extent, military and political prognosis techniques clashed over Vietnam, or whether both were wrong.

4 Whether this was sufficiently the case originally, or later became so through the "local" war in Vietnam, I cannot judge; those better qualified, however, are not convinced. In any event, the fact that this has definitely *not* happened for decades in the unstable, explosive Middle East situation scarcely needs argument.

Chapter 13

1 Literature references very seldom go beyond the year 1960.

2 To some extent this may be a wise and cautious diplomatic gambit aimed at taking the wind out of the sails of the strong resistance the idea can expect. Being personally familiar with De Jouvenel's integrity, however, I am of the opinion that this accords entirely with his actual views.

3 The special future-number of Daedalus, summer 1967, gave a survey of this recent activity.

4 It could hardly be otherwise, since he had taken material for his study mainly from articles which had previously appeared in the French Futuribles and Sedeis publications, and future-research in America was still rather obscure in the Fifties.

5 Especially since Dr. Jantsch informs me that the OECD has now officially decided to publish the report in a number of languages. It is not impossible that the version ultimately published will differ in some points of detail from the document in my possession. The pages quoted in the following discussion may in that case also have a slightly different numbering from that stated here. I hope the reader will bear with this minor degree of inaccuracy.

6 Cf. Chapter 1, 3, and Chapter 11, 2.

7 Jantsch's report, hereafter referred to as Report, p. 22 et seq.

8 Cf. Report, p. 26 et seq.

9 Cf. Report, p. 33 et seq.

10 Cf. Report, p. 15 et seq.

11 Cf. Report, pp. 7-15.

Chapter 14

1 Report, pp. 278, 139 and 33 et seq.

2 Report, p. 113.

3 I already pointed out in Chapter 13, 1, that, by contrast, De Jouvenel seems to me to rely over-much on purely numerical, mainly quantitative-economic, prognostic techniques. The old need for *certainty* plays him false here.

4 Report, pp. 115, 135, 137 et seq.

5 Report, p. 120.

6 Cf. also Robert Jungk's excellent argument in "Modelle für eine neue Welt, der Griff nach der Zukunft", Munich 1964, p. 23 et seq.

7 Report, p. 3.

8 Report, pp. 120, 126, 146-7.

9 Cf. R. Bretnor, Modern Science Fiction, its Meaning and its Future, N.Y., 1953.

Also Patrick Moore, Science and Fiction, London, 1957; B. Davenport, Inquiry into Science Fiction, N.Y., 1955; M. Schonke, Vom Staatsroman zur Science Fiction, Stuttgart, 1957; and finally, my own TIF.

[10] For that matter, the interest (possibly even the priority value) of a fictive world was given prominence over a century and a half ago by Hans Vaihinger in his "Philosophie des Als-Ob".

[11] Report, p. 57.

[12] Report, p. 137 et seq.

[13] Cf. Chapter 26, 2, for a more detailed treatment.

[14] Cf. my TIF and, in a more popularized form, HTP.

[15] Report, pp. 120, 128 and 146 et seq.

[16] Report, pp. 11, 31, 110, 115, 120 et seq., 127-8, 131, 188.

[17] Cf. particularly Vol. IIA of the Commission on the year 2000 of the American Academy of Arts and Sciences: Scenarios of the Hudson Institute: The next thirty-three years, a framework for speculation.

[18] To the extensive bibliography in my book TIF I would particularly like to add here the following works: R. Gerber, Utopian Fantasy, London, 1955. M. L. Berneri, Journey through Utopia, Boston, 1951. R. Ruyer, L'Utopie et les Utopies, Paris, 1950. R. Muchielli, Le Mythe de la Cité Idéale, Paris, 1960. E. M. Cioran, Histoire et Utopie, Paris, 1960. And Utopias and Utopian Thought, ed. F. E. Manuel, Daedalus, Boston, Beacon paperback, 1967, which also lists the most important literature.

[19] Cf., inter alia, Chapter 25, 3.

[20] Report, pp. 110, 120, 126, 128, 131, 140 et seq.

[21] Cf. the Rand Report by Gordon and Helmer already cited, and Jantsch's Report, p. 119-120 et seq., 130 et seq., 142 et seq.

[22] Report, p. 7.

[23] Report, pp. 22 et seq., 44 et seq., 114 et seq., and 222 et seq.

[24] Cf. particularly TIF on this point.

[25] Cf. also Chapter 22.

[26] On the one hand Thomas S. Kuhn, The Structure of Scientific Revolutions, Chicago, Phoenix, 1964 (value-free); on the other, R. G. H. Siu, The Tao of Science, M. I. T. Paperback, 1964, (normative).

[27] Report, pp. 8-9, 55 et seq., 303, 340, 352.

[28] The recent report of the American Academy of Political and Social Science (included in the Annals for 1967) on "Social Goals and Indications for American Society" has already done pioneering work in this sphere.

[29] Report, p. 99 et seq.

[30] It was the Dutchman H. Theil who laid the methodological foundations for this ex-post prediction in the field of economics. Cf. his "Economic Forecasts and Policy", Amsterdam, 1961.

[31] Report, p. 135.

[32] Report, p. 108.

[33] Economics alone, under the pressure of economic-political crises, has apparently managed to free itself at length from this dogmatic strait-jacket. Using the "ruse of reason" it has stated as its "given" goals the simple objectives of stable values, a high level of employment, economic expansion and so on. Only when it comes to defining the complex goal of "welfare" has it inevitably got into enormous difficulties, because this cannot be done without the addition of normative evaluation. One has only to compare the associative contrast in sound between e.g. "welfare economics" and "the affluent society". The same is true of the correct meaning of "development planning" and the like. Economic planning and forecasting, unorthodox in themselves,

were of course nonsensical without alternative criteria, however much the evaluative presuppositions and normative objectives in a complicated and imposing mathematical-statistical model or economic calculation set-up might seem obscure, or at any rate less than crystal-clear. The extent to which the other social sciences have followed suit or otherwise is discussed at greater length in the chapters which follow.

[34] Report, pp. 63 et seq., 71 et seq., 80 et seq., 270 et seq., 280 et seq., 292 et seq.

[35] Report, pp. 55 et seq., 96 et seq., 118 et seq., 262 et seq.

[36] Report, pp. 84 et seq., 252 et seq., 263 et seq., 290 et seq., 313 et seq., 323 et seq., 336 et seq.

[37] Report, pp. 296 et seq., 323 et seq., 336 et seq.

[38] One example will suffice. Americans are now beginning to realize that even the wealthiest country in the world can be manoeuvered into the embarrassing position of having to choose between "guns and butter". Looking at the longer term, the constructive idea is also spreading that the underdeveloped areas at home, especially where racial discrimination and starving sections of the community are concerned, *must* be fully developed as fast as possible.

[39] Report, pp. 14, 30-31, 90, 262, 297, 306, 308, 344 et seq.

[40] Olaf Helmer, "Social Technology", R.C., Feb. 1965.

[41] Hasan Ozbekhan, "The Idea of a Look-Out Institution", SDC, March 1965, and a more advanced view by the same author in "Technology and Man's Future", SDC, May 1966.

[42] Cf. also Chapter 21.

[43] In America, it is mostly the social critics like Galbraith and Riesman who receive attention. The focus of renewal in Europe lies mainly with French thinkers like Raymond Aron (Essai sur les Libertés, Paris, 1965) and Jean Fourastié (Essais de Morale Prospective, Paris, 1966).

[44] Report, pp. 10-11, 48, 70 et seq., 124-125, 231, 262.

[45] Report, pp. 126 et seq., 131 et seq.

[46] Report Part III, "The Organization of Technological Forecasting", pp. 266-309, with four appendices, pp. 309-347.

[47] Report, p. 278.

[48] Report, pp. 138-9.

[49] Helmer, loc. cit., p. 16 et seq.

[50] Cf. Chapter 25, 3.

[51] "Formeln zur Macht", Deutsche Verlagsanstalt, Stuttgart, 1965.

Chapter 15

[1] See Chapter 10 et seq.

[2] See Chapter 13 et seq.

[3] This opinion differs from that of Hannah Arendt, "On Revolution", N.Y., 1963, who claims that the treasure of revolutionary tradition has been lost forever.

[4] To be fair, it must be pointed out that many contemporary prognosticians do not feel quite the same way about this acceleration principle. Obviously, their *evaluations* of it differ! The views reproduced above are roughly the same as those of Dennis Gabor. His conclusion (which I cannot accept) is that we must artificially retard and contain this ever-accelerating, ultimately dangerous process of development. However, there are other viewpoints differing more extremely from each other. At one end of the spectrum for instance, we find De Solla Price and with him many others (e.g. the Rand Report; Plat, "The Step to Man'"; etc.) who are convinced that the acceleration process, especially as it relates to the growth of

science and the population explosion, will eventually level out after the pattern of an S-curve. At the other extreme, Bertaux states that we will not stabilize, but always move higher and faster, that the existing S-curve is only one of a never-ending series of S-curves, ever ascending in the direction of infinity. I myself hold a middle position for the time being.

5 Their report is entitled "Government, Science and Public Policy", U.S. House of Representatives, Washington, 1966.

Chapter 16

1 The first publications of the British Royal Society appeared 300 years ago, in 1665.
2 Besides the well-known standard works on the historical roots of sociology and its development from social philosophy, politics, history and ethics, cf. also Derek J. de Solla Price's "Science since Babylon", New Haven, 1962.
3 Diagnosis of our Time, 1950, p. 54 et seq.
4 The Sociological Imagination, N.Y., 1959.
5 The New Sociology, ed. I. L. Horowitz, N.Y., 1964.
6 Cf. Chapter 9, 2.
7 Cf. Chapter 8, sections 4, 5 and 6.

Chapter 17

1 Since the Forties, about 50% of all Nobel Prizes have gone to America.
2 See J. J. Servan-Schreiber, Le Défi Américain, Paris, 1967.
3 So the term is confusing. This gap is not technological in the narrower sense, but rather a mental one.
4 Cf. Chapters 12, 13, 14 and Appendix.
5 Cf. Chapter 14, 2.
6 This point is further elaborated in Chapter 23.
7 Social Technology, 1965.
8 Technology and Man's Future, 1966.

Chapter 18

1 Founded by G. H. Mead, "Mind, Self and Society", Chicago, 1934.
2 An interesting exception to this rule is "The Passing of Traditional Society", Chicago, 1958 – worth reading, altough slanted rather more historically than towards the future (authors, Daniel Lerner and Lucille Pevsner).
3 Cf. A. L. Strauss, "Mirrors and Masks", N.Y., 1959.

Chapter 19

1 Cf. Chapter 4.
2 TIF discusses this at length.
3 Probably a condensed rhyming version of revolutionary ideas voiced by Langland

and Chaucer and most vividly expressed by the rebellious John Ball, nicknamed "the mad priest of Kent". For a fuller treatment, see G. Dudok, "Sir Thomas More and his Utopia", Amsterdam, 1923.

[4] Cf. Hans Meyerhoff, "Time in Literature", Berkeley, 1955.

[5] Cf. Chapter 5.

Chapter 20

[1] Cf. Chapter 1, 2, sub B.

[2] Cf. especially my book "Hoopvolle Toekomst Perspectieven" (HTP).

[3] Cf. TIF.

[4] Cf. for example the American Academy of Arts and Sciences publication "Utopias and Utopian Thought", ed. Frank Manuel, Boston, 1966, which contains a contribution of my own entitled "Utopia and Cultural Renewal", Daedalus Library, Vol. No. 5; paperback edition 1967.

[5] This is clearly perceived and analysed by Hasan Ozbekhan and Jantsch in their publications quoted earlier.

[6] This really goes right back to the German philosopher Hans Vaihinger ("Die Philosophie des 'Als-Ob' ", 1911), who was imperfectly understood at the time. He considered a fictitious world of the imagination to have greater value than reality in certain respects. What *is* objective reality, in fact? Recent advances in the new science of biotics and the astonishing results it has produced on the phenomenal powers that animals have of perceiving colors, smells, shapes, phenomena, radiation, sounds, figures etc., throw justifiable doubt on this once again – for the first time since Kant.

[7] The deliberate nonsense, which was not of course aimed at any kind of future social reform but simply an example of the light-hearted, relaxed literary genre then current, must not be thought of as part this phenomenon.

[8] Cf. Lamartine: "Les utopies ne sont souvent que des vérités prématurées". Aldous Huxley took as motto for his "Brave New World" a saying of Berdyaev: "Les utopies sont réalisables. La vie marche vers les utopies".

Chapter 21

[1] E. G. Veblen, Alfred Kroeber, Florian Znaniecki, Adolf Löwe, Alfred Schütz, Felix Kaufmann, Myrdal, Sorokin, etc.

[2] E.g. writers like Bell, Lipset, Daniel Lerner, Riesman, Goffmann – a rather arbitrary selection which omits equally meritorious names.

[3] Cf. Berger, Invitation to Sociology, p. 49.

[4] Berger's Chapter 7: Excursion: Sociological Machiavellianism and Ethics (or: How to Acquire Scruples and Keep on Cheating). This is a digression which again illustrates all the traditional merits of the sociologist and defends them, in an exclusively authoritarian way, against the possible accusation of "cynical opportunism". Thanks for the invitation, but the real accusation is of course the passive abstinence towards social events which is defended here too. One cannot say that of Machiavelli!

[5] Diagnosis of our Time, 1950, p. 54 et seq.

419

Chapter 22

[1] Kennen en Keuren in de Sociale Wetenschappen, Leyden, 1947.

[2] Economics has been virtually alone in managing, particularly since the Second World War, increasingly and gratifyingly to escape from it by adding more and more important new branches of economic science.

[3] Cf. Chapter 5, 2 and 6.

[4] Cf. Chapter 13, 2, and Chapter 14, 3.

[5] Daniel Bell (Twelve Modes of Prediction, p. 19) seems to me to go even a little too far when he says: "... decision-theory is not predictive because it is normative". It always continues to indicate what will probably happen if a particular decision is taken.

[6] This has already been argued in the case of economic forecasting by Modigliani and Cohen: "The role of anticipations and plants in economic behavior and their use in economic analysis and forecasting", University of Illinois, 1961. And on a broader base, Fred C. Ikle "On the Epistemology of Forecasting for Our Society", American Academy of Arts & Sciences, Commission on the Year 2000, Vol. III, p. 1 et seq.

[7] "Society", New York, 1935. McIver it attached to New York's Columbia University.

[8] Even the first chapter of Berger's recent "Invitation to Sociology" is still entirely devoted to it, using completely traditional arguments.

[9] Cf. Chapter 8, 3, and Chapter 12.

[10] See the publications of Ozbekhan and Ikle (already cited).

[11] "Prediction and Optimal Decision", Prentice-Hall, 1961.

[12] "Toward the Measurement of Social Change: Implications for Social Progress", Am. Ac. of Arts & Sciences, Commission on the Year 2000, Vol. III, p. 1 et seq.

[13] Cf. his oft-quoted "Invitation to Sociology", an invitation that holds very little attraction for our own time. One is inclined to wonder how on earth it is possible, in this agonized age when the world is faced with shocking social problems, for serious sociology to offer itself to future practitioners in a popular and rather boastful, even clownish way as a sort of amusement industry or entertainment. Its self-affixed label "pastime" is open and unashamed evidence of an escapism which, in flight from the future, delights solely in a close observance of the second-hand and in the immediate, short-lived pleasures of varied forms of relaxation. It is a totally egocentric activity, concerned only with its own hedonism, with "carpe diem" the motto of a day well spent, its eyes deliberately shut to the needs of mankind and its fellow-men in our, literally and figuratively, very disturbed society.

Chapter 23

[1] All my quotations are taken from the Introduction on page 1.

[2] "Illustrative procedural sketches", loc. cit., p. 23 et seq.

[3] Loc. cit., p. 27 et seq. and p. 37 et seq.

[4] Loc. cit., p. 39.

[5] Loc. cit., p. 39.

Chapter 24

[1] The reader is referred to Parts One and Two, where Dogmatics and Continuous Dogmatics are considered in detail.

[2] Compare the fervent homilies of Karl Popper in his "The Free Society and its Enemies" (in two volumes).

[3] Cf. Chapter 8, 3.

[4] In this respect the pioneering work of William Ogburn, Recent Social Trends, N.Y., 1933, is still as valuable as ever, even taking into consideration the hidden influence exerted on it by the Great Depression of the Thirties.

[5] Loc. cit., p. 5.

[6] Loc. cit., p. 6.

[7] Loc. cit., p. 7.

[8] Loc. cit., p. 7.

[9] Cf. Chapter 23.

[10] Cf. particularly Chapters 8, 16, 17, 21, 22 and 23.

[11] See also Chapter 9 in particular.

[12] Cf. Chapter 1, 3.

[13] Cf. Chapter 14, 3.

[14] See Chapters 25 and 26.

[15] This is derived from the proof copy I received of his "Zukunftsforschung als Voraussetzung und Grundlage der Zukunftsplanung", a lecture held in Basle and due to be published by Regio-Verlag, Basle.

Chapter 25

[1] Just before the Dutch edition of this book went to press, I learnt that the Max Planckgesellschaft intends to set up an "Institut für Zukunftsforschung" under the direction of Professor C. F. von Weizsaecker.

[2] It seems that plans for this are at present in an advanced state of development. Olaf Helmer, inter alia, has drawn up an appropriate scheme.

[3] Cf. Chapter 1, 3, and Chapter 17.

[4] Horizon, Summer 1965.

[5] Also referred to as C.A.I., or computer-assisted instruction.

[6] The reader will have gathered that some instruction in historical dogmatics or specific future-dogmatics can, in the author's opinion, have a particularly broadening and liberating influence on the student's mental horizons!

[7] Cf. my TIF and HTP.

[8] A number of such scenarios have been published by Kahn, together with Wiener, in "The Year 2000", New York, 1967.

[9] Science and Social Change, in Vol. IV of "the Working Papers of the Commission on the year 2000", p. 13.

[10] The Israeli kibbutzim, for example, provide for this approach a remarkably good training. It would seem to me too that the Russian education system, among others, also contains similar elements.

[11] Cf. Utopias and Utopia Thought, ed. Frank Manuel, Daedalus Vol. 5, initiated by the American Academy of Arts and Sciences.

[12] Herman Kahn of the Hudson institute also calls this the "alternative worlds future approach". Cf. on this Commission Year 2000, Am. Ac. of Arts and Sciences, Vol. IIA, 1967.

[13] This idea was aired earlier in Chapter 1, 3.

[14] Cf. Chapter 24, 3.

[15] The well-known American sociologist C. Wright Mills has already pointed in this direction with his "The Power Elite". J. K. Galbraith does so again in his recent book "The New Industrial State", though with a number of different nuances and stresses. Cf. Chapter 24, 3.

[16] At present this task is further aggravated by a universally deservable conservatism among large sections of the working classes.

[17] The symbolic number 2000 is of course only an eye-catching date aimed at existing emotional associations – a focus for the *present* time, A.D. 1968. As time rushes past, however, we are compelled to prolong the period of any adequate vision of the future. Thus the present dividing line represented by the year 2000 will soon be replaced by 2050 or 2100, and then 2500, and so on. This is clear if one realizes that the children born today and in the years to come will not have had their first social, and possibly professional, experience until about the year 2000, and that – partly through the longer average life expectancy – the greater part of their adult existence will then lie before them, in still further changing society.

Chapter 26

[1] Cf. Chapter 15.

Appendix

[1] Vol. II-A of the Working Papers of the "Commission on the Year 2000" (Am. Ac. of Arts and Sciences) contains an interesting account by Robert U. Ayres of technological forecasting, which it has not been possible to examine here.

[2] OECD Working Document, Oct. 1966, pp. 10, 113, hereafter referred to as the Report.

[3] Report, p. 120 et seq.

[4] Report, p. 109.

[5] I gladly take this opportunity of thanking Professor J. Koerts of the Netherlands School of Economics, Rotterdam, for his invaluable help with the composition and especially the mathematical infrastructure of this Appendix; any errors there may be are of course entirely my own responsibility.

[6] Stouffer's standard work The American Soldier dates from as far back as the end of the Second World War. The fourth and last part, "Measurement and Prediction", remains important from the methodological point of view. More recent literature in this connection includes: J. W. N. Sullivan, The Limitations of Science, Mentor, 1956, N.Y.; L. C. Lastrucci, The Scientific Approach, Cambridge Mass., 1967; K. E. Boulding, The Impact of the Social Sciences, New Brunswick, 1966. Books specially concerned with mathematical models in sociology are: James Coleman, Introduction to mathematical sociology, Glencoe, 1964, and Raymond Boudon, L'Analyse mathématique des faits sociaux, Plon, 1967.

[7] For a systematic introduction to these branches together, easily followed by the Layman, see Cooper, Leavitt and Shelly, New Perspectives in Organisation Research, N.Y., 1964, and Kast and Rosenzweig, Science, Technology and Management, N.Y., 1962.

[8] Report, p. 2.

[9] The copious literature on it includes W. Feller, An Introduction to Probability Theory and its Applications, Parts I and II, John Wiley, New York, 1957 and 1960.

[10] For this reason Quételet enjoys greater esteem, precisely in sociological matters, than Comte, who regarded him with contempt.

[11] John Wiley, New York, 1954.

[12] Report, p. 196 et seq.

[13] Report, p. 196 et seq.

[14] Report, p. 199.

[15] I have tried to avoid mathematical formulae wherever possible in this Appendix. A linear equation is a first order equation ($y = a + bx$) represented by a straight line. A second order equation ($y = a + bx + cx^2$) is represented by a curve.

[16] Report, p. 222 et seq.

[17] Report, p. 224.

[18] Cf. Chapter 14, section 3.

[19] Report, p. 281 et seq., p. 298.

[20] Cf. Chapter 22, and the concluding chapters 25 and 26.

[21] In fact this method is a refined form of practical "trend fitting".

[22] Report, pp. 39, 168/9.

[23] Report, p. 175 et seq. The name may well lead to confusion with the "curve-following technique", which, however, is concerned with electronic apparatus deciphering handwritten information by using light rays to scan and follow the script to an accuracy of hundredths of millimeters, and so "reading" is.

[24] Report, p. 150 et seq.

[25] Here I differ somewhat with Jantsch's description, which he entitles "Extra polation of time-series on a phenomenological basis". The American term "phenomenolical" means purely factual, i.e. "in abstraction from evaluation", which seems obliged here, however, to make its entrance by the back door.

[26] On this and other pitfalls, cf. especially R. U. Ayres, On Technological Forecasting, Hudson Institute Report 1966, included in Vol. II-A of the Commission on the Year 2000, already quoted.

[27] Abt Associates embarked in late 1965 on an extensive and interesting study, for the American National Commission on Technology, Automation and Economic Progress, of the American model-building techniques, so far developed. The report is entitled "Survey of the State of the Art: Social, political and economic models and simulations", Cambridge, Mass., Nov. 1965. It contains a typology of over 50 models and deals especially with their ties with new computer and prognosis techniques on the one hand, and with an interdisciplinary system on the other. It is interesting to note the repeatedly apparent qualitative aspects of "feeling" evaluation, choice, weighing of alternatives, optimum target definition, checking of plausibility, and so on.

[28] Prof. H. H. Koelle of the Institut für Raumfahrttechnik, Technische Universität Berlin, has tried to construct a "civilization model" of the planet Earth in accordance with selected socio-economic indicators and measurements; published in June 1966 as SEMPE (Socio-economic Model of the Planet Earth).

[29] Cf. also A. Battersby, Network Analysis for Planning and Scheduling, London, 1964, and Brandenberger and Konrad, Netzplantechnik, eine Einführung, Zürich, 1965.

[30] Report, p. 249 et seq.

[31] Report, pp. 249/50.

[32] Report, p. 251.

[33] Cf. especially Chapter 26, 3.

[34] Dr. Alexander King (Director, Scientific Affairs, OECD), paints a similar picture in his simultaneously ironic and serious account of the quasi-report 1983/84 of the "British Government's Council for Scientific Policy", The World of 1984, Pelican, Vol. 2, p. 57 et seq.

[35] Theory of Games and Economic Behavior, Princeton, rev. ed. 1955.

[36] Report, p. 210 et seq.

[37] Cf. Greene and Sisson, Dynamic Management Decision Games, N.Y., 1959.

[38] Report, p. 253. The greatest common divisor is not necessarily identical with the

greatest probability. On the other hand, overwhelming insight can play an active role in the direction of the "self-fulfilling prophecy".

[39] Report, pp. 57/8, 117 et seq., 229 et seq., 294 et seq.

[40] Report, pp. 11, 248/49.

[41] Report, p. 181 et seq.

[42] Cf. also Fritz Zwicky's Entdecken, Erfinden, Forschen im Morphologischen Weltbild, Munich, 1966.

[43] Report, p. 187.

[44] Report, p. 215 et seq.

[45] Expressed somewhat irreverently, this approach evokes associations with the collages of pop art.

[46] Report, p. 221. Particularly in his remark in parentheses on p. 219 regarding the input/output systems named MAPTEK produced by the Quantum Science Corp.: "Input/output is linear, the world is not."

[47] Cf. Chapter 10, 2.

[48] Report, pp. 125, 255 et seq., 317.

[49] Report, p. 178 et seq.

[50] Report, p. 292 et seq., 323 et seq., 336 et seq.

[51] To this extent, therefore, there is a similarity with the application of modern Bayesian statistical methods. So here again we find the systematically required pairing of prevision and revision.

[52] Report, pp. 11, 142 et seq.

[53] Cf. especially Chapter 13, 2.

[54] As to the predicted development and consequences of the process of automation, the agreement with my own view was spectacular. This is not true, however, of a definitely more pessimistic attitude than mine to the likelihood of a third world war, thought to be quite probable but, to my mind, an area in which this very automation could constitute a significant counteracting force.

[55] Report, p. 31.

[56] Cf. Chapter 24, 2.

[57] On Alternative World Futures, Issues and Themes, N.Y., 1965. I have been unable to obtain another revised but still confidential report of his on Some Basic Techniques, Issues, Themes and Variables, Chicago, 1966. According to Jantsch (p. 406) it deals with "technological forecasting" methods in all their cultural, political, social, economic and technical aspects and potential. Much of it will presumably be found in "The Next Thirty-Three Years: A Framework for Speculation", a joint publication by Kahn, W. Pfaff and A. J. Wiener containing a collection of views included in Vol. II-A of the Commission on the Year 2000, already quoted. Vol. II, which is much enlarged, reached me too late for consideration here. It is to be published by Macmillan Cy N.Y., with a foreword by Daniel Bell, under the title The Year 2000.

[58] Report, pp. 188 et seq., 311/12.

[59] This same procedure has of course been followed by earlier imaginative utopists, e.g. Bellamy in his "Looking Backward" (1888).

[60] They come very close, therefore, to the purposive "self-destroying prophecy" here.

[61] Report, p. 128, 131, 309.

[62] Cf. the Abt Associates publications: Great World Issues of 1980, Cambridge, 1965, and Survey of the State of the Art: Social, Political and Economic Models and Simulations, Cambridge, 1965.

[63] Report, p. 320.

[64] Report, p. 140.

[65] It is Jantsch's opinion that biological evolution may provide support for it in accordance with the law "ontology recapitulates philogeny", or historical reality

repeats intuitively anticipated objectives in the phases of its development.

[66] Cf. especially Chapters 21, 22 and 23. I was unable to incorporate here Ozbekhan's article "The Triumph of Technology: "can" implies "ought", of 6th June 1967, SDC, Santa Monica, which also clearly adopts the same line.

[67] Cf. Chapter 26, 2. See also H. Afheldt. Infrastrukturbedarf bis 1980, Prognos Studien, Stuttgart, 1967.

[68] Report, pp. 31, 91 et seq., 258 et seq.

[69] Report, p. 361.

[70] Report, p. 135.

[71] Report, p. 118 et seq.

[72] Report, p. 265.